Case Studies in Family Violence

Second Edition

Case Studies in Family Violence
Second Edition

Edited by
Robert T. Ammerman
Children's Hospital Medical Center
Cincinnati, Ohio

and
Michel Hersen
Pacific University
Forest Grove, Oregon

Kluwer Academic / Plenum Publishers
New York, Boston, Dordrecht, London, Moscow

ISBN 0-306-46247-8 (hardbound)
ISBN 0-306-46248-6 (paperback)

©2000 Kluwer Academic / Plenum Publishers, New York
233 Spring Street, New York, N.Y. 10013

http://www.wkap.nl/

10 9 8 7 6 5 4 3 2 1

A C.I.P. record for this book is available from the Library of Congress

Printed in the United States of America

To Opa
　—RTA

To Victoria
　—MH

Contributors

Michelle Acker, Professional School of Psychology, University of Denver, Denver, Colorado 80208

Robert T. Ammerman, Division of Psychology, Children's Hospital Medical Center, Cincinnati, Ohio 45229

Susan M. Andersen, Department of Psychology, New York University, New York, New York 10003

Suzette M. Booth, Royal Alexandra Hospital for Children, Westmead, New South Wales, Australia 2145

Teresa Ramirez Boulette, Santa Barbara County Mental Health Care Services, Santa Barbara, California 93110

Marla R. Brassard, Faculty of Health and Behavioral Studies, Teachers College, Columbia University, New York, New York 10027

Susan M. Briggs, Massachusetts General Hospital, Harvard Medical School, Boston, Massachusetts 02114

Elissa J. Brown, NYU Child Study Center, NYU School of Medicine, New York, New York 10016

Angela Browne, Harvard Injury Control Center, Harvard School of Public Health, Boston, Massachusetts, 02115

Robert L. Burgess, Department of Human Development and Family Studies, Pennsylvania State University, University Park, Pennsylvania 16802

Shawn P. Cahill, Department of Psychiatry and Behavioral Sciences, National Crime Victims Research and Treatment Center, Medical University of South Carolina, Charleston, South Carolina 29425-0742

Naomi R. Cahn, George Washington University Law School, Washington, DC 20052

Barbara A. Carson, Department of Sociology and Corrections, Minnesota State University, Mankato, Minnesota 56002

Judith A. Cohen, Department of Psychiatry, Allegheny General Hospital, Pittsburgh, Pennsylvania 15212

Mary Ann Dutton, Bethesda, Maryland 20814

Sherry A. Falsetti, Department of Psychiatry and Behavioral Sciences, National Crime Victims Research and Treatment Center, Medical University of South Carolina, Charleston, South Carolina 29425-0742

Paul J. Gearan, Department of Psychiatry, University of Massachusetts Medical School, Worcester, Massachusetts 01655

Ronita S. Giberson, Graham B. Dimmick Child Guidance Services, Lexington, Kentucky 40507

Edward W. Gondolf, Mid-Atlantic Addiction Training Institute, Indiana University of Pennsylvania, Indiana, Pennsylvania 15705

Arthur H. Green[†], Department of Psychiatry, Columbia University College of Physicians and Surgeons, Presbyterian Hospital, New York, New York 10032

Stuart N. Hart, Department of Counseling and Educational Psychology, School of Education, Indiana University-Purdue University, Indianapolis, Indiana 46202

David B. Hardy, Tri-County Youth Program, Greenfield, Massachusetts 01301

Michel Hersen, School of Professional Psychology, Pacific University, Forest Grove, Oregon 97116

Richard L. Judd, Office of the President, Central Connecticut State University, New Britain, Connecticut 06050; and New Britain General Hospital, New Britain, Connecticut 06050

Stacey M. Kleinbaum, Department of Human Development and Family Studies, Pennsylvania State University, University Park, Pennsylvania 16802

David J. Kolko, Department of Psychiatry, University of Pittsburgh School of Medicine, Western Psychiatric Institute and Clinic, Pittsburgh, Pennsylvania 15213

[†]Deceased.

Janel M. Leone, Department of Human Development and Family Studies, Pennsylvania State University, University Park, Pennsylvania 16802

Lisa G. Lerman, Columbus School of Law, Catholic University of America, Washington, DC 20064

Martin J. Lubetsky, University of Pittsburgh School of Medicine, Western Psychiatric Institute and Clinic, Pittsburgh, Pennsylvania 15213

Bruce K. Mac Murray, Department of Sociology, Social Work, and Criminal Justice, Anderson University, Anderson, Indiana 46012

Anthony P. Mannarino, Department of Psychiatry, Allegheny General Hospital, Pittsburgh, Pennsylvania 15212

R. Kim Oates, Royal Alexandra Hospital for Children, Westmead, New South Wales, Australia 2145

Heidi S. Resnick, Department of Psychiatry and Behavioral Sciences, National Crime Victims Research and Treatment Center, Medical University of South Carolina, Charleston, South Carolina 29425-0742

Alan Rosenbaum, Department of Psychiatry, University of Massachusetts Medical School, Worcester, Massachusetts 01655

Mindy S. Rosenberg, Sausalito, California 94965

B. B. Robbie Rossman, Department of Psychology, University of Denver, Denver, Colorado 80208

Michael G. Ryan, Royal Alexandra Hospital for Children, Westmead, New South Wales, Australia 2145

Daniel G. Saunders, School of Social Work, University of Michigan, Ann Arbor, Michigan 48109

Amy H. Schwartz, Department of Psychology, New York University, New York, New York 10003

Tracey J. Strasser, Department of Psychology, New York University, New York, New York 10003

Karen F. Stubenbort, Department of Psychiatry, Allegheny General Hospital, Pittsburgh, PA 15212

William Warnken, Department of Psychiatry, University of Massachusetts Medical School, Worcester, Massachusetts 01655

Preface to the First Edition

The past 20 years have seen the emergence of family violence as one of the most critical problems facing society. The alarming incidence figures of abuse and neglect directed toward family members justify this attention. For example, over 1 million children are thought to be abused and neglected each year. Similarly, almost 2 million women are victims of battering each year. Annual rates of elderly mistreatment are thought to be as high as 32 per 1,000 population. Accurate epidemiological data only now are being compiled on more recently recognized forms of mistreatment, such as psychological abuse, ritualistic abuse of children, and child witnessing of adult violence. The pervasiveness of domestic mistreatment makes it a priority for clinicians and researchers alike.

For clinicians, intrafamilial violence represents a formidable challenge with respect to assessment and treatment. The etiology of abuse and neglect is multidetermined. There are numerous pathways in the development of family violence, and these interact and converge in a nonlinear fashion. The consequences of family violence are equally complex and divergent. Victims of mistreatment can display a variety of physical injuries and psychological disturbances. No single psychiatric syndrome or symptom constellation has been consistently implicated in any form of family mistreatment. The perpetrators of family violence are equally heterogeneous in their clinical presentations. Illustrative dysfunctions in perpetrators include skill deficits, substance abuse, mental illness, and impulse-control disorders. The clinician must administer a comprehensive assessment battery, select the level of intervention (i.e., individual, family, or group therapy), and choose the appropriate treatment. This is conducted within the context of the involvement of other professionals and organizations, including medical, legal, and social services. Balancing the clinical needs of the family with the sometimes competing interests of other disciplines requires extensive and polished case-management skills.

The purpose of this book is to elucidate and highlight the complex and multidisciplinary issues that face the clinician working with family violence cases. It is our contention that most clinicians will confront families engaged in domestic violence at some point, and it is imperative that they be prepared for the maze of issues and problems encountered in intervening with both victims and perpetrators. The empirical literature in family violence rarely reveals the underlying complications in intervening with such families. Therefore, we determined that a collection of case examples describing the different forms of family violence and the many problems with which the clinician must contend would fill a significant gap in the field. The heterogeneity of family violence precludes any one case from being fully representative of each form of abuse or neglect. Therefore, each chapter in this book combines an illustrative case with a broader discussion of the issues encountered by clinicians working with families that engage in abuse or neglect.

This book is divided into three parts. Part I includes chapters that address the ecological, legal, and medical issues encountered in family violence involving children and adults. The various forms of violence toward children are detailed in Part II. Several types of maltreatment that have only recently been identified or scrutinized are represented in this section, including abuse and neglect of handicapped children, the child witness of family violence, psychological and emotional abuse, and ritual abuse. Family violence toward adults is discussed in Part III. Wife battering and elder maltreatment are addressed here, in addition to psychological mistreatment of spouses, marital rape, and domestic homicide. In order to elucidate the many issues encountered by clinicians, the chapters in Parts II and III follow identical formats, in that medical issues, legal issues, social and family issues, assessment of psychopathology, and treatment options are reviewed.

We wish to acknowledge the help provided to us by many individuals in bringing this book to fruition. We are especially grateful to the contributors for sharing with us their knowledge and expertise. We also thank our editor, Eliot Werner, for his valuable support and encouragement. Special mention is due to Mary Jo Horgan, whose day-to-day assistance greatly facilitated the publication process. Several of our support staff also provided considerable assistance, including Karen Drudy, Mary Anne Frederick, Cheryl Huttenhower, Jennifer McKelvey, Louise Moore, and Mary Newell. Finally, we extend our gratitude to our wives, Caroline and Victoria, for their continued faith and support in our endeavors.

Robert T. Ammerman
Michel Hersen

Pittsburgh, Pennsylvania

Preface

The past 25 years have seen the emergence of family violence as one of the most critical problems facing society. The alarming incidence figures of abuse and neglect directed toward family members justify this attention. For example, over 1 million children are thought to be abused and neglected each year. Similarly, almost 2 million women are victims of battering each year. Annual rates of elder mistreatment are thought to be as high as 32 per 1,000 population. Accurate epidemiological data only now are being compiled on more recently recognized forms of mistreatment, such as psychological abuse and child witnessing of adult violence. The pervasiveness of domestic mistreatment makes it a priority for clinicians and researchers alike.

For clinicians, intrafamilial violence represents a formidable challenge with respect to assessment and treatment. The etiology of abuse and neglect is multidetermined. There are numerous pathways in the development of family violence, and these interact and converge in a nonlinear fashion. The consequences of family violence are equally complex and divergent. Victims of mistreatment can display a variety of physical injuries and psychological disturbances. No single psychiatric syndrome or symptom constellation has been consistently implicated in any form of family mistreatment. The perpetrators of family violence are equally heterogeneous in their clinical presentations. Illustrative dysfunctions in perpetrators include skill deficits, substance abuse, mental illness, and impulse-control disorders. The clinician must administer a comprehensive assessment battery, select the level of intervention (i.e., individual family, or group therapy), and choose the appropriate treatment. This is conducted within the context of the involvement of other professionals and systems including medical, legal, and social services. Balancing the clinical needs of the family with the sometimes competing interests of other disciplines requires extensive and polished case-management skills.

In the 9 years since the publication of the first edition of this book, there has been substantial progress made in our understanding of the etiology and associated features of domestic violence. There has also been a growing appreciation for the recalcitrant nature of these problems. As in the first edition, the purpose of this book is to elucidate and highlight the complex multidisciplinary issues that face the clinician working with family violence cases. It is our contention that most clinicians will confront families engaged in domestic violence at some point, and it is imperative that they be prepared for the maze of issues and problems encountered in intervening with both victims and perpetrators. The empirical literature in family violence rarely reveals the underlying complications in intervening with such families. Therefore, we determined that a collection of case examples describing the different forms of family violence and the many problems with which the clinician must contend would fill a significant gap in the field. The heterogeneity of family violence precludes any one case from being fully representative of each form of abuse or neglect. Thus, each chapter in this book combines *two* illustrative cases with a broader discussion of the issues encountered by clinicians working with families that engage in abuse or neglect.

This book is divided into three parts. Part I includes chapters that address the ecological, legal, and medical issues encountered in family violence involving children and adults. The various forms of violence toward children are detailed in Part II. Several types of maltreatment that have only recently been identified or scrutinized are represented in this section, including abuse and neglect of children with disabilities, the child witness of family violence, and psychological and emotional abuse. Family violence toward adults is discussed in Part III. Couples battering and elder maltreatment are addressed here in addition to psychological mistreatment of partners, marital rape, and homicide. In order to elucidate the many issues encountered by clinicians, the chapters in Parts II and III follow identical formats, in that medical issues, legal issues, social and family issues, assessment of psychopathology, and treatment options are reviewed.

We wish to acknowledge the help provided to us by many individuals in bringing this book to fruition. We are especially grateful to the contributors for sharing with us their knowledge and expertise. We also thank our editor, Eliot Werner, for his valuable support and encouragement. Special mention is due to Cindy DeLuca, whose day-to-day assistance greatly facilitated the publication process. Considerable assistance was also provided by Eleanor Gil, Carole Londeree, and Erika Qualls. Finally, we extend our gratitude to our wives, Caroline and Victoria, for their continued faith and support in our endeavors.

We also wish to express our sadness at the untimely death of Arthur Green, a contributor to both editions of the book. Dr. Green was a major figure in the family violence field and his efforts on behalf of maltreated children and their families have left a lasting imprint on the discipline. We extend our condolences to his family, as well as to his many friends and colleagues.

Robert T. Ammerman
Michel Hersen

Cincinnati, Ohio
Forest Grove, Oregon

Contents

PART II.   VIOLENCE TOWARD CHILDREN

PART III.   VIOLENCE TOWARD ADULTS

†Deceased.

I

General Issues

1

Family Violence: A Clinical Overview

Robert T. Ammerman and Michel Hersen

Few topics have elicited such public and professional interest in recent years as family violence. Although the abuse and neglect of other family members has been with us for centuries—and during that time often received tacit societal approval—only recently has the outcry against domestic violence resulted in a significant allocation of resources directed toward intervention and research. The expanded awareness of the extent of maltreatment has also led to a dramatic increase in the reported incidence of abuse and neglect. In turn, clinical intervention with family violence is no longer a specialty practiced by a few professionals. Rather, family violence is so pervasive that most clinicians will confront it at some point in their career. Indeed, family violence has been linked with such diverse phenomena as physical trauma, dental injuries, depression, anxiety disorders, conduct problems in children, sexual dysfunctions, and multiple personality disorder (see Kaplan, 1996). Moreover, several relatively common conditions are associated with family violence, including substance abuse, poverty, unemployment, and stress (see Ammerman & Galvin, 1998; Wolfe, 1987). It is evident that every clinician must be familiar with the indicators, etiology, and treatment of intrafamilial abuse and neglect.

Robert T. Ammerman • Division of Psychology, Children's Hospital Medical Center, Cincinnati, Ohio 45229.   **Michel Hersen** • School of Professional Psychology, Pacific University, Forest Grove, Oregon 97116.

Case Studies in Family Violence, Second Edition, edited by Ammerman and Hersen. Kluwer Academic / Plenum Publishers, New York, 2000.

The likelihood of having professional contact with victims or perpetrators of family violence is great and is underscored by the high incidence of abuse and neglect in the population. For example, in the case of child maltreatment, it is estimated that almost 1 million children were abused and neglected in 1996 (U.S. Department of Health and Human Services, 1998). Woman battering also occurs at alarming rates, with an estimated 2 million women battered each year (see Gelles, 1997). Approximately 20% of children are victims of sexual abuse (see Wurtele, 1997). This, in turn, has focused attention on the large number of adults who were sexually mistreated as children, often by other family members (Gold & Brown, 1999). More recently, recognized forms of family maltreatment have eluded precise epidemiological description, although data are now emerging about such areas as elder abuse and neglect, psychological mistreatment, and child witnessing of intrafamilial adult violence. In fact, evidence suggests that some nonphysical forms of maltreatment (psychological abuse, witnessing adult violence) may have deleterious consequences similar to physically traumatic mistreatment (see Fantuzzo, McDermott, & Noone, 1999).

In addition to the varied types of family violence facing the clinician, the cases are further compounded by the many etiologic influences operating in maltreatment. It is universally acknowledged that causative factors in abuse and neglect interact with each other and can be manifested via multiple pathways. Etiological models in which societal, cultural, family, individual, and contextual variables are represented as contributing factors have predominated in the field. Also, these factors are often thought to combine in nonlinear ways to bring about maltreatment (Ammerman, 1990). Indeed, the search for risk factors in maltreatment that are both sensitive and specific has yielded few consistent findings. There is no variable that significantly accounts for the development and maintenance of maltreatment. Because intervention should follow directly from etiology, problems have been encountered in designing clinical treatments that are useful for *all* families involved in each type of maltreatment. Finally, a growing literature attests to the divergent causes of various forms of abuse and neglect. For example, although past experience of maltreatment as a child is implicated in subsequent child abuse (Kaufman & Zigler, 1987), no such relationship has been found to date for elder abuse and neglect. Likewise, alcohol abuse is strongly associated with woman battering, although its role in other forms of maltreatment is less well understood. A unifying theory tying together the various types of family violence under one conceptual umbrella is unavailable, and it is unlikely that such a model can be constructed given the qualitatively unique developmental and life-span issues associated with violence directed toward children, adults, and the elderly.

Numerous factors mediate the extent, severity, and impact of abuse and neglect. These, in turn, determine the level of intervention required for treatment. For example, in the case of child abuse, the following topographical characteristics of abuse are relevant: age of child, age of first abuse, seriousness of abuse, type and frequency of abuse, and duration of abuse. Number of perpetrators, the addition of psychological abuse, whether or not the child is the sole recipient of mistreatment in families with other children, and the medical status of the child further complicate the clinical picture. Indeed, the differential effects of abuse on child victims as a function of past or current abuse and severity of mistreatment has been demonstrated (see Ammerman & Galvin, 1998). Descriptions of the characteristics of abuse and neglect are only now becoming standard practice in the empirical literature. Incidence of concurrent forms of maltreatment, however, has been documented for some time. Thus, almost half of all child maltreatment cases included both physical abuse and neglect (U.S. Department of Health and Human Services, 1998). An analogous elucidation of those factors influencing the extent and severity of mistreatment involving adult victims of family violence is clearly needed.

Cases of family violence are among the most challenging a clinician will ever face. Few conditions elicit such powerful emotional responses from professionals. It is difficult to imagine other clinical presentations that so clearly require multidisciplinary intervention. These families cannot be treated in isolation; to the contrary, the active participation of medical, legal, and social services is an essential (if complicating) feature of family violence. Clinicians, therefore, not only must be careful assessors and effective therapists but also need to balance the always present (and sometimes competing) interests of other professionals. Skills in case management are, therefore, crucial ingredients in interventions with family violence.

Medical Issues

Physicians, nurses, and emergency medical personnel are the first line in the identification and, in many instances, treatment of family violence. Physical trauma is not a necessary consequence of mistreatment of adults and children, but serious injury often brings the victim to the attention of medical services. For example, up to 25% of abused and neglected children suffered physical injuries (American Humane Association, 1984) as a result of abuse. In the case of woman battering, one study found that 42% of victims in a shelter had sought medical care for injuries sustained secondary to maltreatment (Gondolf & Fisher, 1988).

Emergency intervention is the first task of the medical professional who treats victims of family violence. The possible injuries that are sustained as a result of abuse and neglect are limitless. In physically abused children these range from bruises and abrasions to broken bones (see Wissow, 1995). These children also may display severe burns, organ damage, head injuries, internal damages, malnutrition, failure to thrive, and developmental delays. Likewise, battered adults may sustain bruises, dental trauma, broken bones, burns, and severe multisystemic injuries. Neglected elderly persons often exhibit poor nutrition and open sores, and they may take inadequate or inappropriate medications. All of these conditions require prompt medical attention and treatment. Nonmedical professionals who work with victims of family violence (e.g., shelter workers, social workers, family counselors) must be familiar with the physical signs and consequences of abuse and neglect so that appropriate referrals can be made.

The second role of medical personnel in family violence is the identification of maltreatment. For many victims, their first contact with health and social services is via private or emergency room physicians and other medical professionals. Indeed, up to 20% of battered women are seen in emergency rooms at some point for injuries secondary to domestic violence (Stark, Flitcraft, & Frazier, 1979). Similarly, a significant proportion of physically abused children are seen in emergency settings. Less seriously injured children and adults may be seen in outpatient clinics or in the offices of private physicians. In all of these instances, medical professionals must be familiar with the telltale signs of mistreatment. Certain injuries are clearly indicative of abuse (e.g., cigarette burns, welts from an electric cord). Others, however, are more elusive. Signs of abuse and neglect include (1) implausible or inconsistent accounts of how the injury occurred, and (2) a pattern of poorly explained injuries and accidents over a period of time.

A medical examination may also be important in the identification of child sexual abuse. Tissue damage and the presence of sexually transmitted diseases are compelling evidence for sexual mistreatment. However, absence of such findings does not preclude occurrence of sexual abuse.

Medical personnel must be vigilant for signs of abuse or neglect in patients that are at high risk for maltreatment. These consist of medically fragile or handicapped and multihandicapped populations that sometimes exhibit difficult to manage or "abuse-provoking" behaviors (Ammerman & Patz, 1996). Individuals who significantly add to family stress (and, therefore, may contribute to the development of abuse in already at-risk families) are children with attention-deficit/hyperactivity disorder and elderly adults with dementia. Because these populations often need to be followed by health-care professionals continually, medical personnel are in the best position to recognize early indicators of maltreatment.

Legal and Systems Issues

Legal and criminal justice systems are involved with family violence at several levels. Child protective service agencies exist in every state of the United States and in many other countries to investigate allegations of child abuse and neglect. In addition, these organizations typically provide emergency shelter to maltreated children, offer remedial programs for families engaged in abuse and neglect, and arrange for foster placement and adoption. Child protection laws vary considerably between states and countries, but most mandate reporting of suspected incidents of maltreatment by professionals who work with children.

Although child protective service agencies provide nonmedical intervention for maltreated children, several problems plague these systems. In general, they suffer from too few resources, too many cases, and overworked staffs with an inordinately high turnover in personnel. These issues are further compounded in developing counties, in which structured child service organizations may be severely compromised or nonexistent. Child protective services have come under increasing criticism in recent years, although it is widely acknowledged that they face a formidable task with limited resources and support.

In family violence directed toward adults, no analogous agency exists similar to that mandated to protect children (although there are county and state organizations in the United States that serve battered wives and mistreated elders). Rather, interactions between families and members of the legal and criminal justice systems occur through law enforcement responses to domestic violence and criminal prosecution of perpetrators. Thus, the police may be the first involved with wife battering in reaction to incidents of domestic assault. In the past, law enforcement personnel infrequently arrested the batterer and pursued the case only if the wife pressed charges. Now, however, numerous police departments utilize a protective strategy in which arrests are usually made. This, in turn, has led to a dramatic reduction in recidivism rates (Sherman & Berk, 1984). Court injunctions of protection orders have also been used to restrict contact between the perpetrator and the woman. Unfortunately, these are often difficult to enforce and are of questionable efficacy.

An additional legal issue for clinicians seeing families engaged in domestic violence is the duty-to-warn requirement. Specifically, recent court decisions (see Koocher, 1988) have stipulated the clinicians must notify potential victims of harmful threats made by clients. Even when such threats are made in the context of therapy, these regulations limit therapist–client confidentiality in favor of notifying the potential victim. The importance of the duty-to-warn requirement is underscored by the alarming number of fatalities in battered women in which numerous indications of abuse existed prior to their death (Saunders, 1999).

Because of its relative newness, formal recommendations for law enforcement responses to elder abuse and neglect have not yet emerged. As with wife battering, arrest of the perpetrator and subsequent prosecution are often carried out. Likewise, protection orders may be utilized by victims or legal guardians of the elderly person. These procedures, however, can be difficult for the elderly victim to initiate because of "loyalty" to the perpetrator, dependence on the perpetrator for care and companionship, or confusion and impaired judgments resulting from disease or medication. Many of those impediments also influence arrest and prosecution in wife battering. In such instances, social services, advocacy, and therapeutic interventions are important in using the legal system to the maximum benefit of victims and their families.

Family and Social Issues

Family violence is best understood within the context in which abuse and neglect take place. Indeed, family violence is a symptom of deeper and more extensive problems in the individual (i.e., perpetrator), family, and society. Thus, ecological models describing multilevel contributions to the development and maintenance of abuse and neglect abound. For example, Belsky (1993) and others propose conceptualizations of child abuse and neglect that posit four strata of causative influence: ontogenetic, microsystemic, exosystemic, and macrosystemic. Ontogenetic factors consist of individual personality and behavior characteristics (e.g., low intelligence). Microsystemic elements compromise family variables that mediate the probability of maltreatment (e.g., marital discord). Exosystemic factors pertain to social influence, including unemployment and social isolation. Finally, at the macrosystemic level, cultural factors affect the likelihood of abuse and neglect (e.g., cultural acceptance of corporal punishment). Similar multilevel ecological formulations have been proposed for family violence with adults (see O'Leary, 1988).

Pervasive dysfunction is found in many families plagued with family violence. Coercive family processes, marital distress, and maladaptive parent–child interactions have repeatedly been documented in child abuse and neglect, child sexual abuse, and wife battering. For many authors, family violence is viewed as an expression of more intensive and ingrained family pathology (Brunk, Hengeller, & Whelan, 1987). Interventions, therefore, frequently target deficiencies in the family system rather than abuse or neglect per se.

Social and societal factors also must be considered when working with families engaged in domestic violence. Social isolation or inadequate social supports have been found in perpetrators of child abuse and neglect (see Wolfe, 1987) as well as wife battering. Likewise, economic underprivilege and unemployment also have been linked to family violence.

Assessment of Psychopathology

The prevalence of specific psychiatric disorders is relatively infrequent in perpetrators of family violence and their victims. For example, in child maltreatment, only 10% of abusive parents suffer from a diagnosable mental illness (see Wolfe, 1985). Substance abuse, in particular alcoholism, is often associated with woman battering, although spousal mistreatment in the absence of substance abuse is also common. Similarly, no specific pathological syndrome has been consistently found to result from being the victim of physical abuse, sexual abuse, or neglect. However, both perpetrators and victims display a variety of symptoms and psychopathologies indicative of maladjustment and disturbance. These may contribute to the etiology or maintenance of maltreatment (e.g., marital conflict), precede family maltreatment (e.g., poor parenting skills), or result from abuse or neglect (e.g., depression).

Because so many aspects of family and individual dysfunction can play a role in family violence, it is necessary to administer a comprehensive assessment battery. The purposes of assessment are twofold: (1) to screen for severe forms of psychopathology that may require separate treatment either preceding or in conjunction with interventions for maltreatment, and (2) to identify targets for treatment. There are three assessment strategies that are typically employed. First, a clinical interview of the perpetrator and the victim is required. Second, individual maladjustment is examined using self-report questionnaires. And third, simulated or naturalistic interactions between family members are observed. Time, resources, and other clinical limitations may preclude implementation of all of these assessment approaches.

The objectives of the clinical interview are to determine mental status, diagnose psychiatric disorders, and gather information about maltreatment. Regarding the latter, specific details about the abuse and neglect should be delineated, including frequency, severity, and situational precipitants. Formats of the interview vary widely. For example, an unstructured play session is often most appropriate for a young abused child. For adults, formal structured or semistructured interviews are available. In general, the clinical interview will form the basis of continued assessment and subsequent treatment planning.

Self-report questionnaires in family violence abound. Most of these instruments are borrowed from other specialties, and they are used to evaluate psychopathology, social network, parenting stress, anger responsivity, and knowledge of child development. Several inventories, however, are designed specifically for families engaged in maltreatment. The benefits of utilizing self-report measures are that they are relatively easy to administer and can be completed in a short amount of time, and that they allow for comparisons between the respondent and the normative sample used to develop the measure. On the other hand, the primary drawback of self-report assessments is that they are prone to distortion and fabrication, and thus should be interpreted cautiously.

Interactional dysfunction is a universal characteristic of violent families. Indeed, maltreatment is often symptomatic of more pervasive family distress. Observation of family interactions permits identification of maladaptive patterns that may contribute to the occurrence of maltreatment. These are best conducted in the natural environment (i.e., the home). However, this is often impossible, necessitating simulated interactions (i.e., mother and child playing together, husband and wife discussing a problem) in the clinical setting. Of course, the private and socially undesirable nature of maltreatment makes it unlikely that specific abusive acts will be observed by the clinician (indeed, eliciting maltreatment is clearly unethical). Rather, the goal of the observational assessment is to identify styles of interactions that may serve to escalate conflict or promote neglectful behavior.

Treatment Options

Given the nascent stage of empirical research in family violence, it is not surprising that treatment strategies have only recently come under careful scrutiny. Recent developments in this area are promising, however. Advances have been made in designing treatments for perpetrators of child abuse, spouse batterers, and victims of child maltreatment. No single theoretical approach or intervention has emerged as the treatment of choice in any area of family violence. However, it is evident that interventions targeting multiple areas of change are most efficacious. In addition, at least with child maltreatment, skills-based programs appear to be important components of interventions (see Donahue, Miller, Van Hasselt, & Hersen, 1998).

The first decision to be made concerns the level of treatment that should be implemented. Choices include individual treatment, couples therapy, or group therapy. In some cases, combinations of these approaches are required. Little consensus has been reached about the optimal format of treatment. There is some indication, however, that group interventions are especially helpful for wife batterers (Gondolf, 1985) and sexually abused children (Cohen & Mannarino, 1999).

The primary goal of treatment is to stop and prevent further instances of maltreatment. The secondary goal is to remediate individual and family dysfunction. It is imperative that the victim receive individual treatment in conjunction with other interventions. The long-term negative impact of maltreatment on victims is well documented, and the victims' need for extensive treatment is evident.

Summary

The wide prevalence of family violence all but ensures that clinicians will be faced with maltreatment directed toward children or adults. Few clinical phenomena are as complex as family violence. By necessity, it elicits multidisciplinary involvement and intervention. Effective case management is required to balance the often competing needs of the medical, legal, and social systems working with the family. In addition, familiarity with a variety of assessment strategies and treatment approaches is paramount. Above all, the heterogeneity and complexity of family violence requires creativity, flexibility, and patience. These qualities should be apparent in the case descriptions that follow.

Acknowledgments

Preparation of this chapter was facilitated in part by grant nos. G008720109 and H133A40007 from the National Institute on Disabilities and Rehabilitation Research and the Vira I. Heinz Endowment. However, the opinions reflected herein do not necessarily reflect the position policy of the U.S. Department of Education or the Vira I. Heinz Endowment, and no official endorsement should be inferred.

References

American Humane Association. (1984). *Highlights of official child neglect and abuse reporting 1982*. Denver: Author.

Ammerman, R. T. (1990). Etiological models of maltreatment: A behavioral perspective. *Behavior Modification, 14*, 230–254.

Ammerman, R. T., & Galvin, M. R. (1998). Child maltreatment. In R. T. Ammerman & J. V. Campo (Eds.), *Handbook of pediatric psychology and psychiatry: Vol. 2* (pp. 31–69). Boston: Allyn & Bacon.

Ammerman, R. T., & Patz, R. J. (1996). Determinants of child abuse potential: Contribution of parent and child factors. *Journal of Clinical Child Psychology, 25*, 300–307.

Belsky, J. (1993). Etiology of child maltreatment: A developmental-ecological analysis. *Psychological Bulletin, 114*, 413–434.

Brunk, M., Hengeller, S. W., & Whelan, J. P. (1987). Comparison of multisystemic therapy and parent training in the brief treatment of child abuse and neglect. *Journal of Consulting and Clinical Psychology, 55*, 171–178.

Cohen, J. A., & Mannarino, A. P. (1999). Sexual abuse. In R. T. Ammerman, M. Hersen, & C. G. Last (Eds.), *Handbook of prescriptive treatments for children and adolescents* (2nd ed., pp. 308–328). Boston: Allyn & Bacon.

Donahue, B., Miller, E. R., Van Hasselt, V. B., & Hersen, M. (1998). An echobehavioral approach to child maltreatment. In V. B. Van Hasselt & M. Hersen (Eds.), *Handbook of psychological treatment protocols for children and adolescents*. Mahwah, NJ: Erlbaum.

Fantuzzo, J. W., McDermott, P., & Noone, M. (1999). Clinical issues in the assessment of family violence involving children. In R. T. Ammerman & M. Hersen (Eds.), *Assessment of family violence* (2nd ed.). New York: Wiley.

Gelles, R. J. (1997). *Intimate violence in families* (3rd ed.). Thousand Oaks, CA: Sage.

Gold, S. N., & Brown, L. S. (1999). Adult survivors of sexual abuse. In R. T. Ammerman & M. Hersen (Eds.), *Assessment of family violence* (2nd ed.). New York: Wiley.

Gondolf, E. W. (1985). *Men who batter: An integrated approach to stopping wife abuse*. Holmes Beach, FL: Learning Publication.

Gondolf, E. W., & Fisher, E. R. (1988). *Battered women as survivors: An alternative to treatment learned helplessness*. Lexington, MA: Lexington Books.

Kaplan, S. J. (Eds.). (1996). *Family violence: A clinical and legal guide*. Washington, DC: American Psychiatric Press.

Kaufman, J., & Zigler, E. (1987). Do abusive children become abusive parents? *American Journal of Orthopsychiatry, 57*, 186–192.

Koocher, G. P. (1988). A thumbnail guide to "duty to warn" cases. *Clinical Psychologist, 41*, 22–25.

O'Leary, K. D. (1988). Physical aggression between spouses: A social learning theory perspective. In V. B. Van Hasselt, R. L. Morrison, A. S. Bellack, & M. Hersen (Eds.), *Handbook of family violence* (pp. 31–55). New York: Plenum Press.

Saunders, D. G. (1999). Woman battering. In R. T. Ammerman & M. Hersen (Eds.), *Assessment of family violence* (2nd ed.). New York: Wiley.

Sherman, L., & Berk, R. (1984). The deterrent effects of arrest for domestic assault. *American Sociological Review, 49*, 261–272.

Stark, E., Flitcraft, A., & Frazier, W. (1979). Medicine and patriarchal violence: The social construction of a private event. *International Journal of Health Services, 9*, 461–493.

U.S. Department of Health and Human Services. (1998). *Child maltreatment 1996: Reports from the states to the National Child Abuse and Neglect Data System*. Washington, DC: U.S. Government Printing Office.

Wissow, L. S. (1995). Child abuse and neglect. *The New England Journal of Medicine, 332*, 1425–1431.

Wolfe, D. A. (1985). Child abusive parents: An empirical review and analysis. *Psychological Bulletin, 97*, 462–482.

Wolfe, D. A. (1987). *Child abuse: Implications for child development and psychopathology*. Newbury Park, CA: Sage.

Wurtele, S. K. (1997). Sexual abuse. In R. T. Ammerman & M. Hersen (Eds.), *Handbook of prevention and treatment with children and adolescents: Intervention in the real world context* (pp. 357–384). New York: Wiley.

2

Social and Ecological Issues in Violence toward Children

Robert L. Burgess, Janel M. Leone, and Stacey M. Kleinbaum

Introduction

In the first edition of this book, Burgess (1991) described a biosocial approach to an analysis of the social and ecological issues involved in child maltreatment. Since the publication of that edition, research and theoretical developments have continued at an ever accelerating pace. On the one hand, there has been the expansion of evolutionary-based studies that have led to a renewed consideration of our fundamental nature as humans and the role that evolution by natural selection has played in designing our pan-specific nature (e.g., Barkow, Cosmides, & Tooby, 1992; Buss, 1994; Wright, 1994). On the other hand, there has been an explosion of research from the perspective of developmental behavior genetics, where the issue has centered around the joint contribution of the environment and a person's genetic endowment to the socialization of children and development over the life span (e.g., Rowe, 1994; Sulloway, 1996). Consequently, in the present chapter, we will once again examine social and ecological

Robert L. Burgess, Janel M. Leone, and Stacey M. Kleinbaum • Department of Human Development and Family Studies, Pennsylvania State University, University Park, Pennsylvania 16802.

Case Studies in Family Violence, Second Edition, edited by Ammerman and Hersen. Kluwer Academic / Plenum Publishers, New York, 2000.

issues as they bear upon the maltreatment of children from a biosocial perspective.

Life History Theory

Ecology is that branch of biology that examines the complex relations between living organisms and their environment. In this chapter, we will make use of life history theory in our effort to understand the causal role of social and ecological factors in the maltreatment of children, either from abuse or neglect. Life history theory is a "middle-range" application of general evolutionary theory. Life history theory begins with the assumption that any evolutionarily successful organism must balance its allocation of time, energy, risk, and other resources to itself—its own growth and maintenance (somatic effort)—versus commitment to finding a mate and beginning reproduction (reproductive effort), (Pianka, 1970; Stearns, 1992). Similarly, with respect to offspring, "decisions" are made between strategies that lead to having many offspring, who necessarily receive lower levels of parental investment, and strategies that involve having fewer offspring, each of whom is capable of being more intensively nurtured.

Evolution-based research has made it clear that reproductive effort is strategic. For example, we neither choose our mates randomly nor attract them indiscriminately (Buss, 1994). An increasing body of research has documented that human mating and parenting are governed by a complex combination of domain-general and domain-specific mechanisms that represent evolved solutions to adaptive problems faced by our human ancestors over tens of thousands of years. From the perspective of Darwinian evolution, an *adaptive problem* is any problem whose solution contributes to an individual's survival and ultimately to successful reproduction.

In recognition of the strategic decisions just mentioned, evolutionary ecologists have distinguished between r and K *reproductive strategies*. Organisms that are usually faced with transient, unstable, and unpredictable environments typically pursue strategies that permit them to reproduce prolifically to take advantage of those times when resources are in relative abundance. Such organisms are referred to as *r-strategists* because they manifest traits associated with a high r, the intrinsic rate of increase of a population conforming to the logistic growth equation. *K-strategists* display evolved traits that are associated with alterations in the maximum population size that can be accommodated by organisms interacting with the environment: that is, the "carrying capacity" of logistic population growth, symbolized by K. These organisms are faced with predictably adverse ecological or competitive environments. Under these circumstances, high levels of parental investment are typically critical in order to successfully produce offspring that, themselves, will reach reproductive maturity. These terms are relative; for example, the dandelions in your yard are r-strategists when compared with your apple tree, but they are K-strategists when compared with the prodigious output of a chestnut oak. Among mammals, primates are K-strategists, but among primates, humans are rather extreme K-strategists (although, given the current population explosion, our closest living animal relative, the chimpanzee, is even more of a K-strategist than we are).

For our purposes, the key distinction between r- and K-strategists is the low level of parental investment of the former and the relatively higher level of parental effort of the latter. However, even if we accept the premise that there has been natural selection for high-investment parenting in humans (e.g., Lancaster & Lancaster, 1983), there are undoubtedly individual differences in reproductive strategies (Draper & Harpending, 1988). Some individuals allocate more energy in the pursuit of finding a mate, sometimes producing offspring from several different mates (a mating or r-strategy), than to high-investment parenting. Conversely, there are individuals who devote more of their time and energy and other resources to intensively nurturing their offspring (a parenting or K-strategy). Looked at over a person's entire life span, it is probably the case that most of us pursue a mixed strategy. Nonetheless, there are those who, on a mating- or parenting-effort continuum, can be found at either extreme.

This discussion leads to two observations. First, whichever strategy a person follows, costs and trade-offs must be made. Second, these two alternative strategies may be incompatible at the extremes of the reproductive effort continuum. For example, high-investment parents (those employing the K-strategy) incur considerable costs in providing their children with the high-quality experiences and environments that eventually contribute to the children's success in ecologically adverse and competitive environments. Indeed, research by child developmentalists suggests that an effective high-investment parenting strategy involves a complex of costly and coordinated activities, including feeling and expressing love toward one's offspring, possessing a strong emotional attachment to one's child, talking to the child often, reading to the child, playing with the child, actively listening to the child, being empathic, providing emotional support for the child, imparting values such as cooperativeness, honesty, and self-control, monitoring the child's behavior, enforcing rules in a consistent but flexible manner, providing for the child's nourishment and physical health, and attempting to keep the child from harm (Maccoby & Martin, 1983).

An extreme mating or r-strategy is also costly in time and energy and has its own set of coordinated activities, such as competing intensely for mates, being on the alert for new sexual partners, making oneself attrac-

tive to potential mates, exaggerating one's unique qualities, using deception, denigrating rivals, using coercive tactics for purposes of mate retention, attending inordinately to relationship-repair tactics, becoming sexually
active early in life, being promiscuous, being manipulative, being aggressive, having low empathy, and being impulsive (Draper & Harpending,
1988). The particular set of coordinated activities that are functional can
vary, of course, depending on whether a person's strategy is focused on
short-term sex (an unadulterated mating strategy) or on simply having
many offspring with minimal parental investment (a classic r-strategy). In
both cases, low-investment parenting is likely, and the possession of traits
like those listed here can easily set the stage for child maltreatment,
whether abuse or neglect.

In summary, in order to lay the groundwork for explaining why
certain social and ecological circumstances are associated with child maltreatment, we have described the core elements of life-history theory and
how it has identified two distinct reproductive strategies that explain
different orientations toward the production and care of offspring between
and within species. Our next task is to identify the conditions under which
particular strategies are pursued. Three possibilities appear most plausible. Although it is useful to distinguish between these analytically, they
should not be seen as incompatible explanations. The most reasonable
position is to see them as complementary processes that influence alternative reproductive strategies, including those that can be harmful to children.

The Capacity for Child Maltreatment as a Pan-Human Characteristic

According to a pan-human view, we all have the capacity under
certain contextual conditions to behave in ways that are seriously harmful
to our children. Technically, this is a *conditional-facultative* explanation for
the pursuit of alternative reproductive strategies. Traits or dispositions
that have been selected to take different states as a function of the environments in which they develop are referred to as *facultative* adaptations. In
contrast, there are the relatively fixed polymorphic traits of classical genetics, such as eye color or blood type, which are referred to as *obligate*
adaptations. To the extent that an adaptation is facultative, it responds
readily to environmental influence (i.e., its expression is conditional on the
presence of particular environmental circumstances). To the extent that it
is obligate, it resists such influences (Alcock, 1989). So what kinds of
environmental circumstances are consistent with this explanatory model?

Cultural Norms and Values

One of the important characteristics of a life-history perspective is that it is sensitive to historical and cultural diversity. In this way, it quickly becomes apparent that the relations between parents and offspring display a great deal more variability than is apparent to social and behavioral scientists, whose fields of analysis are limited to complex stratified Western societies. When considered from our current moral values, behaviors such as child abuse and neglect appear to be profoundly pathological. However, our values are entrenched in a stable, centralized political and economic system that distributes huge surpluses with a surprising degree of equity among individuals who are no longer connected to each other by longstanding ties of shared residence and kinship. Because of the rapidity of technological advances and the geometric increase in the world population in the last few hundred years, it is easy to forget that social relationships, including family relationships, were typically structured in a manner different from the ways to which we have become accustomed.

Throughout most of history, the individual's right to life and to some measure of satisfaction was a function of being born into an established group based on kinship ties. This pre-existing group provided economic and political security for new members; it was also a buffer against other similarly structured groups that, depending on circumstances, could constitute a serious competitive threat. For our ancestors, families were a necessity for survival and reproduction (van den Berghe, 1979). In order to maintain a competitive advantage or to expand against the interests of other groups, families (particularly their senior members) were required to allocate resources efficiently among kin and other individuals related by marriage. Families both nurtured members and culled from them. Numerous examples come from European traditions in the form of primogeniture, of sending surplus children into monasteries and convents, of "selling" children into indentured servitude, and of apprenticing children for periods of years to nonfamily members (Dickemann, 1979). In other, more final ways, parents discriminated among children, keeping some and letting others go to distant wet-nurses in the notorious rural baby farms of 17th- and 18th-century Europe (Aries, 1970; DeMause, 1974; Langer, 1972).

We mention these historically recent practices (which seem abhorrent by modern standards), because on the following pages we will argue that human family relationships cannot be assumed to be inevitably benign. Competition for access to scare resources is a fact within as well as between families (Trivers, 1974). It is in this context that the cross-cultural record is most valuable. For example, the socioeconomic conditions found in tribal hunting and gathering societies in resource-rich environments in the Pacific Rim and Polynesia, in low-intensity gardening societies in much of sub-Sahara Africa, and in the "underclass" of technologically advanced societies are associated with especially low male parental effort and high male competition (Harpending & Draper, 1988). Similarly, women in male competitive societies exhibit a pattern of lowered parental care marked by intense care to infants but early weaning followed by little or no direct care and reliance upon parent surrogates, such as older siblings or older relatives (e.g., Gallimore, Boggs, & Jordon, 1974; Hippler, 1974). While this child care arrangement clearly can work, it can also set the stage for behavior that we associate with child abuse or neglect.

When examining cultural norms that influence the amount and kind of parental effort, we must recognize that customs we define as being harmful to children are often benign from the parents' perspectives; they are simply following practices that form a part of the traditional ways in which a child becomes a member of the social group. Cassidy (1980), for example, has used the concept of benign neglect to emphasize that many weaning customs of nonindustrialized people potentiate malnutrition. Ethnographic studies indicate that many customs contribute to the malnutrition and associated secondary infections of children. Some parenting customs do this indirectly, by permitting or encouraging caretakers and toddlers to engage in interpersonal relationships that exacerbate the psychological stress associated with weaning, or directly, by permitting or encouraging the imposition of dietary restrictions and food competition between age and sex groups (Cassidy, 1980).

Food competition takes many different forms. In some societies, a newly weaned toddler is expected to compete on an equal basis with older siblings and even adults. In Malaya, for example, parents attribute independence and responsibility to young children and explain their extreme thinness by simply saying that the children "refuse to eat" (Wolff, 1965). Wolff attributes high toddler malnutrition and mortality to these practices. In many societies, it is common for toddlers to receive a disproportionately small share of the family's food because the traditional food-flow patterns favor adults, especially economically productive males (e.g., Cuthbertson, 1967). These dietary practices usually assume certain predictable patterns. For example, in most societies, the weaning customs favor males (Cassidy, 1980). It is important to note that the child who is weaned later is less at risk of malnutrition.

Several theoretical approaches have been employed to explain these fairly common practices. It has been suggested, for example, that the experience of malnutrition in early childhood may actually be biologically adaptive because it biases developmental plasticity toward hunger resistance in societies where food is often scarce. It has been found that individuals from societies where malnutrition is common grow more slowly, are shorter, and generally require less food (Newman, 1961). Thus, in this case, long-term advantage may accrue despite the short-term damage of malnutrition. Another explanation of these practices is that toddler malnutrition and associated higher mortality rates function as population control mechanisms in that they remove individuals from the population directly by causing their deaths (Scrimshaw, Taylor, & Gordon, 1968). This is perhaps best seen in cases where preferential treatment (better or more nutritious foods and delayed weaning) is given to males. Given the "normally" higher mortality rate of male children, such special favors may serve the function of creating adaptive sex ratios (Fisher, 1958; Trivers, 1985) without implying unlikely group-selection mechanisms (Williams, 1966).

An interesting feature of harmful dietary and weaning customs is the way in which they illustrate that cultural practices can interpose time and space between actions that are harmful to a child's welfare and the child's actual death. Because of this, the relationship between cause and effect can be circuitous and not apparent. For example, systematically denying children access to protein-rich food may produce subclinical malnutrition that may weaken them so that they fall victim to severe diarrhea. In these cases, gastrointestinal disease and dehydration will be recorded as the cause of death instead of the predisposing malnutrition and food practices that are due to parental neglect. Similarly, severe infections may appear several days after puberty rites that ritually inflict wounds. These infections may result in death, especially when ashes or other substances are rubbed into wounds for desired cosmetic effects (Linton, 1936). In addition, Scrimshaw (1984) notes that seeking psychological distance through temporal and spatial distance occurs even among infanticidal parents who often abandon rather than directly murder their children.

There is a considerable amount of evidence that progenicide—action that selectively reduces the probability of survival of children of all ages (McKee, 1984)—has been widely practiced throughout history in many societies. For example, in much of Western Europe throughout the 15th to the 19th centuries, it was customary to send newborn infants to live with rural wet-nurses for 9 months to a year or more. Some of these wet-nurses were reported to nurse two or three infants at once (Sussman, 1975). Mortality rates for these infants were appallingly high. In Britain in the 1870s, the overall infant mortality rate was approximately 15%, but the mortality rates of infants living with "baby farmers" reached 90% (Sauer, 1978).

The phenomenon of progenicide makes it clear that actions harmful to children are found throughout the historical and cultural record, that such practices do not necessarily imply individual or cultural pathology, and that these practices can be adaptive from an evolutionary perspective (that is, they may contribute to parental inclusive fitness under the ecological conditions in which they find themselves). It should not be assumed, however, that we make conscious calculated assessments of actions that may affect our reproductive success. This is probably seldom if ever the case. Instead, a multitude of proximate mechanisms undoubtedly bridge the gap between changing ecological conditions and patterns of child rearing. Social norms, values, and beliefs may well rank among these mechanisms. An example would be cultural norms prescribing that male infants should be breast-fed longer than female infants. Beliefs may develop around such rules. For instance, in rural Taiwan, mothers apparently believe that earlier weaning assures their daughters of an earlier menopause and a welcome end to the round of childbearing (Wolf, 1972). In the Ecuadorian highlands, there is a widespread belief that if a girl is nursed past 1 year she will, at sexual maturity, become "boy-crazy" and rebellious (McKee, 1977).

The role of such cultural norms and beliefs may be most useful in explaining normative child maltreatment. It may be of less importance when looking at harm to children that is culturally proscribed. It is important to recognize, however, that cultures are not monolithic and that individuals as well as groups of individuals may deviate from established cultural standards and norms. In the next section, we will examine the role of economic hardship as a cause of low-investment parenting and child maltreatment.

Poverty

Human groups have historically been exposed to ecological changes that signal improvement or degradation of their life situation. Such signals include changes in the availability of food resources, changes in climatological conditions, and the differential risks associated with war and peace. Given the length of time and amount of effort required for child care, human parents especially should be sensitive to turbulence in their environment. Thus, it can be predicted that transition states marked by instability in the environment in which families live will affect the behavioral systems associated with mating and parental effort.

This argument can be appreciated best by viewing the family as an ecosystem—that is, a group interacting with its habitat (Burgess & Youngblade, 1988). Under optimal conditions, an ecosystem will be in a state of dynamic equilibrium so that there is a fairly equal balance, or even an excess, of resources relative to the problems with which the family must cope. To the extent that resources a family can marshal decrease or are perceived to decrease in proportion to the problems it must solve, stress will occur and the likelihood of conflict and violence will also increase. Actual or perceived decreases in individual and family resources are often observed during transitional periods marked by rapid social change. During these times, there is increased uncertainty and an associated disintegration of normal social control mechanisms (Erlich, 1966).

Dickemann (1979), in her analysis of infanticide, has also recognized the importance of drastic changes in ecology. She has argued that periodic catastrophes and resource scarcities usually raise mortality rates for males because of their increased susceptibility to life-threatening birth defects and infectious diseases, particularly those of the digestive and respiratory tracts. Because infant mortality rates of males are especially sensitive to economic conditions, females tend to become the more numerous sex whenever environmental conditions for child rearing are less than optimal (Preston, 1976). Under these conditions, preferential treatment for males arises. Thus, male preference may have been the preferred parental strategy for humans given the general unpredictability of the environment (Dickemann, 1979). As McKee (1984) comments, "It is ironic that female biological strength may be one factor promoting the development of social systems oppressive to women" (p. 95). In any case, conditions of ecological instability may produce a postcatastrophe sex ratio highly favoring males because of more intense female infanticide. This in turn may lead to the subsequent need for males to colonize less populated areas, which in turn can lead to ecological instability in the new areas (Bigelow, 1969).

From a life history perspective, ecological instability refers to situations in which levels of stress exceed the family's resources. Poverty has been identified as a major cause of stress among maltreating families. For impoverished families, stress is a part of everyday life. There is substantial empirical support for the assertion that poverty is associated with infant mortality as well as physical abuse and neglect of children (Coulton, Korbin, Su, & Chow, 1995; Drake & Pandey, 1996; Garbarino & Sherman, 1980; Pelton, 1978, Polansky, Gavdin, Ammons, & Davis, 1985). While it is true that child maltreatment has been found to occur across all social classes, it is equally true that it is disproportionately represented in lower socioeconomic classes. Resistance by professionals and academicians to recognize this fact simply perpetuates a myth of classlessness (Pelton, 1978). It has been thirty years since Giovannoni and Billingsley (1970) reported that, even among poor families, the highest incidence of child maltreatment occurs when conditions of poverty are most profound. Such circumstances act to create an environment of severe stress, dependency, and hardship, which have been found to play an important role in child maltreatment (Garbarino & Gilliam, 1980; Vondra, 1990). Ecological instability, marked by joblessness and low income, is most likely to exist in families suffering from poverty. Research by Krugman, Lenherr, Betz, and Fryer (1986) suggests a very high correlation between physical abuse reports and unemployment rates. Furthermore, according to Garbarino (1997), the relationship between unemployment and child maltreatment is grounded in the idea that unemployment diminishes financial resources within the family and can negatively affect the providers' mental health. Because parental status, most notably male identity, is so strongly defined by occupational achievement, joblessness can lead to diminished identity, uncertainty, and conflict within the family. This situation provides the opportunity for child maltreatment to occur. Garbarino (1997) also explains that a provider's employment is most often the primary source of health care for the family. Once this resource no longer exists, risks for child neglect rise due to the inability to attend financially to the child's needs.

According to Gelles (1992), severe violence toward children is most likely to occur in families where the annual income is below the poverty line. The second national Family Violence Survey, conducted in 1985, found that in families where incomes were below the poverty line, overall violence toward children was 4% higher, severe violence was 46% higher, and very severe violence was 100% higher than in families living above the poverty line (Gelles, 1992). Increased irritability, conflict, and punitive behavior are all found to be typical parental responses to economic stressors (Vondra, 1990). In addition, the stress incurred by lack of resources can ultimately lead to the child becoming a deliberate focus of frustration and rage, often in the form of abuse and neglect (Garbarino, 1997).

It is important to note that while physical abuse and violence receive more attention in the media, the neglect of children is much more common in high poverty areas, accounting for approximately 60–65% of all cases of maltreatment (Drake & Pandey, 1996). Furthermore, instances of child neglect such as failing to provide immunizations, regular medication, medical examinations, necessary hospitalizations and surgery, and prosthetic care can be just as harmful to a child as direct physical abuse.

Poverty, of course, exists within a social context, and the community context within which a family resides is similarly associated with stress if it is accompanied by the lack of social organization, social support, social cohesion, and social control. Low income joined with poor demographic factors allows for the generation of stress that can contribute to child maltreatment (Garbarino & Crouter, 1978; Justice & Duncan, 1976). Factors such as social isolation (Drake & Pandey, 1996; Wilson, 1987), community norms (Drake & Pandey, 1996; Belsky, 1993), and lack of resources (Drake & Pandey, 1996; Vondra, 1990) have also been associated with increased levels of child maltreatment. If child maltreatment was simply a result of the increased stress surrounding impoverished areas, it would not exist within areas of moderate to low poverty. However, this is not the case. Thus, it is important to examine the characteristics of impoverished neighborhoods in an attempt to identify causal factors that link poverty to child maltreatment.

Child maltreatment has been identified as a product of deficient social networks within a community. According to Belsky (1993), the social support found within a strong social network in a community can act as a stress buffer in that it contributes to physical and psychological well-being. Garbarino and Sherman (1980) found that when comparing two communities of equal social class, families in the community characterized by weak social networks had higher incidences of child maltreatment. Social relationships provide parents with emotional support needed to confront the stress caused by poverty. Social networking within a community also acts as a means of social control; it can set limits on parents' behavior toward their children. In the absence of social exchanges and social visits, community members have fewer opportunities to observe family life in other members' homes (Vondra 1990; Garbarino & Sherman, 1980). Furthermore, Vondra argues that these networks also provide child-care resources for parents in need. Commonly, when social networks are not available to parents, children are often left home alone and neglected.

A lack of social networking can result in social isolation for families in poverty-stricken communities. Social isolation is characterized by having few friends, engaging in short-term friendships, and experiencing unsatisfactory relations with family members (Vondra, 1990; Crittenden, 1985). Such isolation has been identified as the single most common component of maltreating impoverished families when compared to nonmaltreating impoverished families (Vondra, 1990). Similar to the findings by Vondra, Polansky, Chalmers, Buttenweiser, and Williams (1981) found that among neglecting parents the level of social isolation was found to exceed the levels found in nonneglectful parents in similar demographic conditions.

Communities characterized by social isolation among their members and an overall lack of social control have been found to experience much more social disorganization. Such neighborhood conditions have definite implications for the degree of child maltreatment that occurs. Research by Garbarino and Kostelny (1991) clearly establishes this. In studying 27 communities in Chicago, the investigators found that the social climate in areas with high rates of child maltreatment differed from that in areas with lower rates. In the north, where abuse appeared more prevalent, "the tone ... was depressed; people had a hard time thinking of good things to say about the situation.... The physical spaces seemed dark and depressed.... The extremity of the negative features of the environment—poverty, violence, poor housing—seem to be matched by negative community climate" (p. 461). Conversely, in the west, where child maltreatment rates were not as high, "people seemed more eager to talk about their community.... Most felt that their communities were poor but decent places to live" (p. 461). This study illustrates how even among poverty-stricken communities where child maltreatment is prevalent, those areas characterized as having less social cohesion and more social disorganization are more likely to have significantly higher instances of child maltreatment.

In summary, a conditional-facultative explanation is based upon the assumption that, under theoretically specified conditions, all parents are susceptible to courses of action that can threaten the welfare of their child. We have examined two such conditions. The first derived from cultural norms and values; we presented examples of cultural practices that are often harmful to children. These data imply that child rearing must be viewed within the social and historical context in which it is found. The second condition that we examined derived from economic deprivation or poverty, which we showed as a cause of low-investment parenting that is harmful to children. As we have seen, studies over the past thirty years have documented that the maltreatment of children is strongly associated with poverty. For example, the 1986 replication of the National Incidence Study reported that rate of abuse and neglect for families with incomes under $15,000 was five times that for families with incomes above that level. In fact, only 6% of maltreating families had incomes above the national median.

The association of poverty with child abuse and neglect is familiar to everyone. Yet, poverty by itself is just a marker variable; we need to know more about *why* poverty is associated with punitive and neglectful parenting. To be sure, there are special stresses and strains experienced by families living in poverty, and perhaps especially those living in communities deficient in social supports. For example, the purchase of children's books may be virtually impossible because of the expense. Parents may be overwhelmed by difficulties in making ends meet. Living conditions may be cramped. Diets may be bland and not particularly nutritious. It should not be overlooked, however, that much of human history has been characterized by levels of material deprivation and hardship that far exceed our current definition of living in poverty. There is no evidence that such adverse conditions were uniformly associated with low-investment parenting or child maltreatment. Indeed, as noted earlier, ecologically challenging environments are precisely those that are postulated to have led to selection for high-investment parenting strategies.

So it may not be poverty itself that is important but instead the correlates of poverty today. Several of these stand out. One is the structural changes that have been taking place in the U.S. economy, with the shutting down of manufacturing plants and assembly lines, the devaluation of physical labor, and the undercutting of union pay scales. Such circumstances have clearly affected economic prospects, contributed to increasing social inequality, and rightly or wrongly, led many to conclude that upward social mobility is virtually impossible. As described by MacDonald (1997), there have been other occasions in Western history when the lack of hope for upward mobility was associated with early mating, high fertility, and a low-investment parental strategy.

A second correlate of poverty today is the high frequency of female-headed families. For families headed by a single woman, the poverty rate in 1991 was 36%. For all others, it was only 6% (U.S. Bureau of the Census, 1992). What is significant about these statistics is that the frequency of reported maltreatment cases in female-headed households is more than twice that for two-parent households (American Humane Association, 1985).

The third important correlate of poverty today that bears on child welfare is living in high-crime neighborhoods. For example, Simon and Burns (1997), in a fascinating ethnography of a year in the life of an inner-city neighborhood, provide a chilling account of the spread of cocaine use in our urban ghettos. When heroin was the main drug of choice, there was at least a network of single mothers who managed somehow to keep families together. With the influx of cheap cocaine (and later, crack cocaine) in the 1980s, many inner-city families were battered beyond recognition. Where we were once concerned about single-parent families, now loomed the specter of children who were functionally parentless.

But there may be more to it than this. While social and economic stresses and strains are among the best documented correlates of child maltreatment, the presumed causal sequence from poverty to parental behavior has limitations as a causal inference, based as it is on cross-sectional research designs. Cross-sectional designs typically cannot distinguish social causation from social selection. Does economic deprivation lead to the neglect and abuse of children? Or are there personal characteristics that lead both to downward mobility (or economic deprivation) *and* low-investment parenting? This is the issue we explore in our second model for explaining different reproductive strategies.

The Capacity for Child Maltreatment as a Heritable Predisposition

According to this model, individuals with certain genotypes may be predisposed to follow a strategy that can be harmful to their children. Technically, from the perspective of life history theory, this is an *alternative-obligate* explanation of different reproductive strategies. An alternative-obligate strategy refers to evolved adaptations that are obligate for an individual but polymorphic in a population (Alcock, 1989). With regard to the issue of child maltreatment, this explanatory model hypothesizes that there are genetically based differences in response to environmental experiences.

A useful way to examine this model is by returning to the issue of poverty and its causal role in the abuse and neglect of children. Because of their longitudinal nature, Elder's (1974) studies of families who experienced the Great Depression provide us with a unique opportunity not only to explore the consequences of economic hardship on parental behavior but also to resolve an important issue in causal inference—the direction of effect. Among his many published findings, we are particularly interested in those relevant to the mating–parenting continuum of reproductive effort. Concerning the former, Elder reported that there was no significant effect of economic decline on age at marriage among the working class. Among women in the middle classes who suffered economic decline, however, it did result in an earlier onset of dating, pre-marital sex, and marriage than for those women who did not experience income loss. He also noted that those evidencing such changes tended to marry men of higher social status than did economically nondeprived women. So, if anything, it appears that these women responded to economic adversity by taking actions to assure their economic stability and by following a high-investment parenting strategy (MacDonald, 1997).

With regard to parenting, Elder, Liker, and Cross (1984) found that economic hardship affected fathers far more than mothers. Moreover, income loss was strongly predictive of arbitrary and explosive parental behavior *only* among those men who exhibited hostility toward their children before the Depression and who were also experiencing marital problems. For previously friendly and accepting fathers, economic deprivation tells us very little about the nature and degree of paternal involvement. Thus, Elder's (1974) data are inconsistent with the assumption that poverty or downward mobility causes low-investment parenting in any simple straightforward way.

So what is going on? Why is poverty today so often associated with child abuse and neglect? One possible answer is that the pool of poor people has changed significantly over the past two generations (Herrnstein & Murray, 1994). As recently as the 1940s, a remarkably large percentage of the U.S. population was poor by anyone's standards. Yet these people, poor as they may have been, were largely indistinguishable from the rest of the population. With the spread of affluence after the end of the Second World War, those who failed to escape from poverty were probably not representative of those who had. The pool of those who were left behind consisted not only of those who were victimized by bad luck or discrimination—although some certainly were—but also those who lacked energy, thrift, conscientiousness, foresightedness, determination, and intellectual competence (Herrnstein & Murray, 1994). Data indicate that whites with IQs in the bottom 5% of the distribution of intellectual competence are 15 times more likely to be poor than those in the upper 5% (Herrnstein & Murray, 1974). In a study of social mobility, Waller (1971) found that the IQ scores of upwardly mobile sons were consistently higher than those of their fathers, and those of the downwardly mobile sons were significantly lower.

Consequently, if cognitive ability is associated with poverty, and if poverty is associated with child maltreatment, then cognitive ability may have some role in the abuse and neglect of children. Indeed, Polansky et al. (1981), in his comprehensive study of child neglect, found the typical neglectful mother to have less than an eighth grade education and an IQ below 70. Similarly, below-average cognitive competence has been found to be associated with poor prenatal care, low birth weight, low scores on the HOME (Home Observation for Measurement of the Environment), difficult child temperament, and problem behaviors such as antisocial behavior and hyperactivity. These findings led Herrnstein and Murray (1994) to conclude that, after taking into account the SES (socioeconomic status) background of the parents, the HOME index, and poverty, cognitive competence (IQ) has a strong, independent effect on parenting practices. This does not mean, of course, that a person's socioeconomic background plays no role. It is simply the case that the magnitude of the disadvantage of an economically impoverished background by itself may not be as large as we normally assume.

The obvious implication is that low-investment parenting, including child maltreatment, is not necessarily an automatic reaction to poverty but is instead strongly influenced by intelligence, which is significantly heritable. It is important to emphasize, however, that this argument is not a case of simplistic genetic determinism. The connection between intelligence and poverty and low-investment parenting varies with context. For example, as Herrnstein and Murray's (1994) data show, "marriage is a poverty preventative, and this is true for women even of modest cognitive ability" (pp. 138–139). Simply put, poverty hits unmarried mothers of low levels of intelligence much harder than those at higher levels of cognitive ability.

Viewed through this lens, the connection between poverty, single parenthood, low-investment parenting, and the maltreatment of children takes on new meaning because low cognitive ability is not only associated with the risk of living in poverty today but also with the correlates of poverty such as illegitimacy, marital instability, and serious and chronic criminal activity. With regard to criminal behavior, for instance, Gottfredson and Hirschi (1986) note that the person chronically committing criminal acts tends to be a person who is relatively free of concern for the consequences of his acts: "a person who follows the impulse of the moment" (p. 231). At the individual level, they found academic achievement and cognitive competence to function as predictors that transcend social class and ethnicity.

In summary, we have examined evidence that casts doubt upon the often-held assumption that poverty, by itself, causes child maltreatment or a low-investment parenting strategy. We have seen that poverty does not paint with a broad brush; its effects are mediated by personal traits such as personality and intelligence, both of which are, in part, genetically influenced (Rowe, 1994). Given general acceptance for the premise that there has been selection for high-investment parenting in humans, it is not unreasonable to hypothesize that there might also be significant heritability (genetically based individual differences) of the complex behaviors that are related to parental investment. Unfortunately, there appears to have been resistance by researchers to investigate the role of intelligence and other heritable traits in accounting for the abuse and neglect of children. This brings us to our third explanatory model.

The Capacity for Child Maltreatment as a Stress-Induced Response to Early Developmental Experiences

According to our third model, particularly traumatic early experiences may set a person on a developmental trajectory that culminates in a reproductive strategy potentially harmful to children. The role of critical early experiences for subsequent development has long been of interest to developmental psychologists. So far as human development is concerned, a conservative position is that early experiences *can* have long-term consequences to the extent that later person–environment interactions are consistent with those that occurred earlier. Whatever the case may be, the behavioral biologist's (e.g., Alcock, 1989) distinction between "conditional" and "alternative" adaptations appears to break down when we consider the existence of especially potent early environmental experiences. On the one hand, the effects are presumably the product of unique experiences and are, therefore, "conditional" on those experiences. On the other hand, such experiences are considered special precisely because they lead to constrained development. Thus, they appear to be obligate for the individual experiencing them, resulting in an "alternative" strategy. So we are left with a possibility that might best be termed a *conditional-alternative* explanation of different life histories. However this theoretical or terminological issue is resolved, it certainly suggests, at the very least, that conditional and alternative strategies are not necessarily mutually exclusive.

There are two early experiences that have been proposed to have long-term effects that can affect a person's future performance as a parent. We will look at these briefly. The first is a history of having been maltreated as a child. Recognition that a pattern of child maltreatment is often found in successive generations has been a mainstay of the child abuse literature. In a study of high-risk mothers and children in Minneapolis, Egeland, Jacobvitz, and Papatola (1987) reported that 70% of mothers who had been abused in their childhood were maltreating their children. This figure, however, included mothers who were not currently caring for their children or who were providing borderline care. In fact, of the mothers who had suffered severe physical abuse in childhood, almost as many were providing adequate care for their children (30%) as were clearly maltreating them. Furthermore, only one-half of the nonabused mothers in their low SES families were found to be adequately caring for their children.

In a comprehensive analysis of studies that either used appropriate comparison groups or employed prospective rather than retrospective designs, Kaufman and Zigler (1987) concluded that the best estimate of the rate of intergenerational continuity in maltreatment is approximately 30%. Straus, Gelles, and Steinmetz (1980), in their representative sample survey of the U.S. population, found that 12% of abusing parents reported having been abused as children.

The national incidence study (U.S. Department of Health and Human Services, 1988) supported by the National Center on Child Abuse and Neglect, as well as the American Humane Association's study of child abuse and neglect (Garbarino, 1989), reported a 2.5% incidence rate for all types of child maltreatment in the United States. These figures are based on cases known to someone outside the family and, therefore, probably represent underestimates of the true incidence rate. Whatever the true incidence is, cross-generational rates from 12–30% are clearly above the base rate for the population as a whole.

A reasonable conclusion, then, is that under certain conditions being abused or neglected as a child increases the probability of adopting a similar low-investment parental strategy in adulthood. Unfortunately, research has yet to identify conclusively what the necessary conditions are for such generational continuity to occur. Burgess and Youngblade (1988) suggested that developmental experiences outside the family, such as relationships with peers or other adults, may be critical. Our first explanatory model—that the capacity for child maltreatment is a pan-human characteristic—would apply here. However, given that maltreated children and maltreating parents display similar profiles for personality traits that have significant heritabilities (Burgess, 1997), our second explanatory model—that the capacity for maltreatment is a heritable predisposition for some individuals—might also be involved.

Another set of early childhood experiences that may influence the reproductive strategy a child subsequently pursues in adulthood is exposure to marital conflict and domestic violence. Few family problems are more closely related to a child's poor adjustment than marital conflict. Approximately 40–50% of children exposed to marital violence exhibit extreme behavior problems, a proportion more than five times that for the general population (Jourlies, Barling, & O'Leary, 1987; Wolfe, Jaffe, Wilson, & Zak, 1985).

Most studies on the effects of marital conflict have sampled relatively normal, intact families. Not surprisingly, the links between marital conflict and child difficulties appear to be stronger in samples of families with multiple stressors (Emery & O'Leary, 1982; Hughes, Parkinson, & Vargo, 1989; Sternberg, Lamb, Greenbaum, Chicchetti, Dawud, Cortes, Krispin, & Lorey, 1993). Similarly, children in abusive homes are at increased risk of adjustment problems. Moreover, parental aggression toward children is strongly associated with interspousal aggression (Gelles, 1987; Hughes, 1988; Jourlies et al., 1987; Barling & O'Leary, 1987). Approximately 40% of the children who are victims of physical abuse also witness spousal violence (Straus et al., 1980), which, by itself, may contribute to children's vulnerability. Indeed, children who witness parental violence exhibit problematic behaviors that are similar to those of children who are victims of parental violence (Jaffe, Wolfe, Wilson, & Zak, 1986). In addition, research indicates that children who are both witnesses to marital violence and victims of parental abuse exhibit higher levels of parent-reported problem behaviors than do children who are either witnesses or victims of parental violence (Trickett & Susman, 1989). Thus, effects normally attributed solely to child abuse may also reflect effects of exposure to spousal violence and conflict.

To date, effects of combined child abuse and marital conflict are not well understood (Cummings & Davies, 1994). One possibility is that marital conflict could have a negative impact on children's behavior that is independent of the dangerous effects of child abuse (Hughes et al., 1980). Alternatively, marital conflict combined with child abuse may potentiate children's risk for psychopathology (Rutter, 1990). That is, the co-occurrence of marital conflict and child abuse may have far greater effects than the sum of either stressor considered individually.

Marital conflict alone, as a core feature of family life, has implications for the socialization of children. Between 9 and 25% of the differences between children's disruptive and aggressive behavior is accounted for by marital conflict in the home (Grych & Finchham, 1990). Specifically, these children are especially vulnerable to excessive aggression, unacceptable conduct, vandalism, noncompliance, and delinquency (Grych & Fincham, 1990; Emery & O'Leary, 1984), as well as diminished academic performance manifested by poor grades in school and teacher reports of problems in intellectual achievement and abilities (Long, Forehand, Fauber, & Brody, 1987).

The primary focus of most research on the consequences of marital conflict has been on the indirect effects of parents' fights on children. The stress of interparental conflict can cause parents to become less consistent and less effective in their parenting behavior, thereby increasing the rate of child maltreatment (Fauber & Long, 1991). Marital discord may reduce parental attention to children's emotional needs and signals, thereby diminishing the quality of the emotional relationships or attachments between parents and children (Stevensen-Hinde, 1990) and increasing the rate of various childhood problems (Bretherton, 1985).

More recently, attention has shifted to the direct impact of exposure to and involvement in interparental conflict. Exposure to interparental anger may induce emotional distress in children, enmesh children in their parents' problems, or cause anger and aggression that over time will result in the development of dysfunctional behavior. Furthermore, children who both witness marital violence and are victims of abuse are at an even higher risk for antisocial behavior. Parents who use physically aggressive tactics to resolve spousal disputes also use similar tactics in disciplining their children (O'Keefe, 1995; Rosenbaum & O'Leary, 1981; Straus et al., 1980). Children from maritally violent homes who are victims of child maltreatment are also more likely to live in families where there is a greater frequency and severity of marital violence. As we noted earlier, it is even possible that severe and frequent marital violence permeates parent–child relationships, resulting in child abuse or neglect (O'Keefe, 1995). Whatever the case may be, chronic marital discord and domestic violence clearly affect children in a negative way, and perhaps especially when combined with direct child abuse and neglect, could easily contribute to a cycle of maltreatment from one generation to the next.

In summary, according to this third explanatory model, there may be important early life experiences that affect children to increase significantly the chances that they will themselves eventually adopt a low-investment strategy toward their own children, even to the extent of imposing on their children the very same maltreatment that they experienced. Marital discord, domestic violence, and the transmission of low-investment and maltreating parental styles from one generation to the next constitute social and ecological circumstances deserving of continued research.

Summary

Surely by now it should be evident that social and ecological conditions play important roles in the etiology and persistence of the neglect and abuse of children. In this chapter we have attempted to describe some of the more important social and ecological determinants. We have seen that cultural norms and values play significant roles, as do resource scarcity and poverty. By employing concepts and principles from life history theory, we have examined three analytically separate but empirically complementary explanations for these effects. The first explanatory perspective assumes that the capacity for child maltreatment lies within all of us— it is a pan-human characteristic—whose manifestation depends on certain social and ecological conditions. This is a "conditional" explanation. The second explanatory model addresses the issue of individual differences within societies, cultures, and social class. According to this perspective, the capacity for child maltreatment varies across individuals as a function of genetic variation. This is an "alternative" explanation. The third explanatory position we examined hypothesizes that, in some circumstances, the capacity for maltreatment may be the product of early stress-producing life experiences. This explanation involves both conditional and alternative processes. While it is our view that all three explanatory processes are important, only the first and the third have been seriously considered by child maltreatment professionals and researchers. It is our hope that we have made a case for the importance of including all three of these explanatory models.

References

Alcock, J. (1984). *Animal behavior: An evolutionary approach.* Sunderland, MA: Sinaker Associates.
Alcock, J. (1989). Human biology and health: Intelligence in evolutionary biology. *Quarterly Review of Biology, 64,* 232–233.

American Humane Association. (1985). *Highlights of official child neglect and abuse reporting 1983*. Denver, CO: Author.

Aries, P. (1970). *Centuries of childhood, a social history of family life*. New York: Knopf.

Barkow, J. H., Cosmides, L., & Tooby, J. (Eds.). (1992). *The adopted mind: Evolutionary psychology and the generation of culture*. New York: Oxford University Press.

Belsky, J. (1993). Etiology of child maltreatment: A developmental-ecological analysis. *Psychological Bulletin, 114*, 414–434.

Bigelow, R. (1969). *The dawn warriors: Man's evolution toward peace*. Boston: Little, Brown.

Bretherton, I. (1985). Attachment theory: Retrospect and prospect. In I. Bretherton & E. Waters (Eds.), Growing points of attachment theory and research. *Monographs of the Society for Research in Child Development, 50*(1–2, Serial No. 209), 167–193.

Burgess, R. L. (1991). Social and ecological issues in violence towards children. In R. T. Ammerman & M. Hersen (Eds.), *Case studies in family violence* (pp. 15–38). New York: Plenum Press.

Burgess, R. L. (1997, June). *Behavior genetics and evolutionary psychology: A new look at the transmission of maltreatment across generations*. Paper presented at annual meeting of the Behavior Genetics Association, Toronto, Canada.

Burgess, R. L., & Youngblade, L. M. (1988). Social incompetence and the intergenerational transmission of abusive parental practices. In R. Gelles, G. Hotaling, D. Finkelhor, & M. Straus (Eds.), *New directions in family violence research* (pp. 38–60). Beverly Hills, CA: Sage.

Buss, D. (1994). *The evolution of desire: Strategies of human mating*. New York: Basic Books.

Cassidy, C. M. (1980). *Benign neglect and toddler malnutrition: Social and biological predictors of nutritional status, physical growth, and neurological development*. New York: Academic Press.

Coulton, C. J., Korbin, J. E., Su, M., & Chow, J. (1995). Community level factors and child maltreatment rates. *Child Development, 66*, 1262–1276.

Crittenden, P. M. (1985). Social networks, quality of child rearing and child development. *Child Development, 56*, 1299–1313.

Cummings, E. M., & Davies, P. (1994). *Children and marital conflict: The impact of family dispute and resolution*. New York: Guilford Press.

Cuthbertson, D. P. (1967). Feeding patterns and nutrient utilization [chairman's remarks]. *Proceedings of the Nutrition Society, 26*, 143–144.

DeMause, L. (1974). The evolution of childhood. In L. DeMause (Ed.), *The history of childhood*. New York: Psycho History Press.

Dickman, M. (1979). Female infanticide, reproductive strategies, and social stratification: A preliminary model. In N. Chapman & W. Irans (Eds.), *Evolutionary biology and human behavior* (pp. 321–367). North Saituate, MA: Duxbury Press.

Drake, B., & Pandey, S. (1996). Understanding the relationship between neighborhood, poverty, and specific types of child maltreatment. *Child Abuse and Neglect, 20*, 1003–1018.

Draper, P., & Harpending, H. (1988). A sociobiological perspective on the development of human reproductive strategies. In K. B. MacDonald (Ed.), *Sociobiological perspectives on human development* (pp. 340–372). New York: Springer-Verlag.

Egeland, B., Jacobvitz, D., & Papatola, K. (1987). Intergenerational continuity of abuse. In R. Gelles & J. Lancaster (Eds.), *Child abuse and neglect: Biosocial dimensions*. New York: Aldine de Gruyter.

Elder, G. H. (1974). *Children of the Great Depression: Social change in life experience*. Chicago: University of Chicago Press.

Elder, G. H., Jr., Liker, J. K., & Cross, C. E. (1984). Parent–child behavior in the great depression: Life course and intergenerational influences. In P. Baltes & O. Brien (Eds.), *Life span development and behavior* (Vol. 6, pp. 109–158). New York: Academic Press.

Emery, R. E., & O'Leary, K. D. (1982). Children's perceptions of marital discord and behavior problems of boys and girls. *Journal of Abnormal Child Psychology, 12,* 411–420.

Erlich, R. S. (1966). *Family in transition: A study of 300 Yugoslav villages.* Princeton, NJ: Princeton University Press.

Fauber, R. L., & Long, N. (1991). Children in context: The role of the family in child psychotherapy. *Journal of Consulting and Clinical Psychology, 59,* 813–820.

Fisher, R. A. (1958). *The genetical theory of natural selection.* New York: Dover.

Gallimore, R., Boggs, J., & Jordan, C. (1974). *Culture, behavior, and education: A study of Hawaiian Americans.* Beverly Hills, CA: Sage.

Garbarino, J. (1989). Trouble youths, troubled families: The dynamics of adolescent maltreatment. In D. Cicchetti & A. Toth (Eds.), *Child maltreatment: Theory and research on the causes and consequences of child abuse and neglect* (pp. 685– 706). Cambridge, England: Cambridge University Press.

Garbarino, J. (1997). The role of economic deprivation in the social context of child maltreatment. In M. E. Helfer, R. S. Kempe, & R. D. Krugman (Eds.), *The battered child* (pp. 49–60). Chicago: University of Chicago Press.

Garbarino, J., & Crouter, A. (1978). Defining the community context of parent–child relations: The correlates of child maltreatment. *Child Development, 49,* 604–616.

Garbarino, J., & Gilliam, G. (1980). *Understanding abusive families.* Lexington, MA: Heath.

Garbarino, J., & Kostelny, K. (1991). Child maltreatment as a community problem. *Child Abuse and Neglect, 16,* 455–464.

Garbarino, J., & Sherman, D. (1980). High-risk neighborhoods and high-risk families: The human ecology of child maltreatment. *Child Development, 51,* 188–198.

Gelles, R. J. (1987). *Family violence* (2nd ed.). Newbury Park, CA: Sage.

Gelles, R. J. (1992). Poverty and violence toward children. *American Behavioral Scientist, 35,* 258–274.

Giovannoni, J., & Billingsley, A. (1970). Child neglect among the poor: A study of parental inadequacy in families of three ethnic groups. *Child Welfare, 49,* 196–204.

Gottfredson, M., & Hirschi, T. (1986). The significance of white collar crime for a general theory of crime. *Criminology, 27,* 359–371.

Grych, J. H., & Fincham, F. D. (1990). Marital conflict and children's adjustment: A cognitive-contextual framework. *Psychological Bulletin, 108,* 267–290.

Harpending, H., & Draper, P. (1988). Antisocial behavior and the other side of cultural evolution. In T. E. Moffit & S. A. Mednick (Eds.), *Biological contributions to crime causations* (pp. 293–307). Dordrecht, The Netherlands: Martinus Nijhoff.

Herrnstein, R. J., & Murray, C. M. (1994). *The bell curve: Intelligence and class structure in American life.* New York: Free Press.

Hippler, A. E. (1974). *Hunter's Point: A black ghetto.* New York: Basic Books.

Hughes, H. (1988). Psychological and behavioral correlates of family violence in child witnesses and victims. *American Journal of Orthopsychiatry, 58,* 77–90.

Hughes, H., Parkinson, D., & Vargo, M. (1989). Witnessing spouse abuse and experiencing physical abuse: A "double whammy?" *Journal of Family Violence, 4,* 197–209.

Jaffe, P., Wolfe, D., Wilson, S. K., & Zak, L. (1986). Family violence and child adjustment: A comparative analysis of girls' and boys' behavioral symptoms. *American Journal of Psychiatry, 143,* 74–77.

Jourlies, E. N., Barling, J., & O'Leary, K. G. (1987). Predicting child behavior problems in maritally violent families. *Journal of Abnormal Child Psychology, 15,* 163–173.

Justice, B., & Duncan, D. F. (1976). Life crisis as a precursor to child abuse. *Public Health Reports, 91,* 110–115.

Kaufman, & Zigler, E. (1987). Do abused children become abusive parents? *American Journal of Orthopsychiatry, 57,* 186–192.

Krugman, R., Lenherr, M., Betz, L., & Fryer, G. (1986). The relationship between unemployment and physical abuse of children. *Child Abuse and Neglect, 10,* 415–418.

Lancaster, J., & Lancaster, C. (1983). Parental investment: The Hominid adaptation. In D. J. Ortner (Ed.), *How humans adapt: A biocultural odyssey.* Washington, DC: Smithsonian Institution Press.

Langer, W. L. (1972). Checks on population growth: 1750–1850. *Scientific American, 226,* 92–99.

Linton, R. (1936). *The study of man.* New York: Appleton Century.

Long, N., Forehand, R., Fauber, R., & Brody, G. H. (1987). Self-perceived and independently observed competence of young adolescents as a function of parental marital conflict and recent divorce. *Journal of Abnormal Child Psychology, 15,* 15–27.

Maccoby, E., & Martin, J. (1983). Parent–child relationships. In P. Mussen (Series Ed.) & E. M. Hetherington (Vol. Ed.), *Handbook of child psychology: Vol. 4. Socialization, personality and social development* (pp. 1–101). New York: Wiley.

MacDonald, K. (1997). Life-history theory and human reproductive behavior: Environmental/ contextual influences and heritable variation. *Human Mating, 8,* 327–359.

McKee, L. (1977, April). *Differential weaning and the ideology of gender: Implications for Andean sex ratios.* Paper read at the 76th annual meeting of the American Psychological Association, Houston.

McKee, L. (1984). Sex differentials in survivorship and the customary treatment of infants and children. *Medical Anthropology, 8,* 91–98.

Newman, M. T. (1961). Biological adaptation of man to his environment: Heat, cold, altitude, and nutrition. *Annals of the New York Academy of Sciences, 91,* 617–633.

O'Keefe, M. (1995). Predictors of child abuse in maritally violent families. *Journal of Interpersonal Violence, 10,* 3–25.

Pelton, L. H. (1978). Child abuse and neglect: The myth of classlessness. *American Journal of Orthopsychiatry, 48,* 608–617.

Pianka, E. R. (1970). On r- and k-selection. *American Naturalist, 104,* 592–597.

Polansky, N. A., Chalmers, M. A., Buttenweiser, E., & Williams, D. P. (1981). *Damaged parents: An anatomy of child neglect.* Chicago: University of Chicago Press.

Polansky, N. A., Gaudin, J. M., Ammons, P. W., & Davis, K. B. (1985). The psychological ecology of the neglectful mother. *Child Abuse and Neglect, 9,* 265–275.

Preston, S. (1976). *Mortality patterns in national populations with special reference to recorded causes of death.* New York: Academic Press.

Rosenbaum, A., & O'Leary, K. D. (1981). Marital violence: Characteristics of abusive couples. *Journal of Consulting and Clinical Psychology, 49,* 63–71.

Rowe, D. C. (1994). *The limits of family influence: Genes, experience, and behavior.* New York: The Guilford Press.

Rutter, M. (1990). Psychosocial resilience and protective mechanisms. In J. Rolf, A. S. Masten, D. Cicchetti, K. H. Neuchterlein, & S. Weintraub (Eds.), *Risk and protective factors in the development of psychopathology* (pp. 181–214). Cambridge, England: Cambridge University Press.

Sauer, R. (1978). Infanticide and abortion in nineteenth-century Britain. *Population Studies, 32,* 81–93.

Scrimshaw, N. S. (1984). Infanticide in human populations: Societal and individual concerns. In G. Hausfater & S. Hrdy (Eds.), *Infanticide: Comparative and evolutionary perspectives.* New York: Aldine.

Scrimshaw, N. S., Taylor, C. E., & Gordon, J. E. (1968). *Interactions of nutrition and infection* [Monograph series 57]. Geneva: World Health Organization.

Simon, D., & Burns, E. (1997). *The corner: A year in the life of an inner-city neighborhood.* New York: Broadway Books.

Stearns, S. (1992). *The evolution of life histories.* New York: Oxford University Press.

Sternberg, K. J., Lamb, M. E., Greenbaum, C., Cicchetti, D., Dawud, S., Cortes, R. M., Krispin, O., & Lorey, F. (1993). Effects of domestic violence on children's behavior problems and depression. *Developmental Review, 29,* 44–52.

Stevenson-Hinde, J. (1990). Attachment within the family system: An overview. *Infant Mental Health Journal, 11,* 218–227.

Straus, M. A., Gelles, R., & Steinmetz, S. (1980). *Behind closed doors: Violence in the American family.* New York: Anchor Press.

Sulloway, F. J. (1996). *Born to rebel: Birth order, family dynamics, and creative lives.* New York: Basic Books.

Sussman, G. (1975). The wet-nursing business in nineteenth century France. *French Historical Studies, IX(2),* 304–328.

Trickett, P. K., & Susman, E. J. (1989). Perceived similarities and disagreements about child-rearing practices in abusive and nonabusive families: Intergenerational and concurrent family processes. In D. Cicchetti & V. Carlson (Eds.), *Child maltreatment: Theory and research on the causes and consequences of child abuse and neglect* (pp. 280–301). New York: Cambridge University Press.

Trivers, R. L. (1974). Parent-offspring conflict. *American Zoologist, 14,* 244–264.

Trivers, R. L. (1985). *Social evolution.* Menlo Park, CA: Benjamin-Cummings.

U.S. Bureau of Census (1992). *Poverty in the United States* [Series P-60, annual]. Washington, DC: U.S. Government Printing Office.

U.S. Department of Health and Human Services. (1988). *Study findings: Study of National Incidence and Prevalence of Child Abuse and Neglect, 1988.* Washington, DC: U.S. Department of Health and Human Services.

van den Berghe, P. (1979). *Human family systems: An evolutionary perspective.* New York: Elsevier.

Vondra, J. I. (1990). The community context of child abuse and neglect. *Marriage and Family Review, 15,* 19–39.

Waller, J. H. (1971). Achievement and social mobility: Relationships among IQ score, education, and occupation in two generations. *Social Biology, 18,* 252–259.

Williams, G. C. (1966). Natural selection, the costs of reproduction, and a refinement of Lack's principle. *American Naturalist, 100,* 687–690.

Wilson, W. J. (1987). *The truly disadvantaged: The inner city, the underclass, and public policy.* Chicago: University of Chicago Press.

Wolf, M. (1972). *Women and the family in rural Taiwan.* Stanford, CA: Stanford University Press.

Wolfe, D. A., Jaffe, P., Wilson, S. K., & Zak, L. (1985). Children of battered women: The relation of child behavior to family violence and maternal stress. *Journal of Consulting and Clinical Psychology, 53,* 657–665.

Wolff, R. J. (1965). Meanings of food. *Tropical and Geographical Medicine, 17,* 43–51.

Wright, R. (1994). *The moral animal.* New York: Pantheon.

3

The Ecology of Domestic Aggression toward Adult Victims

Alan Rosenbaum, Paul J. Gearan, and William Warnken

Interpersonal aggression may be the plague of the 1990s. We are assailed on a daily basis with media coverage of violent crime both within and outside familial relationships. We fear for our safety in airports, public buildings, and even schools. Perhaps the fact that societal aggression is often attributed to exposure to violence in the family of origin, or perhaps the efforts of the battered women's movement to compel legislatures, the police, and the courts to treat violence against women as the serious crime that it is, have had an impact. Regardless of the reason, domestic violence has finally been recognized as one of the most serious problems afflicting society, and the resources devoted to understanding and treating it have increased dramatically.

This is a version of a chapter published in the first edition of this book that was originally authored by Alan Rosenbaum, Paul Cohen, and Barbara Forsstrom-Cohen. Some of the contents reflects the contributions of the Cohens and they are hereby acknowledged. The current authors assume all responsibility for the accuracy of the material and the opinions expressed herein.
Preparation of this manuscript was supported in part by NIMH grant no. R01 MH 44812 to the first author.

Alan Rosenbaum, Paul J. Gearan, and William Warnken • Department of Psychiatry, University of Massachusetts Medical School, Worcester, Massachusetts 01655.

Case Studies in Family Violence, Second Edition, edited by Ammerman and Hersen. Kluwer Academic / Plenum Publishers, New York, 2000.

Whether or not human beings are inherently aggressive, as some have asserted (Lorenz, 1966), it appears that we are most likely to behave aggressively in our intimate relationships. Almost a third of female murder victims are killed by their intimate partners, a figure that has remained fairly constant since the mid-1970s (*Bureau of Justice Statistics Factbook*, 1998). Child abuse, spouse abuse, and elder abuse have each become a substantial phenomenon in its own right. Date rape and courtship violence occur with distressing frequency. Violence between homosexual couples has been documented in the literature. No type of interpersonal relationship appears to be immune. Familiarity may breed contempt; intimacy apparently begets aggression.

The search for the causes of domestic aggression has focused largely on sociocultural and psychological factors, and to a lesser extent on biological ones. A primary strategy has been to identify characteristics of the participants that distinguish them from their nonaggressive counterparts. With some exceptions, the research has not been guided by theory, but various theoretical formulations have been invoked, post hoc, to explain one or another research finding. Social learning theory, for example, has been invoked as an explanation for the intergenerational transmission of aggression.

Efforts to understand domestic aggression have focused on four sets of factors: intraindividual (the contributions of the background and personality of the participants), interpersonal (marital and familial dynamics), environmental stressors (financial problems, religious or racial influences), and the cultural context in which aggression occurs (including the legislative, law enforcement, and judicial response, as well as literary and media representations). This chapter will examine the contributions of each of these elements to the development of domestic aggression toward adult victims.

Marital aggression is recognized to occur in no less than one in every three marriages, and some estimate in as many as half (O'Leary, Barling, Arias, Rosenbaum, Malone, & Tyree, 1989; Straus & Gelles, 1986). Rates of intimate aggression in homosexual couples are comparable (Lie & Gentlewarrier, 1991; Lockhart, White, Causby, & Isaac, 1994; Sarantokos, 1996). In both heterosexual and homosexual couples, aggression is often mutual (O'Leary *et al.*, 1989), yet in terms of violence reported to the authorities, women are almost six times more likely to be the victim and three times more likely to be murdered (*Bureau of Justice Statistics Factbook*, 1998). Intimate murder accounts for about 9% of homicides nationwide. The best available estimates of the incidence of elder abuse are that approximately 3% to 5% of the elderly population in the United States is maltreated (Pillemer & Finkelhor, 1988; Podnieks, Pillemer, Nicholson, Shillington, &

Frizzell, 1990), suggesting that it is less common than marital aggression but comparable, in frequency, to child abuse. Incidence figures for all forms of domestic aggression are generally assumed to underestimate the extent of the problem. Fear of reprisals, legal implications, the stigmatizing nature of the offenses, and sampling biases are but a few of the contributors to underreporting.

Definitions

Relationship aggression refers to aggression between intimate partners and includes what has been called spouse abuse, marital violence, dating aggression, etc. It includes physical aggression, verbal and emotional abuse, sexual aggression, and destruction of pets and property. These have collectively been referred to as power and control strategies, as it is widely held that the objective of relationship aggression is coercion and control of the female partner. These strategies are graphically depicted in the "power and control wheel" (Pence & Paymer, 1993). Although many of these same behaviors are perpetrated by females against males, the elements of fear and coercion are generally absent when the male is the victim. Thus, the behaviors may be similar, but the consequences are not.

The term *batterer* is used inconsistently and has become somewhat ambiguous. The term connotes a male who engages in ongoing, severe violence against his partner. Because domestic violence occurs "behind closed doors" and there were few resources available to battered women until recently, the only batterers to come to public attention were so seriously abusive that the term was appropriate. Over time, we have begun to recognize that batterers constitute a diverse population. The severely abusive, psychopathic, controlling, brutal tyrant of the stereotype certainly exists, but represents a minority. More common is the *normal batterer*, so named by Gondolf (1988), who resorts to physical and emotional aggression at times, but whose violence consists largely of pushing and shoving. He may be controlling, but not to the pathological extent of his more severely abusive counterpart. In reading the literature, we must be attentive to the sample being described. The "cobras and pit bulls" recently described by Jacobson and Gottman (1998) may be very different from the batterers typically treated in most programs. Whereas we have tried to use the term *relationship aggression* in preference to *battering*, the term *batterer* is more difficult to circumvent and hence we will use it generically to refer to a male who uses aggression in an intimate relationship.

Further confusion comes from the fact that, when describing the behaviors that are considered abusive, most researchers and clinicians include verbal and emotional abuse, sexual aggression, and destruction of pets and property. Yet, in defining research samples, the criteria usually include only the occurrence of physical aggression (and often the aggression has to have occurred within a recent time period, such as the past year). Thus, males who are emotionally abusive but who have not been recently physically aggressive are often (but not always) excluded from research. In this chapter, except where noted, the term aggression refers to physical aggression.

Elder abuse includes all of the same behaviors as relationship aggression, but adds neglect, which has been defined as depriving the elder of some assistance that is required for important activities of daily living. There is also a substantial overlap between relationship aggression and elder abuse, since approximately 60% of the perpetrators of elder abuse are spouses. The cutoff age for defining relationship aggression as elder abuse is 65 (Pillemer & Finkelhor, 1988).

Intrapersonal Factors

Much of the research in marital aggression has been guided by one question: How are batterers and their victims different from spouses in nonaggressive relationships? The focus has been on differences in upbringing, family environment, personality (broadly defined), and psychopathology (more broadly defined). Although the research in this area is often flawed by a host of methodological problems (see Geffner, Rosenbaum, & Hughes, 1988, Hotaling & Sugarman, 1986, and Rosenbaum, 1988 for reviews of these issues), and the findings have been both inconsistent and inconclusive, numerous studies have found abusive males to have typically come from violent homes (Hotaling & Sugarman, 1986; Murphy, Meyer, & O'Leary, 1993; Rosenbaum & O'Leary, 1981). Several studies have found abusers to have experienced violence (from caregivers) as children (Kalmuss, 1984; Telch & Lindquist, 1984), but it is generally agreed that witnessing interparental aggression is a more significant background factor for batterers (Caesar, 1988; Hotaling & Sugarman, 1986). There is evidence that this may be an important factor for perpetrators of dating aggression (Bernard & Bernard, 1983) and elder abuse (Gold & Gwyther, 1989; Pierce & Trotta, 1986) as well. It should be noted, however, that many batterers do not come from violent backgrounds (Caesar, 1988) and that many nonbatterers do.

The question of whether the wife/victim also experiences a violent family environment is more controversial. The controversy stems in part from dissatisfaction with the concept of victim blaming, and in part from the inconsistencies in the research literature. There appears to be a fine line between blaming an individual for being victimized and suggesting that certain people might be more vulnerable to being victimized. An individual walking through a poorly lit area at night, for example, may be at increased risk of being victimized. This does not justify the attack, nor should the possibility be ignored that this individual may have limited choices concerning where she walks due to social and economic circumstances.

Concerning the research, Hotaling and Sugarman (1986) identify interparental aggression in the wife/victim's family of origin as the only consistent risk marker among female victims of marital aggression. Their conclusion notwithstanding, those studies failing to support this relationship (Rosenbaum & O'Leary, 1981; Telch & Lindquist, 1984) have utilized comparison samples of maritally discordant, nonphysically abused women, suggesting that perhaps such violence is more a feature of severe marital discord than marital aggression. Alternatively, experience of background violence seems to be more commonly found in community samples (such as those employed by Straus, Gelles, & Steinmetz, 1980) than in clinic or agency samples (such as those examined by Rosenbaum & O'Leary, 1981, and Telch & Lindquist, 1984), suggesting perhaps that women who viewed or experienced violence in their parental homes may be more tolerant of it and less likely to seek outside assistance from an agency.

Elder abuse has come into the public spotlight even more recently than the other forms of domestic aggression; consequently there is relatively less empirical research. The relationship between childhood exposure to violence and subsequent approval of violence as an adult (Owens & Straus, 1975), coupled with evidence supportive of intergenerational transmission models for both child and spouse abuse (Straus *et al.*, 1980) prompted Pillemer (1986) to examine this factor in elder abusers. Using a case-control methodology, his data failed to support a relationship between physical punishment as a child and becoming an elder abuser as an adult. Unfortunately, he did not assess whether the abused elder had abused her or his own parent and whether the identified elder abuser might have been exposed to this as a child (corresponding to the more robust of the findings among wife abusers, namely, witnessing interparental aggression).

The notion that violent people are suffering from some form of psychopathology persists, despite empirical evidence to the contrary (Monahan, 1981). So too, in the area of domestic aggression, there has been an effort to assess whether perpetrators can be characterized as exhibiting some particular psychopathology or personality disorder. In an early investigation with a small sample ($N = 23$), Faulk (1974) reported psychopathology in 16 (70%) of the batterers, with depression being the most common diagnosis, followed by delusional jealousy, personality disorder, and anxiety. In an investigation employing the Millon Clinical Multiaxial Inventory (MCMI; Millon, 1983), Hamberger and Hastings (1985, 1986) reported psychopathology in all but 15% of batterers. More recently, Hart, Dutton, & Newlove (1993) found 80% to 90% of their batterers to be personality disordered, with the most common diagnoses being sadistic, antisocial, and borderline personality. Although studies of batterers have failed to reveal a consistent pattern of psychopathology, several pathological features commonly emerge from the various investigations. These include borderline symptomatology (Dutton & Starzomski, 1993; Else, Wonderlich, Beatty, Christie, & Staton, 1993), antisocial personality (Dinwiddie, 1992; Hamberger & Hastings, 1991), passive-aggressive tendencies, dependency, and pathological jealousy. It has also been suggested that batterers demonstrate symptoms consistent with posttraumatic stress disorder (PTSD; Dutton & Golant, 1995). Since these studies are retrospective and correlational, it is unclear whether the findings predate (and possibly contribute to the production of) or result from the aggressive dynamics. Most of the evidence supportive of psychopathology among abusers suggests that, if there is psychopathology, it is typically personality disorder. The high base rate of Axis II symptomatology in the general population—especially in the age range most common to batterers—would advise caution in concluding that this represents a significant etiological factor. In fact, although Hamberger and Hastings (1988) demonstrated significant differences between abusers and controls on the MCMI, the batterers' scores were generally within normal limits.

There have also been numerous attempts to identify psychological disturbances among abused women. It has been reported that victims of marital aggression show elevated Minnesota Multiphasic Personality Inventory (MMPI) profiles and suffer from a host of problems, including depression and anxiety (Margolin, Sibner, & Gleberman, 1988). Again, the similarity of the behaviors shown by abused wives to the symptoms of PTSD suggests that these symptoms are a result of, rather than a cause of, the aggression.

Elder abuse is associated more with problems in the perpetrator than in the victim (Wolf & Pillemer, 1989). Wolf, Godkin, & Pillemer (1984) found that 31% of elder abusers had a history of psychiatric illness. Pillemer (1986) reported that 79% of the elder victims reported mental or emotional problems in their abusers (compared to 24% of controls) and further that 35.7% had been psychiatrically hospitalized (compared to only 7.1% of controls). Since people are rarely hospitalized for the treatment of personality disorders, the high percentage of elder abusers receiving inpatient psychiatric treatment suggests that Axis I diagnoses are probably more common among elder abusers than they are in groups of either spouse or child abusers. Pillemer (1986) suggests that elder abuse is a more deviant behavior than either child abuse or spouse abuse, and thus we might expect perpetrators to be more deviant.

Alcoholism is one form of pathology that consistently emerges in domestic violence research. Although the operative mechanism is uncertain, a large body of research evidence supports the conclusion that alcohol is a "potent causal antecedent of aggressive behavior" in general (Taylor & Leonard, 1983). The evidence for the role of alcohol in relationship aggression remains inconclusive. Tollman and Bennett (1990) reported that batterers drink more than nonbatterers, and Barnett and Fagan (1993) noted excessive alcohol use in both batterers and victims. Wife abusers are frequently alcoholic, and heavy drinkers are 2 to 3 times more likely than moderate drinkers to abuse their wives, yet the majority of alcoholics are not wife abusers and, even among batterers, the majority of abuse incidents are not alcohol related (Kantor & Straus, 1986).

As with relationship aggression, the role of alcohol in elder abuse is complex. Anetzberger, Korbin, and Austin (1994) reported that elder abusers were twice as likely as nonabusers to drink heavily. Hwalek, Neale, Goodrich, and Quinn (1996) noted that physical and emotional abuse (as opposed to neglect or financial exploitation) were more likely to occur when the elder abuser had a substance abuse problem. According to Pillemer (1986), elder abusers were significantly more likely to be identified as alcoholics (45.2% of abusers compared to 7.1% of controls), yet more than half of elder abusers were not identified as alcoholic.

A number of studies have demonstrated that wife-abusive males often have defective self-concepts (Goldstein & Rosenbaum, 1985; Neidig, Friedman, & Collins, 1986), undifferentiated sex-role identities (LaViolette, Barnett, & Miller, 1984; Rosenbaum, 1986), spouse-specific assertion deficits (Dutton & Strachen, 1987; Maiuro, Cahn, & Vitaliano, 1986; Rosenbaum & O'Leary, 1981), and high power needs (Dutton & Strachen, 1987). As Hotaling and Sugarman (1986) demonstrate, however, for each of these (and other) factors, there are studies that fail to support the relationship to marital aggression, suggesting that the phenomenon is multidetermined and stimulating research aimed at identifying subtypes of batterers or other moderator variables. Prince and Arias (1994), for example, reported that the relationship between self-esteem and abuse may be moderated by the desire to control, coupled with degree of perceived control. The combination of low self-esteem, low desire for control, and low perceived control was associated with risk for abusiveness, as was high self-esteem coupled with high need for control and low perceived control.

Initial attempts at subtyping focused on either perpetrator behavior or personality. Shields *et al.* (1988) provided an example of the former, dividing violent men into three categories: those whose violence is restricted to the family, those whose violence is exclusively non-family, and generally violent men. Hamberger and Hastings (1986) exemplifies a personality based strategy. They employed the MCMI to classify batterers and identified three personality factors: narcissistic/antisocial, schizoidal/borderline, and passive-dependent/compulsive. Gondolf (1988) advocates for a behavior-based typology, suggesting that what batterers "do" is more relevant to the prediction and treatment of marital aggression. It is also less complex and easier to measure. He utilized a cluster analysis to generate three subgroups: the sociopathic batterer, the antisocial batterer, and the typical batterer (this is a behavior-based typology, the names of groups 1 and 2 notwithstanding). The sociopathic batterer is extremely abusive of all family members, is likely to have been sexually abusive, is the most likely to have been arrested, and is the most prone to substance abuse. The typical batterer group is the largest of the three, accounting for 51% of the sample and representing the type of batterer most likely to be seen in treatment programs (other than court-mandated programs, which would probably see more antisocial and sociopathic batterers). Verbal abuse and physical abuse are less severe. Sexual abuse and child abuse are less extensive. He is most likely to be apologetic following abusive incidents and more likely to continue in the relationship with his partner.

Most recently, Holtzworth-Munroe and Stuart (1994) presented a comprehensive review of previous batterer typologies and concluded that batterer subtypes can be classified along three descriptive dimensions: (1) the severity and frequency of marital violence and abuse; (2) the generality of violence (i.e., family-only or extrafamilial); and (3) the batterer's psychopathology or personality disorders. They proposed a three-group typology that integrated these dimensions: (1) family-only batterers engage in the least severe marital violence, are the least likely to engage in violence outside the home, and evidence little psychopathology or personality disorder; (2) dysphoric/borderline batterers engage in moderate to severe wife abuse, confine their aggression to the partner, are the most psychologically distressed and emotionally volatile, evidence borderline personality characteristics, and may have problems with substance abuse; and (3) generally violent/antisocial batterers engage in moderate to severe marital violence, engage in the most extrafamilial aggression, have the most extensive history of criminal behavior, and are likely to have problems with alcohol and drug abuse. They are the most likely to have an antisocial personality disorder.

There have been relatively few attempts to develop typologies that consider the pairings between subgroups of husbands and wives. Snyder and Fruchtman (1981) utilized a clustering process to classify abused women into subcategories. Although originally intended as a typology of abuse victims, they included perpetrator behavior, resulting in a typology of couples consisting of five subtypes. Among the factors included in the clustering were the severity and frequency of the abuse, whether there was sexual abuse by the husband, whether the husband had also abused the children, whether there had been aggression by the wife toward the husband, whether there was alcohol use by the husband, and whether the couple was cohabiting. Including both husband and wife characteristics (demographic, personality, and behavioral) would appear to merit further consideration by typologists. Two advantages of the subtyping movement are that it highlights the heterogeneity of this population and the importance of multifactorial theoretical formulations and also that it may help explain the inconsistencies in outcome of batterer treatment programs. Subtype matched interventions might prove more effective than current approaches, which assume that all batterers will benefit from the same treatment package. We are not aware of any attempts to develop typologies of either perpetrators or victims (or the combination) in the elder abuse area.

Although the aggression literature recognizes the importance of biological contributors, only recently has this class of factors received any consideration in the etiology of relationship aggression. Lewis, Pincus, Feldman, Jackson, and Bard (1986) and Lewis, Pincus, Bard, Richardson, Prichep, Feldman, and Yeager (1988) studied samples of convicted murderers and reported a significant relationship between head injury and generalized aggressive behavior, in both juveniles and adults. Rosenbaum and Hoge (1989) reported a history of severe head injury in 61% of the male spouse abusers in their sample, suggesting a potential psychophysiological component. Elliot (1977) proposed that dyscontrol syndrome, which is characterized by explosive rage triggered by minimal provocation, was an important cause of wife and child battery. Interestingly, dyscontrol syndrome often appears as a sequela to head injury, features alcohol intolerance, results in pathological intoxication, and like spouse abuse may run in families. Rosenbaum, Hoge, Adelman, Warnken, Fletcher, and Kane (1994) conducted a controlled investigation of the relationship between head injury and relationship aggression and found that a history of head injury was associated with an almost sixfold increase in the likelihood of relationship aggression.

Similarly provocative is the research indicating a relationship between aggression and neurotransmitters. There is evidence, primarily animal analogue studies, linking both predatory and affective aggression with increased levels of acetylcholine and dopamine and with reduced levels of GABA and serotonin (Eichelman, 1987). Although direct assessment of brain serotonin levels in humans is difficult, a number of studies have linked aggressive and impulsive behavior in humans to reduced levels of serotonin metabolites in the cerebrospinal fluid (Brown, Ballenger, Minichiello, & Goodwin, 1979). Using a fenfluramine challenge methodology, in which changes in serum prolactin levels are used as an index of serotonergic activity, Coccaro (1992) demonstrated serotonin deficiencies to be related to aggressive behavior. Using the same methodology, Rosenbaum, Abend, Gearan, and Fletcher (1997) examined the serotonergic functioning of partner-abusive men and found that absent a history of head injury, batterers showed significant deficits as compared to nonabusive controls.

The question of whether there are intraindividual demographic factors, such as age, race, and religion, associated with wife battering is difficult to answer because of sampling problems. There is general agreement that wife battering cuts across all races, religions, and social classes; however, there is also evidence that age may be an important factor. Straus and Gelles (1986), reporting on the 1985 resurvey of a nationally representative sample, found that wife batterers were significantly younger than nonbatterers. Controlling for age, Gelles (1988) demonstrated that the association of pregnancy and the onset of spousal aggression, which had previously been reported by a number of investigators (Eisenberg & Micklow, 1977; Gelles, 1974; Helton, 1986; Stacy & Shupe, 1983), was artifactual. These recent findings emphasize the importance of age as a factor in the etiology of spousal aggression. With respect to elder abuse, there is some evidence that abusers are more likely to be male, unmarried, and younger than nonabusers (Anetzberger et al., 1994).

Interpersonal Dynamics

Unlike many other forms of aggression, domestic violence by definition assumes a relationship between perpetrator and victim. This has several implications, including differential treatment by law enforcers, the legal system, the helping professions, the media, and the public; increased difficulty of avoiding revictimization for the victim; and a justification for examining victim contribution to the aggressive interaction. It also suggests that we examine the nature of the marital relationship. To begin with, it seems intuitively obvious that abusive couples would report lower levels of marital satisfaction, and there is empirical evidence that this is the case. Research has shown that there is more marital discord, less marital satisfaction, and a less supportive family climate in homes where marital violence has occurred (Resick & Reese, 1986; Rosenbaum & O'Leary, 1981). It is also true, however, that aggression can occur even between relatively satisfied partners. Reporting on a large sample of engaged couples assessed in the month prior to marriage, O'Leary et al. (1989) found 44% of the women and 31% of the men to be physically aggressive with their partners. Although consistently aggressive couples were less maritally satisfied than consistently nonaggressive couples, two-thirds of the men and three-quarters of the women in the stably aggressive group scored in the satisfactory range on a standardized measure of marital satisfaction.

Almost every study that has examined the rates of aggressive behaviors of both partners has reported higher levels of aggression by women toward their partners (O'Leary et al., 1989; Straus et al., 1980; Straus & Gelles, 1986). This is true of dating couples (Elliot, Huizinga, & Morse, 1986; O'Leary et al., 1989) and even among Quakers (Brutz & Allen, 1986). This is consistent with reports of abusive husbands in treatment who frequently offer the excuse, "She hit me first" (Rosenbaum & Maiuro, 1990). Researchers reporting such statistics are quick to point out that the aggression of women toward men is different and less physically and emotionally damaging. Morse (1995), for example, reported that women are equally often perpetrators of minor assaults but more likely the victims of repeated beatings. Women are also more likely to be physically injured. While this is no doubt true, it may also be true that aggression by the woman is relevant to the development of the aggressive dynamics of the relationship, which eventuate in violence by her partner. This is, in fact, supported by the literature on youth and dating aggression, which suggests that grade school age girls are much more likely to aggress against boys than vice versa, and that as children age the gap narrows. This line of inquiry is not intended to excuse male aggression but only to suggest that we not ignore the potential importance of this factor for fear that it will deflect responsibility away from the abuser.

There is some evidence that ideological and racial differences may be associated with marital aggression. Hotaling and Sugarman (1986) report that religious incompatibility is a consistent risk marker of husband-to-wife aggression. In their study of Quaker families, Brutz and Allen (1986) concluded that religious commitment was a better indicator of the influence of religion on couple aggression. Interestingly, they reported that religious commitment was associated with low levels of marital aggression for wives but with high levels for husbands. There is also some evidence that abusive couples are more likely to be interracial (Wasileski, Callaghan-Chaffee, & Chaffee, 1982).

Hornung, McCullough, and Sugimoto (1981) offer status inconsistency and status incompatibility as couple factors productive of aggression. They suggest that wife abuse is more probable when the wife is better educated or employed in a higher-status occupation than her husband. Whereas the ideological and racial differences might operate through increased stress and by contributing more serious (and intense) arguments with a higher probability of provoking an aggressive response, status incompatibility and inconsistency would appear to potentiate the perpetrator's defective sense of self-esteem, perhaps contributing to a shame-induced rage.

A number of investigators have examined components of the marital interaction itself. Margolin, John, and Gleberman (1988) analyzed taped interactions between physically aggressive couples as well as couples in three comparison groups, and they reported that husbands in the aggressive group exhibited more overtly negative behaviors, more negative affect, and higher levels of physiological arousal. It has been suggested that couples characterized by physical aggression exhibit marked communications deficits (Neidig & Friedman, 1984); however, these have not been empirically demonstrated.

There is some evidence that communication deficits may play a role in elder abuse as well. Hirst and Miller (1986) offer a profile of the individual at high risk to be an elder abuser. According to their profile, the person at high risk is a daughter, experiences marital conflict, and has a lack of communication skills.

Marital dependency has been implicated in the development and maintenance of relationship aggression. Kalmuss and Straus (1982) reported that a wife's dependency on her husband was positively related to the extent to which she experienced violence. They defined dependency both objectively (financial dependency and the presence of young children) and subjectively (whether she perceived things would deteriorate if the marriage broke up). According to Margolin et al. (1988), batterers have also been characterized as dependent on their wives. Dependency among abusers is less likely to be financial but rather may derive from the sense that his wife and family are "all he has." Holtzworth-Munroe et al. (1997) studied attachment patterns, dependency, and jealousy and found batterers to have more anxiety about abandonment and more anxious attachment than nonbatterers. Others have similarly reported batterers to show higher interpersonal dependency, higher spouse-specific dependency, and lower self-esteem (Murphy, Meyer, & O'Leary, 1994). Batterers, however, were not found to differ from discordant nonbatterers in terms of jealousy (Barnett et al., 1995; Murphy et al., 1994).

Dependency is widely believed to be an important factor in elder abuse; however, the directionality of the dependency may be different. The notion of generational inversion, wherein the parent–child roles are reversed and the elderly parent becomes dependent on the children, has been advocated by some (Steinmetz, 1983). According to this model, aggression erupts when the caretaker cannot cope with the stress of providing care to the elderly parent. This may interact with the guilt evoked by the perceived obligation, coupled with the financial strain of providing adequate care. The family disruption engendered by the intrusion of an elderly parent into the home and the diversion of temporal and emotional resources from the children of the caretaker to the parent of the caretaker can be a further source of stress, guilt, and, consequently, anger.

Although the generational inversion model has face validity, there is evidence that it is the dependency of the abuser on the abused that is more relevant to the production of aggression. According to Wolf, Strugnell, and Godkin (1982), the abuser was financially dependent on the abused elder in two-thirds of their sample, a finding supported by Hwalek, Sengstock, and Lawrence (1984). Pillemer (1986) reported that elder abusers were significantly more dependent on the elder in the areas of housing, household repair, finances, and transportation than were the nonabusive controls. He found fewer than 36% of elder abusers to be financially independent of their elderly victims and concluded that financial dependence of an adult child on an elderly parent "may be an important predictor of violence" (p. 254). In their article on the abuse and neglect of elderly persons, Lachs and Pillemer (1995) noted increased dependency to be a risk factor for both victims and perpetrators.

It has been suggested that powerlessness or perceived powerlessness may be causal factors common to all forms of family violence (Finkelhor, 1983). According to Pillemer (1986), "It may be that the feeling of powerlessness experienced by an adult child who is still dependent on an elderly parent is especially acute, because it goes so strongly against society's expectations for normal adult behavior" (p. 244).

Environmental Stressors

If financial dependence of abuser on victim is an important cause of elder abuse, it suggests that factors that produce economic stress would promote elder abuse. Since it has been established that both child abuse and spouse abuse are associated with unemployment and economic stress (Straus & Gelles, 1986), the addition of elder abuse means that this factor is common to all forms of domestic aggression. Despite the earlier statement that marital aggression cuts across all socioeconomic strata, every study that has shown a relationship between social class and aggression has shown it to be a negative one. Even taking sampling problems into account, it seems clear that there is more marital aggression among the poorer socioeconomic groups.

Job dissatisfaction and work stress have also been associated with marital violence. Barling and Rosenbaum (1986) examined work involvement, organizational commitment, job satisfaction, and work stress in three groups of men: wife abusers, nonabusive maritally dissatisfied, and satisfactorily married. The results indicated that the occurrence of stressful work events and their negative impact were related to wife abuse. This is consistent with studies indicating a relationship between parental work stress and child abuse (Agathanos & Stathakopoulo, 1983). In addition to work stress, it has been reported that life stress in general is strongly related to marital aggression. Straus et al. (1980) counted the number of life (including work) stressors experienced by their subjects and reported that, as the number of stressors increased, so did the probability of marital abuse. Women reporting the occurrence of 10 or more life stressors were husband-abusive more than 50% of the time. Husbands reporting 10 or more life stressors were wife-abusive about 25% of the time.

Many of the stressors experienced by couples and families may be moderated by social support networks. The stress of multiple children, for example, can be reduced by the availability of extended-family caretakers. Similarly, close relatives can often be counted on for financial support (sometimes in the form of a free meal or the "goody bag" of groceries), a place to stay (if the wife has to leave), moral support, and even as an insurance policy against aggression (negative consequences threatened if you "touch my sister/daughter again"). It is not surprising that domestic aggression is often characterized by social isolation. There is research supporting the relationship between social isolation and both marital aggression (Stark et al., 1981) and elder abuse (Pillemer, 1986). In the case of wife abuse, social isolation may be both a cause and an effect of aggression. Abused wives often withdraw from social interaction because of the stigma attached to being victimized, the embarrassment of visible injuries, or constant scrutiny by the husband on how they spend their time. It has been suggested that the husband may inflict visible injuries in order to isolate his wife from others, especially other men, who he fears may be more desirable mates than he is.

Cultural Context

Several years ago a superior court judge in Massachusetts heard a case involving a battered woman who was seeking protection from a severely abusive husband. The judge rebuked the woman, in the presence of the husband, for wasting the court's time. A short time later the woman was murdered by her husband. The judge was blamed by feminist groups for the woman's death and criticized by the media. The chief justice promised an inquiry, and under intense pressure, initiated a program of educating the Massachusetts judiciary with regard to domestic violence. The judge was not removed from the bench, although he was, at least temporarily, prevented from hearing marital aggression cases. This is but one example of the way society legitimizes and thereby perpetuates domestic aggression.

Numerous writers have chronicled the historical legitimization of domestic aggression (see, for example, Pleck, 1987). Only recently has society proscribed the use of aggression between family members. Increasingly, states are passing domestic violence legislation that may provide for mandatory arrest of perpetrators and the use of diversionary programs, including batterers' treatment, as a term of probation. Many states have established certification standards for batterers' treatment programs. The issuance of court orders of protection (e.g., restraining orders) has also increased dramatically in recent years. In many jurisdictions, police officers as well as judges are required to attend domestic violence training.

Although the battered women's movement has lobbied for the arrest and prosecution of batterers, initial optimism that arresting the abuser effectively reduces the recurrence of battering (Sherman & Berk, 1984) has been replaced by concerns that arrest alone does not deter subsequent aggression (Dunford, Huizinga, & Elliot, 1990; Hirschel, Hutchinson, & Dean, 1992; Sherman, Smith, Schmidt, & Rogan, 1992). Arrest in combination with other interventions (e.g., sheltering of victims, mandated batterers' treatment, prosecution, and incarceration), however, may be more effective. Rosenbaum, Gearan, and Ondovic (in press) conducted an outcome evaluation of a batterers' treatment program and reported that both a court mandate and treatment completion were necessary to significantly reduce rates of recidivism.

Another manifestation of society's increasing intolerance of relationship aggression is the proliferation of antistalking statutes. The first antistalking laws were passed in 1990 and there are today such laws in every state and the District of Columbia. Although no state currently has a mandated reporting statute for relationship aggression (there are mandated reporting statutes for both child abuse and elder abuse), California has come the closest to establishing a mandate for reporting possible spousal violence.

Sociocultural factors contribute to family violence in other ways as well. Pornography sexualizes aggression toward women and may promote their victimization by strangers and within the family. Sommers and Check (1987) found that abusive husbands read more pornography than nonabusive husbands (according to wife report). Abused wives also reported that their husbands were more likely to ask them to perform sexual acts depicted in the pornography. Sexual aggression is characteristic of the more severe cases of marital aggression and has been identified as a risk marker for interspousal homicide (Browne, 1987).

There has been a very gradual change in the marital norm from a traditional male-dominated structure to a more egalitarian one (Thornton, Alwin, & Camburn, 1983). This change is also evident in the television and cinematic representations of the typical American family, as dramatized by the differences in the family structure depicted in *Father Knows Best* (1950s) and *The Cosby Show* (1990s). According to Straus and Gelles (1986), male-dominant marriages are the most violent and egalitarian marriages the least violent. They attribute the observed decreases in rates of marital aggression from 1975 to 1985, in part, to this social change.

Another important social change concerns the number of women employed outside the home. Although far from equality with men in terms of salary, women are increasingly likely to be employed outside the home, and the two-income household is becoming the norm. Since full-time housewives are more likely to be abused (Straus et al., 1980) and more likely to remain in an abusive relationship (Gelles, 1976), changes in cultural norms that encourage women to pursue careers and paid employment should decrease rates of marital aggression. On the other hand, batterers having poor self-esteem may be threatened by a woman's independence and exposure to "more desirable" males and become increasingly controlling and abusive.

Elder abuse flourishes in a sociocultural environment that glorifies youth and treats aging as a disease. Studies have shown that young people have generally negative views of the elderly. Children tend to describe older people as tired, ill, and ugly (Seefeldt, 1984). In today's mobile society, children are often cut off from contact with aging grandparents and are unable to develop positive relationships with the elderly, reducing the likelihood of their learning to care for, care about, or learn from the older generation. Ageism, the age equivalence of racism, is a serious problem and one which may contribute to elder abuse (Galbraith, 1986). According to a 1975 Harris poll, the public image of the elderly is negative and possibly damaging. Media coverage of the elderly poor, the elderly sick, the elderly institutionalized, and the elderly unemployed or retired, reinforces distorted stereotypes of the elderly. The significance of this negative image for elder abuse can be better appreciated if we consider de Beauvoir's (1973) historical, cross-cultural observation that nations and cultures that perceive the elderly negatively tend to treat them accordingly. According to Viano (1983), "There is no doubt that in American society becoming old means becoming less of something on the way to losing everything. If, in the eyes of many, becoming old means becoming less human, it is easy to see how a wide spectrum of victimization of the elderly can take place and be justified" (p. 13).

One reason for the sudden emergence of elder abuse as a significant problem concerns a phenomenon known as the graying of America (Quinn & Tomita, 1986). This refers to the fact that as the life expectancy of Americans increases, the elderly make up an increasing proportion of the population. This strains a host of social institutions and has a dramatic economic impact on the nation. In recent years this has been seen most clearly in the form of threats to the economic stability of the social security system, a shortage of nursing home beds, dramatic increases in health insurance costs, and the portion of the economy devoted to health care, Medicare, and other services to the elderly. Burdened with a national deficit that threatens the fiscal foundations of the country, the federal government has been cutting the funds and services provided to the elderly. In 1985, the House Select Committee on Aging prepared a report entitled *Elder Abuse: A National Disgrace.* In that report they noted that while 40% of reported abuse cases involve adults and elderly adults, only 4.7% of state budgets for protective services are devoted to elderly protective services. Since 1981, the primary source of federal funding for protective services has been cut by nearly a fifth. Three-quarters of the states reported that elderly abuse is increasing, yet in the face of a clear need to increase services the federal government is, instead, doing considerably less.

With the federal and state governments doing less, the burden of caring for the elderly falls to their families. This not only increases stress on the family system, which as we have discussed is a major contributor to all forms of domestic violence, but also represents a societal devaluation of the elderly. It would be unfair to close this section without mentioning that governmental support for shelters and other programs for battered women, batterers' treatment programs, and services to families afflicted by violence is also inadequate. Shelters, in particular, are more and more often forced to appeal to the private sector for needed operating funds or to compete for an ever-shrinking pool of resources. Lack of services for abuse victims and their children forces many victims to remain in abusive situations and perpetuates the aggression.

Summary

Knowledge of the causes of domestic aggression has been increasing exponentially over the past 20 years, yet there are still many unanswered questions. Early studies called it *wife abuse*, a testament to the notion that this was thought to be a phenomenon of married adult couples. The choice of the term *relationship aggression* in the present chapter acknowledges the sad fact that researchers are describing similar behaviors in dating populations and even among grade school age children (Connolly, McMaster, Craig, & Pepler, 1997), while at the other end of the age spectrum Pillemer and Finkelhor (1988) suggest that "the largest proportion of elder abuse is, in fact, spouse abuse" (p. 56). Continuities between the various developmental manifestations of relationship aggression are unknown. Of course, the ultimate objective is to use our knowledge of the etiology of relationship aggression to prevent its occurrence in future generations. We are beginning to see experimental prevention programs, mostly at the high school and college levels, but the long-term effectiveness of such programs has not been established.

We hope that it is by now clear that domestic aggression is complex and multidetermined. In trying to understand it, we must consider the individuals involved, their histories, and their psychological makeup. We must consider the nature of the relationship between abuser and victim, as well as the family environment. Financial, work, and other life stressors must be taken into account. Finally, we must consider the sociocultural milieu, which either tolerates and legitimizes aggression or prohibits and punishes it, and which either devalues segments of the population (women and the elderly, for example) or preaches and practices respect and equality for everyone.

References

Agathanos, H., & Stathakopolou, N. (1983). Life events and child abuse: A controlled study. In J. Leavitt (Ed.), *Child abuse and neglect: Research and innovations in NATO countries* (pp. 83–91). Netherlands: Kluwer.

Anetzberger, G. J., Korbin, J. E., & Austin, C. (1994). Alcoholism and elder abuse. *Journal of Interpersonal Violence, 9*, 184–193.

Barling, J., & Rosenbaum, A. (1986). Work stressors and wife abuse. *Journal of Applied Psychology, 71*, 346–348.

Barnett, O. W., & Fagan, R. W. (1993). Alcohol use in male spouse abusers and their female partners. *Journal of Family Violence, 8*, 1–25.

Barnett, O. W., Martinez, T. E., Bleustein, B. W. (1995). Jealousy and anxious romantic attachment in maritally violent and nonviolent males. *Journal of Interpersonal Violence, 10*, 473–486.

Bernard, M. L., & Bernard, J. L. (1983). Violent intimacy: The family as a model for love relationships. *Family Relations*, 32, 283–286.

Brown, G. L., Ballenger, J. C., Minichiello, M. D., & Goodwin, F. K. (1979). Human aggression and its relation to cerebrospinal fluid, 5-hydroxyindole acetic acid, 3-methoxy-4-hydroxyphenylglycol and homovanillic acid. In M. Sandier (Ed.), *Psychopharmacology of aggression*. New York: Raven Press.

Browne, A. (1987). *When battered women kill*. New York: Free Press.

Brutz, J. L., & Allen, C. M. (1986). Religious commitment, peace activism, and marital violence in Quaker families. *Journal of Marriage and the Family*, 48, 491–502.

Bureau of justice statistics factbook. (1998). Washington, DC: U.S. Department of Justice, Office of Justice Programs.

Caesar, P. L. (1988). Exposure to violence in the families-of-origin among wife abusers and maritally nonviolent men. *Violence and Victims*, 3, 49–63.

Coccaro, E. F. (1992). Impulsive aggression and central serotonergic system functioning in humans: An example of a dimensional brain–behavior relationship. *International Clinical Psychopharmacology*, 7, 3–12.

Connolly, J., McMaster, L., Craig, W., & Pepler, D. (1997). *Dating, puberty, and sexualized aggression in early adolescence*. Paper presented at the convention of the Association for the Advancement of Behavior Therapy, San Diego, November.

de Beauvoir, S. (1973). *The coming of age*. New York: Warner.

Dinwiddie, S. H. (1992). Psychiatric disorders among wife batterers. *Comprehensive Psychiatry*, 33, 411–416.

Dunford, F. W., Huizinga, D., & Elliott, D. (1990). The role of arrest in domestic assault: The Omaha experiment. *Criminology*, 28, 183–206.

Dutton, D. G., & Golant, S. K. (1995). *The batterer: A psychological profile*. New York: Basic Books.

Dutton, D. G., & Starzomski, A. J. (1993). Borderline personality in perpetrators of psychological and physical abuse. *Violence and Victims*, 8, 327–337.

Dutton, D. G., & Strachen, C. E. (1987). Motivational needs for power and spouse-specific assertiveness in assaultive and nonassaultive men. *Violence and Victims*, 2, 145–156.

Eichelman, B. (1987). Neurochemical bases of aggressive behavior. *Psychiatric Annals*, 17, 371–374.

Eisenberg, S., & Micklow, P. (1977). The assaulted wife: "Catch-22" revisited. *Women's Rights Law Reporter*, 3, 138–161.

Elliott, D. S., Huizinga, D., & Morse, B. J. (1986). Self-reported violent offending: A descriptive analysis of juvenile violent offenders and their offending careers. *Journal of Interpersonal Violence*, 4, 472–514.

Elliott, F. A. (1977). The neurology of explosive rage: The dyscontrol syndrome. In M. Roy (Ed.), *Battered women* (pp. 97–109). New York: Van Nostrand Reinhold.

Else, L., Wonderlich, S. A., Beatty, W. W., Christie, D. W., & Staton, R. D. (1993). Personality characteristics of men who physically abuse women. *Hospital and Community Psychiatry*, 44, 54–58.

Faulk, M. (1974). Men who assault their wives. *Medicine, Science, and the Law*, 14, 180–183.

Finkelhor, D. (1983). Common features of family abuse. In D. Finkelhor, R. J. Gelles, G. Hotaling, & M. A. Straus (Eds.), *The dark side of families: Current family violence research* (pp. 17–26). Beverly Hills, CA: Sage.

Galbraith, M. W. (1986). Elder abuse: An overview. In M. W. Galbraith (Ed.), *Elder abuse: Perspectives on an emerging crisis* (pp. 5–22). Kansas City: Mid-America Conference on Aging.

Geffner, R., Rosenbaum, A., & Hughes, H. (1988). Research issues concerning family violence.

In V. B. Van Hasselt, R. L. Morrison, A. S. Bellack, & M. Hersen (Eds.), *Handbook of family violence* (pp. 457–481). New York: Plenum.

Gelles, R. J. (1974). *The violent home: A study of physical aggression between husbands and wives.* Beverly Hills, CA: Sage.

Gelles, R. J. (1976). Abused wives: Why do they stay? *Journal of Marriage and the Family, 38,* 659–668.

Gelles, R. J. (1988). Violence and pregnancy: Are pregnant women at greater risk of abuse? *Journal of Marriage and the Family, 50,* 841–847.

Gold, D. T., & Gwyther, L. P. (1989). The prevention of elder abuse: An educational model. *Family Relations, 38,* 8–14.

Goldstein, D., & Rosenbaum, A. (1985). An evaluation of the self-esteem of maritally violent men. *Family Relations, 34,* 425–428.

Gondolf, E. W. (1988). Who are those guys? Toward a behavioral typology of batterers. *Violence and Victims, 3,* 187–203.

Hamberger, L. K., & Hastings, J. E. (1985, March). Personality correlates of men who abuse their partners: Some preliminary data. Paper presented at the meeting of the Society of Personality Assessment, Berkeley, CA.

Hamberger, L. K., & Hastings, J. E. (1986). Personality correlates of men who abuse their partners: A cross-validation study. *Journal of Family Violence, 1,* 323–341.

Hamberger, L. K., & Hastings, J. E. (1988). Characteristics of male spouse abusers consistent with personality disorders. *Hospital & Community Psychiatry, 39,* 763–770.

Hamberger, L. K., & Hastings, J. E. (1991). Personality correlates of men who batter and nonviolent men: Some continuities and discontinuities. *Journal of Family Violence, 6,* 131–147.

Hart, S. D., Dutton, D. G., & Newlove, T. (1993). The prevalence of personality disorders among wife assaulters. *Journal of Personality Disorders, 7,* 329–341.

Hastings, J. E., & Hamberger, L. K. (1988). Personality characteristics of spouse abusers: A controlled comparison. *Violence and Victims, 3,* 31–48.

Helton, A. (1986). Battering during pregnancy. *American Journal of Nursing, 86,* 910–913.

Hirschel, D. J., Hutchison, I. W., & Dean, C. W. (1992). The failure of arrest to deter spouse abuse: Experimentation in criminal justice [Special issue]. *Journal of Research in Crime and Delinquency, 29,* 7–33.

Hirst, S. P., & Miller, J. (1986). The abused elderly. *Journal of Psychosocial Nursing and Mental Health Services, 24,* 28–34.

Holtzworth-Munroe, A., & Stuart, G. L. (1994). Typologies of male batterers: Three subtypes and the differences among them. *Psychological Bulletin, 116,* 476–497.

Holtzworth-Munroe, A., Stuart, G. L., & Hutchinson, G. (1997). Violent vs. non-violent husbands: Differences in attachment patterns, dependency, and jealousy. *Journal of Family Psychology, 11,* 314–331.

Hornung, C. A., McCullough, B. C., & Sugimoto, T. (1981). Status relationships in marriage: Risk factors in spouse abuse. *Journal of Marriage and the Family, 43,* 675–692.

Hotaling, G. T., & Sugarman, D. B. (1986). An analysis of risk markers in husband to wife violence: The current state of knowledge. *Violence and Victims, 2,* 101–124.

Hwalek, M. A., Sengstock, M. C., & Lawrence, R. (1984, November). *Assessing the probability of abuse of the elderly.* Paper presented at the annual meeting of the Gerontological Society of America.

Hwalek, M. A., Neale, A. V., Goodrich, C. S., & Quinn, K. (1996). The association of elder abuse and substance abuse in the Illinois elder abuse system. *Gerontologist, 36,* 694–700.

Jacobson, N. S., & Gottman, J. M. (1998). When men batter women: New insights into ending abusive relationships. New York: Simon & Schuster.

Kalmuss, D. (1984). The intergenerational transmission of marital aggression. *Journal of Marriage and the Family, 46*, 11–19.

Kalmuss, D., & Straus, M. A. (1982). Wife's marital dependency and wife abuse. *Journal of Marriage and the Family, 44*, 277–286.

Kantor, G. K., & Straus, M. A. (1986, April). *The drunken bum theory of wife beating.* Paper presented at the National Alcoholism Forum Conference on Alcohol and the Family, San Francisco.

Lachs, M. S., & Pillemer, K. (1995). Abuse and neglect of elderly persons. *New England Journal of Medicine, 42*, 169–173.

LaViolette, A. D., Barnett, O. W., & Miller, C. L. (1984, July). *A classification of wife abusers on the BEM Sex-Role Inventory.* Paper presented at the Second National Conference of Research on Domestic Violence, Durham, NH.

Lewis, D. O., Pincus, J. H., Feldman, M., Jackson, L., & Bard, B. (1986). Psychiatric, neurological, and psychoeducational characteristics of 15 death row inmates in the United States. *American Journal of Psychiatry, 143*, 838–845.

Lewis, D. O., Pincus, J. H., Bard, B., Richardson, E., Prichep, L. S., Feldman, M., & Yeager, C. (1988). Neuropsychiatric, psychoeducational, and family characteristics of 14 juveniles condemned to death in the United States. *American Journal of Psychiatry, 145*, 584–589.

Lie, G., & Gentlewarrier, S. (1991). Intimate violence in lesbian relationships: Discussion of survey findings and practice implications. *Journal of Social Service Research, 15*, 41–59.

Lockhart, L. L., White, B. W., Causby, V., & Isaac, A. (1994). Letting out the secret: Violence in lesbian relationships. *Journal of Interpersonal Violence, 9*, 469–492.

Lorenz, K. (1966). *On aggression.* New York: Harcourt Brace.

Maiuro, R. D., Cahn, T. S., & Vitaliano, P. P. (1986). Assertiveness deficits and hostility in domestically violent men. *Violence and Victims, 1*, 279–289.

Margolin, G., John, R. S., & Gleberman, L. (1988). Affective responses to conflictual discussions in violent and nonviolent couples. *Journal of Consulting and Clinical Psychology, 56*, 24–33.

Margolin, G., Sibner, L. G., & Gleberman, L. (1988). Wife battering. In V. B. Van Hasselt, R. L. Morrison, A. S. Bellack, & M. Hersen (Eds.), *Handbook of family violence* (pp. 89–117). New York: Plenum.

Millon, T. (1983). *Millon Clinical Multiaxial Inventory Manual.* Minneapolis: Interpretive Scoring Systems.

Monahan, J. (1981). *The clinical prediction of violent behavior.* Rockville, MD: National Institute of Mental Health.

Morse, B. J. (1995). Beyond the Conflict Tactics Scale: Assessing gender differences in partner violence. *Violence and Victims, 10*, 251–272.

Murphy, C. M., Meyer, S. L., & O'Leary, D. K. (1993). Family of origin violence and MCMI-II psychopathology among partner assaultive men. *Violence and Victims, 8*, 165–176.

Murphy, C. M., Meyer, S. L., & O'Leary, K. D. (1994). Dependency characteristics of partner assaultive men. *Journal of Abnormal Psychology, 4*, 729–735.

Neidig, P. H., & Friedman, D. H. (1984). *Spouse abuse: A treatment program for couples.* Champaign, IL: Research Press.

Neidig, P. N., Friedman, D. H., & Collins, B. S. (1986). Attitudinal characteristics of males who have engaged in spouse abuse. *Journal of Family Violence, 1*, 223–234.

O'Leary, K. D., Barling, J., Arias, I., Rosenbaum, A., Malone, J., & Tyree, A. (1989). Prevalence and stability of physical aggression between spouses: A longitudinal analysis. *Journal of Consulting and Clinical Psychology, 57*, 263–268.

Owens, D. S., & Straus, M. A. (1975). The social structure of violence and approval of violence as an adult. *Aggressive Behavior, 1,* 193–211.

Pence, E. & Paymer, M. (1993). *Education groups for men who batter: The Duluth model.* New York: Springer.

Pierce, R. L., & Trotta, R. (1986). Abused parents: A hidden family problem. *Journal of Family Violence, 1,* 99–110.

Pillemer, K. A. (1986). Risk factors in elder abuse: Results from a case-control study. In K. A. Pillemer & R. S. Wolf (Eds.), *Elder abuse: Conflict in the family* (pp. 239–263). Dover, MA: Auburn House.

Pillemer, K., & Finkelhor, D. (1988). The prevalence of elder abuse: A random sample survey. *Journal of the Gerontological Society of America, 28,* 51–57.

Pillemer, K. A., & Wolf, R. S. (1986). *Elder abuse: Conflict in the family.* Dover, MA: Auburn House.

Pleck, E. (1987). *Domestic tyranny.* New York: Oxford University Press.

Podnieks, E., Pillemer, K., Nicholson, J.P., Shillington, T., & Frizzell, A. (1990). *National survey on abuse of the elderly in Canada: Final report.* Toronto: Ryerson Technical Institute.

Prince, J. E., & Arias, I. A. (1994). The role of perceived control and the desirability of control among abusive and nonabusive husbands. *The Journal of Family Therapy, 2,* 126–134.

Quinn, M. J., & Tomita, S. K. (1986). *Elder abuse and neglect: Causes, diagnosis, and treatment strategies.* New York: Springer.

Resick, P. A., & Reese, D. (1986). Perception of family social climate and physical aggression in the home. *Journal of Family Violence, 1,* 71–83.

Rosenbaum, A. (1986). Of men, macho, and marital violence. *Journal of Family Violence, 1,* 121–129.

Rosenbaum, A. (1988). Methodological issues in marital violence research. *Journal of Family Violence, 3,* 91–104.

Rosenbaum, A., & Hoge, S. K. (1989). Head injury and marital aggression. *American Journal of Psychiatry, 146,* 1048–1051.

Rosenbaum, A., & Maiuro, R. D. (1990). Treatment of spouse abusers. In R. T. Ammerman & M. Hersen (Eds.), *Treatment of family violence: A sourcebook.* New York: Wiley.

Rosenbaum, A., & O'Leary, K. D. (1981). Marital violence: Characteristics of abusive couples. *Journal of Consulting and Clinical Psychology, 49,* 63–71.

Rosenbaum, A., Hoge, S. K., Adelman, S. A., Warnken, W. J., Fletcher, K. E., & Kane, R. L. (1994). Head injury in partner-abusive men. *Journal of Consulting and Clinical Psychology, 62,* 1187–1193.

Rosenbaum, A., Abend, S. A., Gearan, P. J., & Fletcher, K. (1997). Serotonergic functioning in partner abusive men. In A. Raine, D. Farrington, P. Brennan, & S. A. Mednick (Eds.), *The biosocial bases of violence* (pp. 329–332). New York: Plenum.

Rosenbaum, A., Gearan, P., & Ondovic, C. (in press). Completion and recidivism among court- and self-referred batterers in a psychoeducational group treatment program: Implications for intervention and public policy. *Journal of Aggression, Maltreatment, and Trauma.*

Sarantokos, S. (1996). Same-sex couples: Problems and prospects. *Journal of Family Studies, 2,* 147–163.

Seefeldt, C. (1984). Children's attitudes toward the elderly: A cross-cultural comparison. *International Journal of Aging and Human Development, 19,* 319–328.

Sherman, L. W., & Berk, R. A. (1984). The specific deterrent effects of arrest for domestic assault. *American Sociological Review, 49,* 261–271.

Sherman, L. W., Smith, D. A., Schmidt, J. D., & Rogan, D. P. (1992). Crime, punishment, and stake in conformity: Legal and informal control of domestic violence. *American Sociological Review, 57,* 680–690.

Shields, N. M., McCall, G. J., & Hanneke, C. R. (1988). Patterns of family and nonfamily violence: Violent husbands and violent men. *Violence and Victims, 3*(2), 83–98.

Snyder, D. K., & Fruchtman, L. A. (1981). Differential patterns of wife abuse: A data-based typology. *Journal of Consulting and Clinical Psychology, 49*, 878–885.

Sommers, E. K., & Check, J. V. P. (1987). An empirical investigation of the role of pornography in the verbal and physical abuse of women. *Violence and Victims, 2*, 189–209.

Stacy, W. A., & Shupe, A. (1983). *The family secret: Domestic violence in America*. Boston: Beacon Press.

Stark, E., Flitcraft, A., Zuckerman, D., Gray, A., Robinson, J., & Frazier, W. (1981). *Wife abuse in the medical setting: An introduction to health personnel* [Monograph series no. 7]. Washington, DC: National Clearinghouse on Domestic Violence.

Steinmetz, S. (1983). Dependency, stress and violence between middle-aged caregivers and their elderly parents. In J. I. Kosberg (Ed.), *Abuse and maltreatment of the elderly* (pp. 134–139). Littleton, MA: Wright.

Straus, M. A. (1986). Medical care costs of intrafamily assault and homicide. *Bulletin of the New York Academy of Medicine, 62*, 556–561.

Straus, M. A., Gelles, R. J., & Steinmetz, S. K. (1980). *Behind closed doors: Violence in the American family*. New York: Anchor/Doubleday.

Taylor, S. P., & Leonard, K. E. (1983). Alcohol and human physical aggression. In R. G. Green & E. I. Donnerstein (Eds.), *Aggression: Theoretical and empirical reviews* (pp. 77–101). New York: Academic Press.

Telch, C. F., & Lindquist, C. U. (1984). Violent vs. nonviolent couples: A comparison of patterns. *Psychotherapy, 21*, 242–248.

Thornton, A., Alwin, D. F., & Cambum, D. (1983). Causes and consequences of sex-role attitudes and attitude change. *American Sociology Review, 48*, 211–227.

Tollman, R. M., & Bennett, L. W. (1990) A review of quantitative research on men who batter. *Journal of Interpersonal Violence, 5*, 87–118.

Viano, E. (1983). Victimology: An overview. In J. I. Kosberg (Ed.), *Abuse and maltreatment of the elderly*. Littleton, MA: Wright.

Wasileski, M., Callaghan-Chaffee, M. E., & Chaffee, R. B. (1982). Spousal violence in military homes: An initial study. *Military Medicine, 147*, 761–765.

Wolf, R. S., & Pillemer, K. A. (1989). *Helping elderly victims: The reality of elder abuse*. New York: Columbia University Press.

Wolf, R. S., Strugnell, C., & Godkin, M. (1982). *Preliminary findings from three model projects on elderly abuse*. Worcester: University of Massachusetts, University Center on Aging.

Wolf, R. S., Godkin, M., & Pillemer, K. A. (1984). *Elder abuse and neglect: Report from three model projects*. Worcester: University of Massachusetts, University Center on Aging.

4

Legal Issues in Violence toward Children

Bruce K. Mac Murray and Barbara A. Carson

Legal issues on child maltreatment focus on the role of the state to investigate, adjudicate, and respond to those who maltreat children. In this chapter we will review issues relating to the typical practices and concerns at each stage in the legal processing of child abuse and neglect cases. We will also discuss current controversies in how and when the criminal justice system should intervene in cases of child maltreatment. Finally, we will review innovative approaches and policies that have been proposed, and in some cases implemented, for cases of child maltreatment.

Legal Definitions

Statutes defining child maltreatment vary greatly across the United States (Besharov, 1990; Kalichman, 1993); however, understanding the basic components of the legal definitions in this area will be useful for the remaining discussion. Generally, *physical abuse* is any act that results in a nonaccidental physical injury (Stein, 1991). *Sexual abuse* occurs when a child is used for sexual stimulation by another (*Child Abuse Manual*, 1989). Sexual abuse may involve physical contact, pornographic photography, or

Bruce K. Mac Murray • Department of Sociology, Social Work, and Criminal Justice, Anderson University, Anderson, Indiana 46012.   **Barbara A. Carson** • Department of Sociology and Corrections, Minnesota State University, Mankato, Minnesota 56002.

Case Studies in Family Violence, Second Edition, edited by Ammerman and Hersen. Kluwer Academic / Plenum Publishers, New York, 2000.

coercion to participate in sexual activities. *Emotional abuse* is generally defined to include acts that cause emotional or psychological injury, although this is extremely difficult to operationally define (Gondolf, 1987; McGee & Wolfe, 1991) and it has been argued that there is no consensus on what the legal standard is (Daro, 1988). *Neglect* occurs when a caretaker or guardian fails to provide minimum physical and emotional needs for a child and again, there is disagreement on how to define "minimum needs" (Steinbach, 1989).

There are many legal issues associated with these definitions. For example, there is considerable concern about distinguishing between issues related to poverty and those that involve intentional maltreatment (Giovannoni & Becerra, 1990; Huxtable, 1994; Pelton, 1991). There is also debate about the differentiation between the legal use of physical punishment and illegal physical and emotional abuse (Walsh, 1996). Some of the difficulties in making such fine distinctions regarding these definitions become moot in many jurisdictions because the rates of abuse are so high that only the most serious incidents of alleged maltreatment are ever investigated (Sedlak & Broadhurst, 1996).

Current Prevalence/Incidence Data and Reporting Practices

Recent decades have seen a tremendous increase in the number of cases of alleged child maltreatment reported to official agencies. For 1995, based upon annual surveys from all 50 states and the District of Columbia, the National Committee to Prevent Child Abuse (NCPCA) has estimated that over 3,111,000 children were reported to child protective services as alleged victims (Lung & Daro, 1996). These figures translate to a rate of 46 out of every 1,000 children in the United States (under the age of 18) as reported victims of child maltreatment. This represents a 49% increase in number of reports since 1986 (which itself followed a fourteenfold increase from the time period just prior to mandatory reporting—1963—up to 1987 [Besharov, 1990]). NCPCA further estimates that between 1992 and 1995 approximately 1 million children were not just alleged victims but were involved in cases that were legally substantiated, indicating a rate of 15 per 1,000 children.

The consequences of these abusive acts are serious. The NCPCA continues to state that, in the past decade, more than three children have died every day as a result of parental maltreatment. Most of these child victims are under the age of five at the time of death, with almost one-half under a year old (Lung & Daro, 1996). Even more disturbing for each of these figures is the generally accepted evaluation that they are underestimates. For example, the U.S. Advisory Board on Child Abuse and Neglect estimates that approximately 2,000 child deaths occur from maltreatment per year, making the average 5 deaths per day (U.S. Department of Health and Human Services, Administration for Children and Families, 1995).

The relative frequency of reported cases of child maltreatment according to the four main types of abuse noted above are: neglect (54%), physical abuse (25%), sexual abuse (11%), and emotional maltreatment (3%). In part as a result of the apparent scope of child abuse and maltreatment, the Advisory Board of the National Center on Child Abuse and Neglect (U.S. Department of Health and Human Services, 1990) has declared child maltreatment in the United States a national emergency. While such officially reported figures are significant in and of themselves, community-based incidence studies have indicated that reported cases of child maltreatment may make up only about 40% of all cases that actually occur (National Center on Child Abuse and Neglect, 1988). This is the beginning point for the difficult issues within the legal system for responding to cases of child maltreatment; most cases are not reported.

Since 1964, all U.S. states have enacted laws requiring reports to be made for incidents of suspected child maltreatment, including physical, sexual, and emotional abuse and neglect. All states mandate professionals who work with children, such as physicians, teachers, and social workers, to report suspected cases, and some require additional groups, such as lawyers, therapists, religious leaders, and commercial film processors, also to report. The majority of the states have established criminal penalties for the failure to report, and some attach civil liabilities. Justification for mandatory reporting is based on the view that children, either because of their physical immaturity or because of their relative powerlessness, are unable to make reports for themselves. As such, the burden is placed on adult members of society to notify authorities of improper treatment.

There are ethical and clinical disagreements on appropriateness of mandating reports of child abuse. Counselors are concerned that mandated reporting violates the confidentiality between therapists and clients, whether the clients are victims or offenders (Kalichman, 1993). Others have questioned the justification behind mandated reporting if the abuse has stopped or the offender is undergoing treatment (Miller & Weinstock, 1983; Zellman, 1990). As will be discussed in more detail later, there are also concerns about how mandatory reporting has created a greater emphasis on investigative intervention into cases of child maltreatment, instead of focusing on providing more service and preventative types of intervention. In response to this situation, Finkelhor and Zellman (1991) have proposed a "flexible reporting options" approach where some particular designated mandated reporters would be given broader discretionary latitude in determining what is best for the child.

Reports of child abuse are typically directed toward child protective services (CPS) or police departments. Jurisdictions vary as to who is responsible for determining the immediate safety of the involved children and the investigation of the allegation. While this chapter will primarily deal with the role of the criminal justice system, we would like to review briefly current developments on multidisciplinary investigative teams, an approach that we advocated for in the first edition of this volume (Mac Murray & Carson, 1992).

Multidisciplinary Teams

The necessity of coordination and collaboration of services in responding to allegations of child maltreatment is clearly described in the following portion of a federal government publication directed to professionals working in this area:

> Child abuse is a community problem. No single agency has the training, manpower, resources, or legal mandate to intervene effectively in child abuse cases. No one agency has the sole responsibility for dealing with abused children.
> When a child is physically beaten or sexually abused, the ideal set of events is that doctors treat the injuries, therapists counsel the child, social services works with the family, police arrest the offender, and attorneys prosecute the case. To promote this response, effective community intervention involves the formation of a child protection team that includes professionals from medicine, criminal justice, social work, and education who understand and appreciate the different roles, responsibilities, strengths, and weaknesses of the other team members but cooperate and coordinate their efforts. [Office of Juvenile Justice and Delinquency Prevention (OJJDP), 1997b, p. 1]

At least 33 states and the District of Columbia have laws requiring joint investigations and cooperation between law enforcement and child protection agencies in child abuse cases. Furthermore, 29 U.S. states and 2 U.S. territories have laws in place that mandate or authorize the creation of multidisciplinary and multiagency child protection teams. Other jurisdictions have interagency agreements or informal arrangements for information-gathering and case decision making (U.S. Department of Justice, 1993). In a national study, Sheppard (1992) found that almost all (94%) of more than 600 police and sheriffs' departments surveyed indicated that they conducted some joint investigations with CPS agencies.

Through cooperation and coordination, use of teams for investigation reduces the number of interviews a child victim will undergo (research documenting the harmful effects of multiple interviews will be discussed later in this chapter). Generally, these team efforts also enhance the quality of evidence discovered for civil litigation and criminal prosecution and help minimize the likelihood of conflicts between agencies with different philosophies or mandates (Lanning, 1996; U.S. Department of Justice, 1993).

Throughout the investigation process, team members must balance the needs of the evidence gathering process with the desire to protect the child's best interests (Goldstein, 1987). These goals can be best accomplished when the team is functioning within the parameters of a written investigative protocol—a protocol that provides predictability and direction to the investigation. In most cases of abuse or neglect where a family member or a day care is involved, a civil or administrative investigation will overlap and often complicate matters. Law enforcement and CPS investigators differ in their training, policies, decision-making processes, and goals for intervention. Thus, cooperation and communication between these parties is critical. Because of the potential for conflict and miscommunication, and because the resources of both agencies are necessary for successful intervention, it is helpful to have protocols addressing different areas of responsibility, the issue of timely cross-notification of allegations, and decisions regarding the interviewing of children, other witnesses, and offenders (Walsh, 1996).

Two basic forms for such protocols are currently advocated: (1) those which articulate the nature of the interagency agreement (Pence & Wilson, 1994; see also Martin & Besharov, 1991) and spell out the purpose of the agreement, the types of cases in which it will be used, the nature of cross-reporting between different agencies, and issues of team coordination (e.g., the frequency of team meetings, how the team should function if one member or another is not present, etc.), and (2) those which detail the investigative process and outline the investigative steps to be undertaken and the order in which the team will typically approach these steps. This latter form of protocol provides a framework within which to work by outlining such issues as report taking, background checks, the order of interviews, evidentiary issues, and team decision-making processes (Pence & Wilson, 1994).

We continue to advocate for use of multidisciplinary teams throughout the criminal justice process, and as will be discussed later, we also advocate for multidisciplinary approaches to working with the involved parties after court sentencing. Near the end of this chapter, we will also review some of the controversies surrounding the use of these teams; however, since this chapter focuses on legal issues, much of the following discussion will emphasize the role of the criminal justice system.

Criminal Justice Responses to Child Abuse

Although the particular sequencing and pattern of actions taken by involved agencies may differ across jurisdictions, the primary task of the criminal justice system is as follows: (1) to try to ascertain and establish the "facts" of what did (or did not) take place with respect to the alleged maltreatment; (2) to gather whatever evidence (physical, medical, testimonial by victims, witnesses, and others, etc.) is available, and (3) to determine what legal and child protective actions are necessary and appropriate for the victim, family, and alleged perpetrators. Related to this point, in the 1990s there has increasingly developed a perspective that the criminal justice system shall make all attempts possible to cause victims "no greater harm."

Efforts aimed at reducing injuries to victims are especially relevant in child abuse and maltreatment. First, the victim is a child who may not understand the dynamics of and justifications for the actions and approach of the legal system in her or his case. This confusion is often deepened by the fact that in many cases of child maltreatment, the abuser is a parent, other family member, or close acquaintance. The close relationship that typically exists between the victim and perpetrator also has an impact on relationships between other family members. The network of family relations means that multiple relationships may potentially be harmed by the criminal justice system's intervention. Thus, it is critical for criminal justice practitioners to try to reduce the amount of trauma experienced at every stage of the proceedings, from the investigation to prosecution and disposition.

A focus on reducing such *revictimization* (or secondary victimization) of victims in the area of child maltreatment has worked to eliminate practices such as multiple interviewing or lengthy legal processing in cases. In addition, programs designed to provide assistance through the assignment of victim advocates, guardians *ad litem*, and court-appointed special advocates (CASA) have been successfully implemented in many communities (Leung, 1996; OJJDP, 1997a; see also Whitcomb, 1992).

Law Enforcement

The role of law enforcement is to conduct criminal investigations; interview victims, witnesses, and suspects; and collect evidence. Such professionals also have the legal mandate to execute search warrants and effect arrests and the ultimate responsibility for conducting criminal investigation of suspected abuse and neglect. In addition to this, police in many states have the authority to remove children from the home in a crisis situation, although in many cases this duty is shared with CPS.

The decision to temporarily remove a child from the home is based on a decision about the child's safety in the home or community, and this is not an easy decision. The federal Adoption Assistance Act (P.L. 96-272) mandates that all efforts should be made to prevent removal of children; if they are removed, all efforts should be made to eventually reunite the family. Thus, there must be substantial belief that a child is in danger before he or she is removed. Much of the information needed to make such a determination is gathered from the initial investigation.

Investigation

Whether investigating the current safety of a child or generally investigating allegations of maltreatment, many considerations must be kept in mind. It is crucial at this stage for law enforcement to coordinate with CPS in order not to duplicate or confound the other's efforts. Paramedics, police, nurses, teachers, child care providers, and other persons who may have had contact with the child should be interviewed at this time (Walsh, 1996). Any caretakers for the child should also be interviewed separately from possible victims and other possible offenders (Faller, Froning, & Lipovsky, 1991). All persons interviewed should be encouraged to put their statements in writing on Affidavit in Fact forms when possible, a process that will enhance the quality of formal prosecution, if pursued (see Walsh, 1996).

The actual investigation process, whether team-coordinated or not, begins once an agency has been notified of an alleged incident involving potential abuse or neglect against a child via report. Usually, the first formal stages of the investigation involve interviewing the alleged victim. Considerable attention and controversy has and continues to surround issues of child interviews. Among the main issues that we will address here are concerns about the credibility and truth value of child witness statements, concerns about how the interview should take place procedurally, and the potential for revictimization of the child through this interview process.

Interviewing Children

Among the topics in this area that have remained controversial and received considerable attention from researchers in recent years are: interviewing children generally, and more particularly, the credibility of children's statements and testimony about allegations of abuse, especially sexual abuse. Current research on memory and suggestibility leads to mixed conclusions. First, younger children (especially those who are pre-school age) are more often suggestible than adults and older children (Goodman & Aman, 1991), and younger children spontaneously recall less information than older ones (see Ceci, Ross, & Toglia, 1987). However, research in this area also indicates that even younger children are not necessarily highly suggestible or have poor memories (Saywitz & Good-man, 1996).

Recent work has turned to those factors that can affect memory and suggestibility in children and adults. It is well documented that a child's spontaneous, free-recalled reports are more accurate, although somewhat less complete, than those elicited by specific questioning (see Dent, 1991). Thus, generally, interview guidelines recommend establishing rapport and "warming up" the interview situation in order to increase the amount of information that a child provides spontaneously (see American Profes-sional Society on the Abuse of Children, 1990). Free recall in response to open-ended questions is seen as more helpful in interview situations, because children are susceptible to bias or distortions in an accusatory context or when they are presented with misleading questions repetitively (Dunn, 1995; Warren & McGough, 1996). Similar problems are noted for the use of more detail-oriented specific questions and the use of cues and leading questions when interviewing children (Dunn, 1995).

Another concern deals with developmental issues, especially the child's communication and linguistic skills. Among the common problems here are cases in which either the child being interviewed misunderstands the questions posed by adults or the adults misunderstand the answers provided by the child. The most important guideline here is age-appro-priateness in the type and level of questions asked and in the specific wording used by interviewers (Lamb, Sternberg, & Esplin, 1994; see also Saywitz & Goodman, 1996; Warren & McGough, 1996).

Interviewers need to establish rapport and ask primarily open-ended questions that encourage narrative responses. The hope here is that such an initial interview context will set the stage for more reliable responses to the investigative questions that follow. On this point, the research litera-ture is a bit tricky. There is support for the conclusion that further inter-views with a child involving more specific and direct questions will elicit more depth of information and more complete recall of events; however, such repetitive interviewing also has the potential to bias the child's responses or traumatize the child victim (see Warren & McGough, 1996; Yuille, Hunter, Joffe, & Zaparniuk, 1993).

Similarly, there is not a strong consensus about the wisdom of record-ing or videotaping investigative interviews with children. Some, such as

Warren and McGough (1996) and Dunn (1995) firmly endorse such an approach. Professionals making up the Child Victim Witness Investigative Pilot Project (California Attorney General's Office, 1994) have similarly endorsed the use of videotape at this stage of case investigation. Others, however, have been critical or more cautious in their support (see for example, Lanning, 1996). In general, the literature is full of sources that merely note the major advantages and disadvantages of using videotape in investigative interviews of children without strong endorsement or disapproval (e.g., Dunn, 1995; Myers, 1992; National Center for Prosecution of Child Abuse, 1993). Regardless of whether or not such interviews are videotaped, it is important that they be conducted and documented carefully and thoroughly (Walsh, 1996).

Among the innovations that are being implemented today to try to address some of these concerns are cognitive interviewing techniques that attempt to root memories in contexts (Geiselman, Saywitz, & Bornstein, 1993); the use of a "step-wise interview" method, which is designed to maximize recall while minimizing contamination and other potential problems in interviewing (Yuille et al., 1993); and narrative elaboration techniques (see the review by Saywitz & Goodman, 1996).

The trade-off between completeness (when using specific questions) and accuracy (when using general and free-recall questions) has led to the development of nonverbal means of eliciting information and related interview aids. Most of the attention in the literature has focused on the use of anatomically detailed (AD) dolls. Widespread use and concern about the issue of suggestiveness are raised in this regard. Generally, research is inconclusive on the clear merits or harm resulting from the use of such dolls and other props when interviewing children. Some (see for example, Lamb et al., 1994) have expressed concern that little research is available to help investigators analyze reactions of potentially victimized children to anatomically correct dolls. Skinner's review (1996) of research in this area further suggests that there is no well-grounded empirical support for the basic assumptions behind using AD dolls to validate sexual abuse of children.

Skinner (1996) highlights the important and often overlooked role of the interviewer when using such dolls. She concludes by noting the controversy and contrary statements over the use of AD dolls and calls for caution and considerable care when doing so as well as for further research to document their use more fully. Finally, in their review, Lie and Inman (1991) discuss the controversy surrounding use of AD dolls, the mixture of state courts' rulings on such use, and related expert testimony. They emphasize the potential value of utilizing these aids with special-needs children and the need for training in the proper use of such dolls.

All of the foregoing suggests the importance of using skilled interviewers who have received special training to interview children in these
cases (Dunn, 1995; Warren & McGough, 1996). Many in the field emphasize
that this needs to be especially the case in instances of alleged child sexual
abuse (see Pence & Wilson, 1994). Some practitioners have suggested that
investigators and prosecutors in these cases should be volunteers who
have been carefully selected and trained in this highly specialized work,
recognizing that such work is not for everyone (Lanning, 1996; Smith,
1995). Humphrey (1996) has found that, regardless of level of professional
training, a specific closed unit in a police department that is designated to
work with cases of child abuse is the most effective type of law enforcement organization for responding to such cases.

Besides the focus on how interviews with children should be conducted and by whom, the research literature has also placed particular
emphasis on the manner in which the interview is conducted and the
setting in which it takes place. Regarding the issue of setting, a range of
options appear acceptable and appropriate, according to the literature—
from the child's own home to a school setting to a special interview room
in the prosecutor's office, the police department, or elsewhere in the
community. Although little research work has formally addressed this
question, available data indicate that a comfortable, "child-friendly," supportive atmosphere in which the child feels safe is most conducive both to
eliciting accurate information and to aiding resistance by the child to
suggestive misinformation (see the reviews by Saywitz & Goodman, 1996;
Warren & McGough, 1996).

In recent years, a tentative consensus has begun to develop around
issues of how interviews of children should take place when allegations of
abuse or neglect are involved. First, it is generally recognized that the
number of interviews that the child goes through should be kept to the
practical and necessary *minimum*; this also extends to trying to minimize
the number of court appearances and amount of testimony a child has to
give (Henry, 1997; Runyon, Everson, Edelsohn, Hunter, & Coulter, 1988;
Tedesco & Schnell, 1987; see also, Saywitz & Goodman, 1996; Whitcomb,
1992). This guideline grows out of concerns primarily for the welfare of
the child in relating the details of the abuse, and the trauma or revictimization that might occur with the continual retelling (and thus reliving) of the
abuse experience. Regarding the timing of interviews, generally it is advised that the earlier following the maltreatment the interviewing takes
place, the better, both as a way of inoculating children (and other witnesses) against forgetting and as a means of guarding against suggestibility from other persons with access to the child (see National Center for

Prosecution of Child Abuse, 1993; Tedesco & Schnell, 1987; Warren & McGough, 1996).

In response to these concerns, several different strategies and approaches have been proposed and utilized. For those jurisdictions in which a team approach is in place, common options include either having a joint interview with the child conducted by team members (for example, representing CPS and law enforcement) using a single interviewer with other team members or agency representatives present to observe the interview (Pence & Wilson, 1994; Vogelstanz & Drabman, 1995). There has been less consensus on the use of one-way mirrors, audiotaping, and videotaping as means of allowing such observation of the interview (see Dunn, 1995). Over the past decade, child or family advocacy centers as neutral sites where such interviews of children can be conducted have been created in a number of jurisdictions. These centers streamline investigations and prosecution of child maltreatment cases, particularly those involving sexual abuse, in that often medical exams and collection of evidence are also conducted at the same site (Reichard, 1993; Whitcomb, 1992).

As with the investigation of any alleged crime, there is concern about false or fictitious reports. Research indicates that in cases of child maltreatment, false allegations are relatively uncommon. For example, in regard to sexual assault research, studies finds that only between 2 and 9% of allegations are fictitious (Cantwell, 1981: Jones & McCraw, 1987; Peters, 1976). Indeed, despite popular stereotypes, such false allegations are relatively rare even in cases of divorce or custody and visitation disputes (Faller & DeVoe, 1995; Thoennes & Tjaden, 1989). Surveys of mental health counselors, judges, and police officers indicate that most practitioners are aware of these low percentages (Everson, Boat, Bourg, & Robertson, 1996).

Prosecution Decisions and Actions

Increasingly over the past decade, prosecutorial decision making and the processing of cases in the criminal justice system have become more interrelated with the overall multidisciplinary team approach in many jurisdictions (see for example, Pence & Wilson, 1994; National Center for Prosecution of Child Abuse, 1993). Prosecutors and law enforcement agents are often integrated team members from the early points of investigation in cases of alleged child abuse and neglect today (Lanning, 1996; National Center for Prosecution of Child Abuse, 1993; Walsh, 1996). At the same time, once a CPS or law enforcement investigation of a case is complete, it is the prosecutor who must decide whether or not criminal charges should be pursued, and if so, how to proceed through the criminal justice system.

Earlier work has suggested that most cases involving allegations of child abuse or neglect usually do not make it all the way through the criminal justice system to court hearings or trials (Finkelhor, 1983; Mac Murray, 1988; Rogers, 1982). Tjaden and Thoennes (1992) report more recently that despite reforms in the reporting of child maltreatment and other innovations in the prosecution of such cases, prosecutorial intervention is still the exception, with approximately 20% of all substantiated cases of child maltreatment resulting in abuse and neglect petitions and fewer than 5% of these cases resulting in prosecution in criminal court.

This low percentage does not mean that nothing is being done with the cases, however. Pretrial diversion practices may be useful for intervening in the family unit and preventing recidivism (Mac Murray, 1991). There actually may be benefits of not taking cases to trial, given such issues as potential trauma to children, the difficulty of finding collaborating witnesses and evidence, and a concern about wanting to help the family instead of punishing it. Diversion programs can offer the added benefit of documenting a pretrial admission of guilt by the abuser that can strengthen prosecution if the maltreatment continues and a court hearing is pursued. Unfortunately, Skibinski (1994) found that jurisdictions that emphasize pretrial diversion programs are less likely to conduct thorough investigations, including such things as medical examinations, which may hinder subsequent investigations. In their national study of four counties, Cross, DeVos, and Whitcomb (1994) found that only 2% of the cases that were presented to prosecutors were assigned to diversion programs. Representative studies of the use of diversion practices are needed to document more fully the possible beneficial effects of these practices.

In looking at case factors relevant to case decisions, Cross et al. (1994) found that prosecutors were more likely to accept child sexual abuse cases in which victims were between 7 and 17 years of age, where the relationship between the alleged perpetrator and victim was not biological, and where oral-genital abuse was alleged. Prosecutors were also more likely to accept for prosecution those cases reported first to law enforcement agencies, those where the investigation was shorter in length of time, and when physical evidence, especially a confession, was available. Other research confirms that prosecutors appear more willing to take cases to court if they involve older children (Cross et al., 1994).

In their study, Whitcomb and Hardin (1996) report that although in many cases of alleged child maltreatment law enforcement and child protective services work fairly well together during investigations, cooperation is less common among the attorneys who handle these cases in the criminal and juvenile courts. Despite an overlap of such cases being processed concurrently in both juvenile and criminal courts nationally, Whitcomb and Hardin found little coordination. After an examination of several model jurisdictions working with such coordination problems, they suggest improved communication between legal counsel who are involved in child protection and prosecutors, as well as possible involvement by both attorneys on multidisciplinary teams; additional work to coordinate information and actions between the differing courts; and reform of testimonial immunity statutes that motivate offenders not to testify in juvenile court or take part in therapy because of the potential that such testimony or records will be used against them in subsequent criminal court proceedings.

Court Procedures

The particular type of court that may hear different cases of child maltreatment varies by different states' judicial structures. For example, some states typically hear child maltreatment cases in juvenile courts, while others may try them in domestic or family courts. Even in a given state, portions of the same case may be tried in more than one type of court, as already noted. For example, a serious case might involve criminal court action for prosecution of the offender but also civil court action if the victim is attempting to receive compensation for injuries incurred. Procedures and rules of evidence vary tremendously between these courts, and this can be very confusing to young victims and their families.

Major debates have taken place about court testimony of children in child maltreatment cases. First, there is concern about the trauma that children may experience while testifying in court, and second, there is debate about the impact of alternative forms of testifying on the legal rights of those accused of committing such crimes. Each of these topics requires further attention (see Goodman, Levine, Melton, & Ogden, 1991).

Be it during pretrial investigations or actual court proceedings, there is general agreement in the literature that asking children to testify may cause them considerable trauma. However, there is also strong indication that trauma does not necessarily occur if children are adequately prepared for the courtroom process and only have to testify once (Goodman, Pyle-Taub, Jones, England, Port, Rudy, & Pradeo, 1992; Whitcomb, Shapiro, & Shellwagon, 1985; see also Saywitz & Goodman, 1996; Whitcomb, 1992). For example, Runyon *et al.* (1988) found that the mental health of child victims of sexual abuse actually improved if they were allowed to testify in juvenile court, but that a child's involvement in longer criminal proceedings could have negative effects.

Alternative means for interviewing children in court proceedings have been tried and there have been challenges to their use throughout the past decade. Such challenges stem from primarily the confrontation clause of the Sixth Amendment to the U.S. Constitution. This amendment states that an accused person has a constitutional right to confront the witnesses against him or her. Two cases (*Coy v. Iowa*, 1988; *Maryland v. Craig*, 1990), eventually heard by the U.S. Supreme Court, have laid the foundation for current practice in this area. The outgrowth of these decisions is a legal standard that *allows exceptions* to the defendant's right to confrontation when there is a case specific, individualized finding by a trial judge of emotional trauma on the part of the child witness who is to testify. The U.S. Supreme Court has ruled that under such circumstances, alternatives to in-court testimony—such as one- or two-way closed circuit television procedures and other approaches—may be used (Gordon, 1992; Myers, 1992).

Another challenge involves the role of hearsay testimony, that is, statements made outside of the courtroom that are used as evidence in court. In most criminal proceedings such information is not allowed because there is no opportunity to cross-examine the person who made the statements. However, exceptions are allowable under rules of evidence, and hearsay testimony has been permitted in criminal proceedings in some cases involving child maltreatment allegations (see Myers, 1992; Whitcomb, 1992). For example, in cases where a child who is clearly too young to participate in court proceedings has made statements to others about the abuse, such information may be used as evidence in court. Generally these statements must have been made spontaneously and not as part of any interrogation (*State v. Robinson*, 1987; *White v. Illinois*, 1982; see also Myers, 1992, Whitcomb, 1992, for more discussion of this issue).

Innovations and challenges to these alternatives to traditional court practices continue; however, concerns about potential trauma and other negative effects on children of having to testify are somewhat dampened by the fact that relatively few cases of maltreatment are accepted for prosecution and actually go to trial (Goodman *et al.*, 1992; Whitcomb, 1992).

Legal Responses to Child Abuse Offenders

As described earlier, the criminal justice system is primarily involved in investigating allegations of abuse, charging alleged offenders if sufficient evidence is collected, and then either constructing diversion requirements or prosecuting those charged in court. If offenders are convicted, the criminal justice system is also responsible for determining what happens to them. The system has mixed objectives that influence requirements for diversion or determine sentencing outcomes after conviction. Some efforts are directed toward punishment for wrongdoing (retribution) and others focus on finding interventions for changing the offender's future behavior (rehabilitation). In cases of child maltreatment, punitive responses range from prohibiting contact with the victim to relinquishing parental rights to serving time in jail or prison. These responses may help reduce further abuse if they prohibit contact with victims, but they do not guarantee the safety of either the particular victim of the prior offense or other children in the future. As such, the following section offers a brief description of diversionary or sentencing options that focus on trying to change the offender's abusive behavior—those that attempt rehabilitation.

Prosecutors or judges may recommend community treatment-based programs established to work with adults who are abusive of children. There are many programs nationwide that address an array of issues associated with child maltreatment; these are usually operated by local social services agencies and nonprofit and for-profit organizations.

If there has been a conviction, people who abuse children may also be placed on probation while attending various treatment programs. Unfortunately, probation officers are not always well prepared to work with some types of offenses, such as the sexual abuse of children (Allen & Simonsen, 1995). Besides lacking specific training, often extremely large caseloads prevent them from effective supervision to ensure that all of the conditions of the probation, such as participating in treatment programs, are followed.

In serious cases of child maltreatment, offenders may be sentenced to prison. In these cases, usually children were either sexually abused or received serious physical injuries. In prisons that provide comprehensive treatment services, these individuals may be involved in parenting courses, anger management classes, group or individual therapy, and sex offender rehabilitation programs. However, not all prisons offer these programs, not all judges mandate attendance, and treatment programs can and do reject offenders they deem unsuitable for treatment. Overall, the success of these programs in working with offenders is not good (Allen & Simonsen, 1995).

One legal issue regarding treatment of offenders convicted of child sexual abuse, that has recently emerged is the required registration of sex offenders upon their release into the community. Over 40 states now require some form of police or community notification upon release. There have been constitutional legal challenges to this notification requirement, but it appears that it is considered neither cruel and unusual punishment nor ex post facto punishment (Brooks, 1995). The justification for this policy is that since current methods of rehabilitation for those who sexually abuse children are so often unsuccessful, community notification is essential (Welsh, 1996). To date, there are numerous, important concerns about how community notification should be conducted, and as of yet, little research suggesting answers (Brooks, 1995). In addition, there is no research determining whether or not the policy of requiring registration of sex offenders actually increases the safety of children in the community.

Assessment of a Criminal Justice Approach toward Child Maltreatment

As the preceding review indicates, many changes and adaptations have been made by the criminal justice system in responding to child maltreatment. Yet several overriding controversies still exist. For example, 10 years ago we were advocating for the rights of children to testify about their own victimization. Today, the call for children's rights has increased in part because of the combination of child maltreatment cases and other legal concerns such as divorce, child custody, and delinquency cases. With our increasing knowledge about child maltreatment, we know that it is not a problem that is disassociated from other family pathologies. For example, it is well documented that in families where violence is taking place between the parents, incidents of violence against children are also common (Davidson, 1994). We also know that even if children are not physically beaten in these households, they are at risk of becoming violent adults. We now know that crimes of child maltreatment are frequently found in drug-abusing households (Famularo, Stone, Barnum, & Wharton, 1987; Lung & Daro, 1996). We also know that many adults convicted of physical or sexual assaults were physically or sexually assaulted themselves as youth (Maxfield & Widom, 1995; Widom, 1989). This last correlation makes it even more imperative that criminal justice practitioners take into consideration issues of the victim when responding to child maltreatment so as not to increase future maltreatment and violence in society.

Despite the overlapping nature of these multiple problems, however, the legal process of intervention tends to view each of these behaviors distinctly, with questions arising about the legality of permitting the other related concerns to be considered in formal proceedings. For example, some states will not allow undocumented reports of child abuse to be admissible in child custody cases; however, progress is being made on this issue in that, by 1992, some 33 states had passed legislation requiring the courts to consider marital violence when determining custody of children.

Another, and perhaps the most controversial, legal issue in intervention into child abuse and neglect cases involves the overlapping functions of varying agencies. While use of multidisciplinary terms has been advocated by many scholars and experts in the area, this approach appears to have resulted in a blending of functions by the separate agencies involved in handling the cases. Some multidisciplinary team decisions seem to have emerged as a result of a form of "groupthink" (Janis, 1982), where the blending of each agency's functions has occurred. This has been most thoroughly reviewed in the social work literature, where there is serious concern that the investigation of child abuse cases from a legalistic perspective has overtaken many social welfare agencies' ability to provide prevention and early intervention to troubled families (Huxtable, 1994; Patton, 1992–93; Pelton, 1991). Today, it is rare that troubled families voluntarily seek assistance or advice from public welfare agencies, because they fear being reported for child maltreatment and will not risk the chance that their children will be removed from the home.

Some scholars who are troubled by this situation have suggested that only the most serious cases of maltreatment should be sent on to the legal system and that CPS should be allowed to work with other social agencies in prevention and service provision for families in need and at risk, without legal interference (Pelton, 1991). Similarly, others (e.g., Davidson, 1994; Levesque, 1995) have argued that family preservation, as well as the safety and best interests of children, needs to be given the highest priority by those professionals dealing with child maltreatment cases and that criminalization and formal legal actions may not necessarily best serve these goals in such cases.

Much work remains to be done. To paraphrase the 1995 report "A Nation's Shame" (U.S. Department of Health and Human Services, Administration for Children and Families, 1995), our review suggests that four major steps need to be taken to address the legal issues involved in cases of violence toward children. First, more knowledge is needed, both in the research area and with respect to the training of practicing professionals who respond to cases of child abuse. Second, useful innovations need to be developed and refined to investigate and handle child maltreatment cases, in both the criminal justice and social service spheres. Third, increased coordination and collaboration such as the implementation of a team or multidisciplinary team approach in cases involving allegations or reports of child maltreatment—needs to occur, with each agency maintaining its own distinct role and priorities. And finally, continued work is necessary both to make aggressive efforts to protect children and to facilitate prevention efforts and family services in communities.

Innovations

In conclusion, this chapter will focus on some innovative efforts and programs that begin to address the concerns raised in the previous discussion.

Advocacy Centers

One innovative concept involves family or child advocacy centers, which offer facilities useful both in coordinating the activities and decisions of various professionals involved in handling cases of child maltreatment and in meeting the special needs of the children involved. Perhaps the most famous demonstration of this concept is the National Children's Advocacy Center located in Huntsville, Alabama which has been a model for communities throughout the country. Such centers are designed to facilitate a multidisciplinary team approach, to help make children feel comfortable during interviews, and yet also to permit the collection of quality evidence acceptable for court use (California Attorney General's Office, 1988; see also Whitcomb, 1992).

Another example of this approach is the Marion County Family Advocacy Center (FAC) in Indianapolis, which also houses local and county law enforcement and CPS and prosecutorial staff, all of whom collaborate and adopt a team approach to cases. FAC provides services to families involved in domestic violence and a "peace learning center" program on conflict resolution for elementary schoolchildren throughout the city. This center also offers "child-friendly" interview rooms, specially trained interviewers, and operates a "kids court program" designed to introduce and familiarize children with the courtroom setting and court personnel in order to reduce potential trauma and better prepare children for court proceedings (Marion County Family Advocacy Center, 1997; Reichard, 1993).

Unified Family Courts

Although this term is used differently and somewhat loosely in different contexts, essentially a family court has jurisdiction over *all types* of family dispute cases within a unified court system. Some states have had such courts for several years, but others are only starting to experiment with them of late, particularly now that the need for handling child maltreatment cases is so great. These courts can consolidate virtually all issues of children and families under their jurisdiction, including determination of custody, termination of parental rights, children in need of supervision, criminal charges of child abuse, and civil suits where victims are suing for compensation (Sagatun & Edwards, 1995). Such courts allow a more coordinated, and child- or family-focused, approach to child maltreatment cases.

Restorative Justice Programs

A new paradigm that is being proposed both within the formal criminal justice system and through informal interventions into crime is the perspective of *restorative justice*, a method of responding to conflict and crime that strives to promote healing by both the offender and the victim in a process supported and usually facilitated by community members. It is believed that by working with both victim and offender, the program can help them to assist each other and themselves in resolving the hurt, injury, or conflict caused by the initial offense (Mackey, 1990; Bazemore & Mahoney 1994; Pranis, 1997a; Zehr, 1985).

Examples of the varied types of restorative justice programs currently operating include mediations, victim–offender reconciliations, victim impact panels, family group conferencing, and sentencing circles. Currently, several of these methods are being used to work with issues of violence and in familial contexts (Umbreit, 1972). A primary tenet of restorative justice programs is that no one shall suffer more harm. Thus, safety is a primary concern for all of these programs, as is the belief that participation must be voluntary.

When applying these ideas to cases of child maltreatment, the inability to guarantee safety, be it physical or emotional, as well as the voluntary component, would preclude involving some families in these programs. However, other types of meetings might be encouraged that could help reduce the overall harm suffered by family members, either directly related to the abuse experience or resulting from the criminal justice intervention into the case. For example, in cases where the abuser is removed from the home, reconciliations may be needed between grandparents, other extended family members, the nonabusive parent, and noncustodial parents. There may also be the need for reconciliations between nonvictimized children in the family and the abuser. It would appear that there are many arenas in the network of family relationships where abuse has occurred that could benefit from mediation or reconciliation programs.

Victim impact panels might also be useful in cases where the direct victim of the violence does not wish to participate (or is advised not to). Currently, victim impact panels have been created by local chapters of Mothers Against Drunk Driving (MADD) where victims who want to can share their stories of tragedy to audiences of drunk-driving offenders. Sprang (1997) has found these panels to be effective in getting offenders to consider the consequences of their relevant behavior as well as to reevaluate their own belief system regarding the appropriateness of such behavior. It is also possible that victim impact panels might be useful in getting adults to listen to the stories of other adults describing their childhood experiences of physical, sexual, or emotional abuse or neglect.

There are many creative ways that restorative justice programs can be adapted to respond to child maltreatment. One currently operating project is located in the Hawthorne neighborhood of Minneapolis. Here, sentencing circles, modeled on traditions of Native Americans in the Yukon, are being used as part of legal interventions into child maltreatment cases. These circles are made up of all the relevant family members, as well as judges, police officers, probation officers, social workers, and any other involved persons, such as religions leaders, teachers, or neighbors.

All participants gather in a circle to analyze the dilemma faced by the family and to offer support and suggestions for handling the crises. All have the right to speak, and the group focuses on the problems as a group, not as individuals. Often, multiple circles meet, such as a separate healing circle for the victim and offender, a circle to determine the disposition of the case, and follow-up circles to monitor the progress of the offender (Pranis, 1997b). It is possible for circles to include fairly young children; others include only adults. Typically, multitudes of familial problems surface, conditions that have contributed to the abuse. For the family members to heal, these additional factors must be addressed.

Restorative justice programs may be extremely beneficial to some families involved in child maltreatment. These programs go beyond merely responding to the physical injuries of maltreatment alone, to address the long-term consequences for children of recognizing that it is someone they love or whom they presume is there to care for them who causes the injuries. Currently, our criminal justice system does little to respond to these emotional injuries, and actually, few of our current practices provide much assistance to offenders in stopping the abuse. The reality is that most families where abuse has occurred will eventually be reunited, and the possibility of future abuse is high. There are abused children who would rather live with their abusive parent than be placed out of the home. There are abused children who feel extremely guilty about having their parents arrested and sent to jail. As with many other forms of victimization, the children may blame themselves. Under such circumstances, restorative justice programs may offer the best ideas available to help reduce the trauma of legal intervention as well as the prospects of reducing future maltreatment.

Summary

Legal responses to child maltreatment have undergone tremendous reform and change, particularly in the 1990s. However, important problems and challenges remain. In this chapter, we have sought to review the main legal issues and controversies surrounding violence toward children and have suggested some of the new and promising areas of reform and innovation.

References

Allen, H., & Simonsen, C. (1995). *Corrections in America: An introduction* (7th ed.). Englewood Cliffs, NJ: Prentice-Hall.

American Professional Society on the Abuse of Children. (1990). *Guidelines for psychological evaluation of suspected sexual abuse in young children.* Chicago: Author.

Bazemore, G., & Maloney, D. (1994). Rehabilitating community service: Toward restorative service in a balanced justice system. *Federal Probation, 58,* 24–35.

Besharov, D. J. (1990). *Combating child abuse: Guidelines for cooperation between law enforcement and child protective services.* Washington, DC: American Enterprise Institute Press.

Brooks, A. D. (1995). The legal issues. *Criminal Justice Ethics, 14,* 12–16.

California Attorney General's Office. (1994). *Child victim witness investigative pilot project: Research and evaluation final report.* Sacramento, CA: Author.

California Attorney General's Office. (1988). *California child victim witness judicial advisory committee: Final report.* Sacramento, CA: Author.

Cantwell, H. (1981). Sexual abuse of children in Denver, 1979; revised with implications for pediatric intervention and possible prevention. *Child Abuse & Neglect, 5,* 75–85.

Ceci, S. J., Ross, D. F., & Toglia, M. P. (1987). Age differences in suggestibility: Narrowing the uncertainties. In S. J. Ceci, M. P. Toglia, & D. F. Ross (Eds.), *Children's eyewitness memory* (pp. 79–91) . New York: Springer-Verlag.

Child Abuse Manual. (1989). *Police Academy Training Manual.* Sacramento, CA: Police Training Academy.

Coy v. Iowa, 487 U.S. 1012 (1988).

Cross, T. P., DeVos, E., & Whitcomb, D. (1994). Prosecution of child sexual abuse: Which cases are accepted? *Child Abuse & Neglect, 18,* 663–677.

Daro, D. (1988). *Confronting child abuse: Research for effective program design.* New York: Free Press.

Davidson, H. (1994). *The impact of domestic violence on children: A report to the president of the American Bar Association.* Chicago: American Bar Association.

Dent, H. (1991). Experimental studies of interviewing child witnesses. In J. Doris (Ed.), *The suggestibility of children's recollections: Implications for eyewitness testimony* (pp. 138–146). New York: Springer-Verlag.

Dunn, A. R. (1995). Questioning the reliability of children's testimony: An examination of the problematic elements. *Law and Psychology Review, 19,* 202–215.

Everson, M. D., Boat, B. W., Bourg, S., & Robertson, K. R. (1996). Beliefs among professionals about rates of false allegations of child sexual abuse. *Journal of Interpersonal Violence, 11,* 541–553.

Faller, K. C., & DeVoe, E. (1995). Allegations of sexual abuse. *Journal of Child Sexual Abuse, 4,* 1–25.

Faller, K. C., Froning, M. L., & Lipovsky, J. (1991). The parent–child interview: Use in evaluating child allegations of sexual abuse by the parent. *American Journal of Orthopsychiatry, 61,* 552–557.

Famularo, R., Stone, K., Barnum, R., & Wharton, R. (1987). Alcoholism and severe child maltreatment. *American Journal of Orthopsychiatry, 56,* 481–485.

Finkelhor, D. (1983). Removing the child and prosecuting the offender in cases of sexual abuse: Evidence from the national reporting department for child abuse and neglect. *Child Abuse & Neglect, 7,* 195–205.

Finkelhor, D., & Zellman, G. L. (1991). Flexible reporting options for skilled child abuse professionals. *Child Abuse & Neglect, 15,* 335–341.

Gieselman, R. E., Saywitz, K. J., & Bornstein, G. K. (1993). Effects of cognitive questioning techniques on children's recall performance. In G. S. Goodman & B. L. Bottoms (Eds.),

Child victims, child witnesses: Understanding and improving testimony (pp. 71–94). New York: Guilford.

Giovannoni, J., & Becerra, R. (1990). *Defining child abuse.* New York: Free Press.

Goldstein, S. (1987). *The sexual exploitation of children.* New York: Elsevier.

Gondolf, E. (1987). Evaluating programs for men who batter: Problems perspective. *Journal of Family Violence, 2,* 95–108.

Goodman, G. S., & Aman, C. (1991). Children's use of anatomically detailed dolls to recount an event. *Child Development, 61,* 1859–1871.

Goodman, G. S., Levine, M., Melton, G. B., & Ogden, D. W. (1991). Child witnesses and the confrontation clause. *Law and Human Behavior, 15,* 13–30.

Goodman, G. S., Pyle-Taub, E. P., Jones, D. P. H., England, P., Port, L. K., Rudy, L., & Pradeo, L. (1992). The effects of criminal court testimony on child sexual assault victims. *Monographs of the Society for Research in Child Development, 57,* 1–163.

Gordon, M. A. (1992). Recent supreme court rulings on child testimony in sexual abuse cases. *Journal of Child Sexual Abuse, 1,* 61–73.

Henry, J. (1997). System intervention trauma to child sexual abuse victims following disclosure. *Journal of Interpersonal Violence, 12,* 499–512.

Humphrey, C. (1996). Exploring new territory: Police organizational responses to child sexual abuse. *Child Abuse & Neglect, 20,* 337–344.

Huxtable, M. (1994). Child protection: With liberty and justice for all. *Social Work, 39,* 60–66.

Janis, I. L. (1982). *Groupthink* (2nd ed.). Boston: Houghton Mifflin.

Jones, D., & McCraw, M. J. (1987). Reliable and fictitious accounts of sexual abuse of children. *Journal of Interpersonal Violence, 2,* 27–45.

Kalichman, S. C. (1993). *Mandated reporting of suspected child abuse: Ethics, law, and policy.* Washington, DC: American Psychological Association.

Lamb, M. E., Sternberg, K. J., & Esplin, P. W. (1994). Factors influencing the reliability and validity of statements made by young victims of sexual maltreatment. *Journal of Applied Developmental Psychology, 15,* 255–280.

Lanning, K. V. (1996). Criminal investigations of suspected child abuse: Section 1. Criminal investigation of sexual victimization of children. In J. Briere, L. Berliner, J. A. Bulkley, C. Jenny, & T. Reid (Eds.), *The APSAC Handbook on Child Maltreatment* (pp. 247–264). Thousand Oaks, CA: Sage.

Leung, P. (1996). Is the court-appointed special advocate program effective? A longitudinal analysis of time involvement and case outcomes. *Child Welfare League of America, 75,* 269–284.

Levesque, R. J. R. (1995). Prosecuting sex crimes against children. Time for "outrageous" proposals? *Law and Psychology Review, 19,* 59–91.

Lie, G.-Y., & Inman, A. (1991). The use of anatomical dolls as assessment and evidentiary tools. *Social Work, 36,* 396–399.

Lung, C.-T., & Daro, D. (1996). *Current trends in child abuse reporting and fatalities: The results of the 1995 annual fifty-state survey.* Chicago: National Committee to Prevent Child Abuse.

Mackey, V. (1990). *Restorative justice: Toward nonviolence.* Louisville, KY: Presbyterian Criminal Justice Program, National Ministries Division.

Mac Murray, B. K. (1988). The nonprosecution of sexual abuse and informal justice. *Journal of Interpersonal Violence, 3,* 197–202.

Mac Murray, B. K. (1991). Legal responses of prosecutors to child sexual abuse: A case comparison of two counties. In D. D. Knudsen & J. L. Miller (Eds.), *Abused and battered: Social and legal responses to family violence* (pp. 153–167). New York: Aldine de Gruyter.

Mac Murray, B. K., & Carson, B. A. (1992). Legal issues in violence toward children. In R. T. Ammerman & M. Hersen (Eds.), *Case studies in family violence* (pp. 57–71). New York: Wiley.

Marion County Family Advocacy Center. (1997). *1996 annual report*. Indianapolis, IN: Marion County Family Advocacy Center.

Martin, S. E., & Besharov, D. J. (1991). *Police and child abuse: View and expanded responsibilities*. Washington, DC: U.S. Department of Justice.

Maryland v. Craig, 110 S.Ct. 3157 (1990).

Maxfield, M., & Widom, C. S. (1995, November). *Childhood victimization and patterns of offending through the life cycle: Early onset and continuation*. Paper presented at the American Society of Criminology meeting, Boston.

McGee, R. A., & Wolfe, D. D. (1991). Psychological maltreatment: Toward an operational definition. *Developmental Psychopathology, 3*, 3–18.

Miller, R., & Weinstock, R. (1987). Conflict of interest between therapist-patient confidentiality: Duty to report sexual abuse of children. *Behavioral Sciences and the Law, 5*, 161–174.

Myers, J. E. B. (1992). *Legal issues in child abuse and neglect*. Thousand Oaks, CA: Sage.

National Center for Prosecution of Child Abuse. (1993). *Investigation and prosecution of child abuse* (2nd ed.). Alexandria, VA: American Prosecutors Research Institute, National District Attorneys Association.

National Center on Child Abuse and Neglect. (1988). *Study findings: Study of national incidence and prevalence of child abuse and neglect*. Washington, DC: U.S. Department of Health and Human Services.

Office of Juvenile Justice and Delinquency Prevention. (1997a). *Court-appointed special advocates: A voice for abused and neglected children in court*. Washington, DC: U.S. Department of Justice.

Office of Juvenile Justice and Delinquency Prevention. (1997b). *Law enforcement response to child abuse*. Washington, DC: U.S. Department of Justice.

Patton, W. W. (1992–93). Child abuse: The irreconcilable differences between criminal prosecution and informal dependency court mediation. *Journal of Family Law, 31*, 37–64.

Pelton, L. H. (1991). Beyond permanency planning: Restructuring the public child welfare system. *Social Work, 36*, 337–343.

Pence, D., & Wilson, C. (1994). *Team investigation of child sexual abuse: The uneasy alliance*. Thousand Oaks, CA: Sage.

Peters, J. (1976). Children who are victims of sexual assault and the psychology of offenders. *American Journal of Psychology, 30*, 398–421.

Pranis, K. (1997a). The Minnesota Restorative Justice Initiative: A model experience. *The Crime Victim Report, 1*, 2.

Pranis, K. (June, 1997b). *Restoring community: The process of circle sentencing*. Presentation at Justice Without Violence Conference, Minneapolis, MN, June 6, 1997.

Reichard, R. D. (1993). Dysfunctional families in dysfunctional systems? Why child advocacy centers may not be enough. *Journal of Child Sexual Abuse, 2*, 103–109.

Rogers, C. M. (1982). Child sexual abuse and the courts: Preliminary findings. *Journal of Social Work and Human Sexuality, 1*, 145–153.

Runyan, D. K., Everson, M. D., Edelsohn, G. A., Hunter, W. M., & Coulter, M. L. (1988). Impact of legal intervention on sexually abused children. *Journal of Pediatrics, 113*, 647–563.

Sagatun, I., & Edwards, L. P. (1995). *Child abuse and the legal system*. Chicago: Nelson Hall.

Saywitz, K. J., & Goodman, G. S. (1996). Interviewing children in and out of court: Current research and practice implications. In J. Briere, L. Berliner, J. A. Bulkley, C. Jenny, & T. Reid (Eds.), *The APSAC handbook on child maltreatment* (pp. 297–319). Thousand Oaks, CA: Sage.

Sedlak, A. J., & Broadhurst, D. D. (1996). *Executive summary of the third national incidence study of child abuse and neglect*. Washington, DC: U.S. Department of Health and Human Services.

Sheppard, D. (1992). *Study to improve joint law enforcement and child protective service agency investigations of reported child maltreatment.* Washington, DC: Police Foundation.

Skibinski, G. (1994). Intrafamilial child sexual abuse: Intervention programs for first time offenders and their families. *Child Abuse & Neglect, 18,* 367–375.

Skinner, L. J. (1996). Assumptions and beliefs about the role of AD dolls in child sexual abuse validation interviews: Are they supported empirically? *Behavioral Sciences and the Law, 14,* 167–185.

Smith, B. E. (1995). *Prosecuting child physical abuse cases: A case study in San Diego.* Washington, DC: U.S. Department of Justice.

Sprang, G. (1997). Victim impact panels: An examination of the effectiveness of the program on lowering recidivism: Changing offenders attitudes about drinking and driving. *Journal of Social Service Research, 22,* 73–84.

State v. Robinson, 735 P. 2d 801, 814 (1987).

Stein, R. (1991). *Child welfare and the law.* New York: Longman.

Steinbach, A. (1989, June 25). The neglected child: A quiet crisis. *Baltimore Sun,* p. 1.

Tedesco, J. F., & Schnell, S. V. (1987). Children's reactions to sex abuse investigation and litigation. *Child Abuse & Neglect, 11,* 267–272.

Thoennes, N., & Tjaden, P. G. (1989). The extent, nature, and validity of sexual abuse allegations in custody/visitation disputes. *Child Abuse & Neglect, 14,* 151–163.

Tjaden, P. G., & Thoennes, N. (1992). Predictors of legal intervention in child maltreatment cases. *Child Abuse & Neglect, 16,* 807–821.

Umbreit, M.S. (1992). Victims of violence confront the offender. *National Victims Center, 7,* 1–6.

U.S. Department of Health and Human Services. (1990). *Child abuse and neglect: Critical first steps in response to a national emergency. A report of the U.S. advisory board on child abuse and neglect.* Washington, DC: U.S. Department of Health and Human Services.

U.S. Department of Health and Human Services. (1995). *A nation's shame: Fatal child abuse and neglect in the United States. A report of the U.S. advisory board on child abuse and neglect.* Washington, DC: U.S. Department of Health and Human Services, Administration for Children and Families.

U.S. Department of Justice. (1993). *Joint investigations of child abuse: Report of a symposium.* Washington, DC: National Institute of Justice and National Center on Child Abuse and Neglect.

Vogelstanz, N. D., & Drabman, R. S. (1995). A procedure for evaluating young children suspected of being sexually abused. *Behavior Therapy, 26,* 579–597.

Walsh, B. (1996). Criminal investigation of physical abuse and neglect. In J. Briere, A. Berliner, J. A. Bulkley, C. Jenny, & T. Reid (Eds.), *The APSAC handbook on child maltreatment* (pp. 264–271). Thousand Oaks, CA: Sage.

Warren, A. R., & McGough, L. S. (1996). Research on children's suggestibility. *Criminal Justice and Behavior, 23,* 269–303.

Welsh, M. (1996). *Corrections: A critical approach.* New York: McGraw-Hill.

Whitcomb, D. (1992). *When the victim is a child* (2nd ed.). Washington, DC: U.S. Department of Justice.

Whitcomb, D., & Hardin, M. (1996, October). *Coordinating criminal and juvenile court proceedings in child maltreatment cases.* Washington, DC: U.S. Department of Justice.

Whitcomb, D., Shapiro, E. R., & Shellwagen, L. D. (1985). *When the victim is a child: Issues for judges and prosecutors.* Washington, DC: U.S. Department of Justice.

White v. Illinois, 112 S. Ct. Rpt. 736 (1982).

Widom, C. S. (1989). Child abuse, neglect, and violent criminal behavior. *Criminology, 27,* 251–271.

Yuille, J. C., Hunter, R., Joffe, R., & Zaparniuk, J. (1993). Interviewing children in sexual abuse cases. In G. S. Goodman & B.L. Bottoms (Eds.), *Child victims, child witnesses: Understanding and improving testimony* (pp. 95–115). New York: Guilford Press.

Zehr, H. (1985). Retributive justice, restorative justice. Elkhart, IN: Mennonite Central Committee, Office of Criminal Justice.

Zellman, G. L. (1990). Child abuse reporting and failure to report among mandated reporters: Prevalence, incidence, reasons. *Journal of Interpersonal Violence, 5,* 3–22.

5

Legal Issues in Violence toward Adults

Lisa G. Lerman and Naomi R. Cahn

Introduction

Until the 1970s, family violence was largely ignored by the police, lawyers, judges, and legislators. Law enforcement officials generally refused to intervene in domestic violence cases, viewing them as private matters to be handled within the family. A victim of spouse abuse could get a divorce on the basis of her husband's cruelty, or she could get a piece of paper issued by a court warning her husband not to abuse her again. Mental health professionals responded in a similar fashion by treating violence as a relational problem caused by both parties, rather than as a crime committed by one party against another.

In many places, judges, prosecutors, and police remain reluctant to intervene in family matters. In most states, however, there are some legal tools that a victim of family violence can use to change her situation. Through the courts, she may get a civil protection order to compel the abuser to stop the violence. If the abuser violates the order, he can be jailed. These orders may require the abuser to participate in counseling, to pay financial support to the victim, or to leave the residence. A victim of abuse

Lisa G. Lerman • Columbus School of Law, Catholic University of America, Washington, DC 20064. Naomi R. Cahn • George Washington University Law School, Washington, DC 20052.

Case Studies in Family Violence, Second Edition, edited by Ammerman and Hersen. Kluwer Academic / Plenum Publishers, New York, 2000.

may file criminal assault charges against the abuser; if the abuser is con-victed, he may be put in jail, fined, or ordered into a counseling program.

The primary purpose of these legal tools is to force abusers to take responsibility for stopping their violent conduct. Both criminal prosecu-tion and civil protection orders are intended to punish or rehabilitate the abuser and protect the victim from further violence. Mediation and other informal legal intervention designed to conciliate is ineffective in accom-plishing these goals.

Effective intervention in violent families requires a coordinated re-sponse of the law enforcement system and the mental health system. This partnership is essential. Mental health professionals have a critically im-portant role to play in stopping family violence. The law enforcement system has the police power to enforce the criminal law, which provides that an adult may not commit an act of violence against another. However, the law enforcement system cannot monitor and rehabilitate criminal defendants without the assistance of the mental health system. The mental health system is needed to help implement the law enforcement mandate that the violence must stop. It can do this by informing victims of abuse about legal remedies for domestic violence and by offering treatment to perpetrators of family violence who are referred by the courts.

This chapter examines the role of mental health professionals in stop-ping domestic violence. It first offers an overview of the legal remedies for domestic violence and then discusses the roles that may be played by mental health professionals. Mental health professionals who understand the legal system can be most effective in responding to court-mandated cases and in referring family members for the appropriate legal action.

Legal Responses to Domestic Violence

Each state has its own laws and its own court system. In every state, there are two types of laws—civil laws and criminal laws. Civil and criminal laws usually are enforced in different courts. In many states, an abused woman can choose to initiate both civil and criminal proceedings relating to the abuse she has suffered. Civil proceedings often are quicker and less formal, but they may not be as effective as criminal penalties in deterring future violence. The following is a list of some important differ-ences between civil and criminal proceedings.

Overview of Civil Remedies

Purpose: To settle disputes between individuals and to compensate for injuries.

Remedies: Court may order payment of money to an injured party, or may order a defendant to stop doing certain acts. Court may order counseling.

Proof: Violation of the law must be proven by a "preponderance of evidence," that is, that it is more likely than not that the act occurred.

Lawyers: Both the plaintiff (victim) and the defendant (abuser) may hire private attorneys, or if they qualify, obtain representation from legal services lawyers. Either or both parties may proceed on their own, without a lawyer (*pro se*).

Overview of Criminal Penalties

Purpose: To punish conduct that is disruptive of social order and to deter other similar conduct.

Penalties: Conviction of a crime may result in a jail sentence, a fine, an order to pay money to the victim, or a term of probation during which certain conduct may be required or prohibited. Court may order counseling.

Proof: Violation of the law must be proven "beyond a reasonable doubt." This is a much higher standard of proof than the "preponderance of evidence" needed for a civil suit.

Lawyers: The state hires prosecutors (district attorneys) to enforce criminal law. The prosecutor represents the state and acts on behalf of both the victim and the community. In some places, prosecution may occur even if the victim would prefer to drop the charges because the state has an interest in punishing a criminal even if the victim does not wish to do so (Corsilles, 1994; Hanna, 1996). If the conviction could result in a jail sentence, the defendant has a right to legal representation (paid for by the state if he is indigent).

Civil Remedies

Before 1976, very few jurisdictions had legislation specifically providing civil remedies to victims of domestic violence (Note, 1982). Since then, almost every state has enacted legislation creating new civil relief for domestic violence victims (Lerman, 1984a). Several forms of civil relief are available to battered women. These include protection orders, divorce or separation, child custody and visitation rights, alimony and child support, and money damages for personal injury.

Protection Orders

A protection order (sometimes called a restraining order) is an order from a civil court to an abuser to require him to change his conduct. The order can remain in effect for a period of up to one year (Tracy, 1997). Depending on the state law, the court may order the abuser:

- To refrain from abuse of any household member
- To stay away from the victim
- To move out of a residence shared with the victim even if the title or lease is in the abuser's name
- To make rent or mortgage payments even if he has been evicted from the residence
- To provide alternative housing for the victim
- To pay for the support of the victim and/or of minor children in her custody
- To attend a counseling program designed to stop violence and/or alcohol or drug abuse; in some jurisdictions, both the abuser and the victim may be ordered to participate in counseling
- To pay the victim a sum of money for medical expenses, lost wages, moving expenses, property damage, court costs, or attorneys' fees.

The court also may award temporary custody of children to the victim, and may order visitation with the abuser. In many states, protection orders may be issued on behalf of anyone abused by a spouse, former spouse, family member, household member, or former household member. Some states limit relief to victims who are married to or living with their abusers. A protection order may be obtained by filing a petition in the court that has the authority to issue it. It is useful but not necessary for a victim to be represented by a lawyer when she files a petition. In most states, victims may represent themselves in the hearings. In some cities there are clinics that assist victims in writing their petitions.

When a petition is filed, the court schedules a hearing, usually within two weeks of the date of filing. The abuser is notified of the hearing and asked to appear. The abuser can be represented by a lawyer, but there is no requirement that he have legal counsel. The hearing is before a judge or magistrate; there is no jury. Both parties have an opportunity to testify as to why an order should or should not be issued.

In most states, a victim of abuse who is in immediate danger can get a temporary protection order. Temporary orders are emergency orders that may be issued within a few hours of when requested. They are issued after hearings at which only the victim is present.

To get a protection order (temporary or longer-term), the victim must show that some type of "abuse" has occurred. Abuse for which a protection order is available may include (1) an act causing physical injury, such as hitting, shoving, or use of a weapon; (2) an attempt to cause physical injury, such as raising a fist, pointing a gun; (3) a threat to cause physical injury, such as saying, "I'm going to beat you up"; or (4) sexual abuse of a spouse, partner, or children.

To get some of the types of relief available through a protection order, such as custody or support, a victim of abuse must show more than that violence has occurred. For example, to get temporary custody of children, the woman probably will need to show that this is in the best interests of the child. Some states, such as Florida, require a court to consider spouse abuse as one factor in determining custody (Women's Legal Defense Fund, 1986).

In most states a protection order may last for up to one year. Once a victim of abuse obtains an order, she must provide copies of it to the abuser and the police to ensure enforcement. Many states allow police officers to make an arrest without obtaining a warrant when they respond to calls from victims who have obtained protection orders, if there is evidence of violation of an order. A majority of states allow warrantless arrest in domestic violence cases even if the officer did not witness the abuse and even if there are no visible injuries. The officer must have probable cause to believe either that a protection order was violated or another crime was committed by the person being arrested.

Violation of a protection order is either contempt of court (term used to describe any violation of a court order; it may be treated either as a civil offense or a criminal offense) or a misdemeanor offense, and it is punishable by a jail sentence (in most states, up to six months), a fine (in most states, up to $500), a term of probation, or a combination of any of these. To prove that the protection order has been violated, the victim must return to court for another hearing. She and the abuser will have the opportunity to present evidence. A judge or a commissioner will decide whether there has been a violation and order the appropriate remedy. If the abuser is released on probation, he may be required to attend counseling sessions, to avoid contact with the victim, to refrain from abuse, etc. The abuser must report to a probation officer, who is responsible for ensuring that the abuser complies with the order (Finn & Colson, 1990; Klein & Orloff, 1993).

Mediation

Some domestic violence cases are referred for mediation by responding police officers, court clerks, or prosecutors' offices. In mediation, a neutral third person works with parties to help them reach an agreement about their dispute. While mediation may be a cost-efficient way of handling some disputes, it is inappropriate in domestic violence cases and should not be used (Lerman, 1984b).

Mediation is useful to solve problems if the parties have equal bargaining power, and if both parties make concessions until they reach an agreement. In domestic violence situations, however, a battered woman does not have equal bargaining power with her abuser. Permitting an abuser to mediate about whether he will continue his battering implies that, in the absence of an agreement, he may continue his behavior. Some mediators will not conduct mediation over abuse but will undertake to mediate issues other than violence, such as custody, visitation, or support. Even these other issues cannot be fairly mediated if one party has been violent toward the other, because the implicit ongoing threat of violence creates an atmosphere of coercion. In such circumstances, a victim cannot freely accept or reject proposed terms. Another problem with mediation is that the resulting agreement usually is enforceable only as a contract. It does not become a court order, so it provides no real protection.

Other Civil Remedies

In addition to using civil protection order statutes, victims of family violence may be able to bring other types of lawsuits. In most states, a victim of domestic abuse can sue her abuser to obtain a court order requiring the abuser to pay for any injury to her or to her property. This remedy is not useful unless the abuser has significant financial resources.

Victims of domestic violence have successfully sued police for failure to respond appropriately when the victims called for help. These victims claimed that the police respond less effectively to domestic violence calls than to other requests for police help, and thus have violated their duty of care to victims of domestic violence (*Thurman v. City of Torrington*, 1984; *Watson v. Kansas City*, 1988). Battered women request money damages in these cases for injuries that occurred because of the police failure to act. In several cases, victims negotiated settlements with police departments to provide better response to domestic violence victims (e.g., *Bruno v. Codd*, 1979).

Criminal Prosecution

Assaulting another person is a crime. Every state has laws prohibiting physical assault and threats of assault. These laws apply regardless of whether the assailant and the victim are strangers, friends, or family members. Some states have enacted laws that make spouse abuse a separate criminal offense.

Until the 1970s, and at present in many places, spouse abuse is treated as a family matter, and criminal law is rarely enforced against wife beaters.

Historically, prosecutors have been slow to respond to domestic violence cases. In many (perhaps most) jurisdictions, charges are filed against spouse abusers only in a few extreme cases. One writer estimated that of the cases in which charges are filed, as many as 50% of domestic violence cases are dropped before a disposition is reached (Comment, 1985). Prosecutors often blame battered women for the dropping of charges and use this as an excuse not to pursue domestic violence crimes. Some prosecutors' offices have established special domestic violence units to increase prosecution of domestic violence cases. These offices have developed procedures that ensure victim cooperation in the majority of cases (Lerman, 1980; Waits, 1985).

Many different types of conduct violate state criminal law and may be the basis of criminal complaints. These include hitting, slapping, shoving, or other physical assault; sexual assault, rape, or attempted rape; threat of physical assault; any act causing the death of another; destruction or theft of private property belonging to another; kidnaping or confining another against his or her will; and violation of the terms of a protection order.

There are two ways in which a criminal action against an abuser may be started. First, the police may make an arrest after being called for assistance. Second, the victim may go to a prosecutor's office or to an intake unit in criminal or family court to file a criminal complaint. In over half the states, police may make arrests without warrants in domestic violence cases, even if no weapons are used and there are no serious injuries. Some of these laws allow warrantless arrest only if a protection order has been violated. In some states, there are mandatory arrest laws that may require police to make an arrest in certain situations in which domestic violence has occurred (Note, 1988).

Arrest of an abuser may be a deterrent to further violence, even if there are no other legal proceedings. In one study that set out to measure the effectiveness of different types of police response, researchers found that subsequent violence was more effectively prevented by police arrest than by attempting to counsel both parties or by sending the abuser away from the home for a few hours (Sherman & Berk, 1984). Subsequent research on the deterrent effect of arrest produced more ambiguous results ("Symposium on Domestic Violence," 1992).

A criminal charge may be filed after an arrest is made. In some cases, charges are filed by the police; in others, the police send a report to the prosecutor's office and the prosecutor files charges.

A victim of domestic abuse may file a criminal complaint if the police were not called after the abuse occurred, of if they were called but failed to appear or did not make an arrest. After a complaint is filed, the prosecutor's office will conduct an investigation and decide whether criminal charges should be filed. If charges are filed, the court will issue a warrant for the arrest of the abuser or a summons directing him to appear in court on a certain date.

The arrest of the abuser and the filing of the criminal charge begins the process of prosecution. The next step is an arraignment or bail hearing, at which time the abuser may be required to submit a sum of money (bail or bond) to the court to ensure that he will reappear for his trial. Other conditions may be imposed on the abuser's pretrial release, such as participation in counseling, avoiding contact with the victim, or terminating the abuse. If the terms are violated, the abuser may be taken into custody until the prosecution is completed. Criminal charges may reach disposition through diversion or a plea bargain, or they may go to trial.

Diversion

In cases in which injuries are not severe and the abuser is a first-time offender, prosecution may be suspended after charges are filed for a period during which the abuser is required to comply with certain conditions. He may be required to avoid any violence, attend counseling, avoid contact with the victim, or move out of a shared residence. The prosecutor (or a probation officer) is responsible for making sure that the abuser complies with the agreement. If the abuser agrees to attend counseling, the prosecutor may ask the mental health professional to report on the abuser's attendance and progress. If the abuser complies with the agreement for the specified period, charges will be dropped. If he violates the order, prosecution will be resumed.

Some battered women's advocates oppose the use of diversion because the abuser may not be convicted of the crimes he has committed. Others, however, endorse the use of diversion because it can offer more immediate intervention and closer supervision than traditional prosecution.

Plea Bargaining

In the majority of criminal cases, the prosecutor, the defense attorney, and the defendant (the person charged with a crime) make an agreement in which the defendant agrees to plead guilty to charges and the prosecutor agrees to request a less severe penalty than might be imposed by a court after a trial. A judge must approve each plea bargain before it takes effect.

Plea bargaining in spouse abuse cases usually results in a sentence of a period of probation. During probation, just as during diversion, the abuser may be required to refrain from abuse, to attend counseling, to move out of a shared residence, or stay away from the victim. If the abuser violates the terms of probation, he may be put in jail without a trial because he has already agreed to his conviction by admitting guilt during the plea bargaining.

Trial

If the abuser pleads innocent to the charges against him and refuses to negotiate a plea bargain, he will be tried on the offenses charged. If convicted, he may be jailed, fined, or placed on probation. Jail sentences are rarely imposed in domestic assault cases and when they are, they are seldom longer than one year. The possible terms of probation are the same as those available through plea bargaining.

If a victim of abuse is required to testify at a trial, she may be able to get help either from the prosecutor's office or from another agency. She may need someone to go to hearings with her, or to explain the court system to her. She may need child care while she goes to court. She may need assistance in getting housing, public benefits, a divorce, or a protection order.

Sometimes, battered women become defendants in the criminal justice system. Battered women who kill their husbands usually face criminal charges and must defend their actions (Browne, 1987). If the prosecutor finds that a woman acted in self-defense, this may lead to a decision not to file charges. Those who are charged have the options, as discussed earlier, of diversion, plea bargain, or trial (Buzawa & Buzawa, 1992).

Role of Mental Health Professionals

As the preceding discussion indicates, there are many circumstances in which the legal and mental health systems should work together. In both civil and criminal cases—before, during, and after adjudication— mental health professionals have an important role to play. A fundamental issue for mental health professionals who work with the legal system is their attitude toward abuse. Therapists who treat family violence as a crime can help end the violence. Therapists who attempt to reconcile the parties without addressing the issue of violence may only perpetuate the cycle of violence, because in most cases if the relationship continues the violence continues. To intervene and treat violent families effectively, mental health professionals need special training on the psychology of battering and the legal resources available within the community. With special training, they can make appropriate referrals for their patients, seek out involvement in court-mandated treatment programs, and play many other roles.

Referrals to the Legal System

Initially, mental health professionals need to recognize the occurrence of violence in the families of their patients. They should routinely ask their patients whether there is violence in their families, regardless of whether they observe signs of possible abuse. If they are aware that both victims and abusers tend to minimize the violence, mental health professionals are more likely to understand the existence and possible extent of the abuse (Goolkasian, 1986).

Therapists who learn of family violence can help family members stop the violence by referring them to the legal system. Mental health professionals who understand the differences between civil and criminal remedies can inform either victims or abusers of what the law requires or permits. In many jurisdictions, brochures are available on remedies for domestic abuse. These could be placed in a reception area or given to selected individuals. Because patients may be unfamiliar with the legal system, the therapist may be an important source of information on what behavior is a crime, and how the abuse can be stopped. Simply sharing information about existing remedies may deter abusive behavior or may motivate remedial action.

When mental health professionals see patients who are involved in civil or criminal cases, they can provide counseling and support at each stage of the legal action. Mental health professionals can help victims with the trauma of testifying against their abusers. They also can provide referrals for shelter, medical services, or financial aid. Similarly, mental heath professionals who work in shelters or at other social service agencies that deal with domestic violence can provide victim assistance.

Court-Mandated Treatment

Once a criminal case has been adjudicated, a defendant who has been placed on probation remains accountable to the court for his conduct. A probation officer often is responsible for developing a comprehensive treatment plan and for monitoring the abuser's treatment and his compliance with any court orders. The officer may develop a plan requiring the abuser to attend individual or group counseling, such as a batterers' group, or an alcohol or drug treatment program.

The best treatment programs focus on stopping the violence and holding abusers responsible for their conduct. A court-mandated treatment program, in conjunction with monitoring by a probation officer, becomes the eyes and ears of the law enforcement system. Communication between the different service providers and the courts is essential to ensure that the abuser is being treated effectively and that the abuse is not recurring. Generally, the court must arrange for continued contact with victims to learn of any new incidents of violence.

If the abuser fails to appear for counseling, or if violence recurs, the therapist must report back to the court so law enforcement action can be taken against the abuser. Many court systems do not monitor cases effectively, so the therapist must take an active role to ensure that the information gets back to the appropriate official and is acted upon. Every professional who works with members of violent families must become an advocate.

In many other areas of mental health, it is generally agreed that patients respond best to treatment undertaken voluntarily. In treatment of spouse abusers, the opposite is usually true. Most abusers will not accept any form of treatment unless mandated by a court, and many respond well to compulsory treatment (Dutton, 1995; Ganley, 1981).

Individual and group treatment of abusers is likely to be more effective than couples counseling or family therapy because the latter focus on the collective responsibility of all parties instead of primarily on the abuser's responsibility for his own conduct. For the purpose of stopping the violence, it is necessary to require that the person committing the acts of violence stop using physical coercion to get what he wants. This requirement must be unconditional; any intervention that treats the victim as being partly responsible for the violence undercuts this message.

Mental health professionals who are specially trained in domestic violence issues should seek referrals from the court. They need to become familiar with how the legal system refers abusers for treatment. Once mental health professionals begin to treat abusers referred by the courts, they should work with the legal system to develop an effective monitoring program.

Other Roles

Another important role of mental health professionals is to testify in spouse abuse cases. Where child custody is an issue, the victim may need psychological evidence showing the detrimental effect of battering on children to help her secure custody and obtain visitation arrangements that will not endanger either her or the children (Cahn, 1991).

In cases in which a victim of abuse has been accused of killing the abuser, the victim may need expert testimony by a psychologist. Some battered women kill their mates in self-defense after being battered repeatedly. To prove self-defense, a woman must show that at the time of the homicide she reasonably believed she was in danger of serious bodily harm and that she used reasonable force to prevent this harm. Many courts allow women to use expert witnesses to support their arguments. Mental health expert witnesses can be very useful in informing the jury about the psychological impact of spouse abuse on a woman and explaining why a woman has been unable to leave the relationship.

Summary

In many states, a battered woman can use one or more of the legal remedies described in this chapter. For example, a protection order is often useful to a woman who files criminal charges against her husband. The victim's decision about legal action should depend on her goals. Most victims want to end the violence. Some also may want to punish the abuser, get help for him, end the relationship, or all of these.

Mental health professionals and the legal system can work together to end the violence. But cooperation will be effective only if the legal and mental health systems have the same goals. The best responses of the mental health system are those that support the legal system in communicating that domestic violence is wrong and that those who commit acts of violence may suffer severe consequences.

References

Browne, A. (1987). *When battered women kill*. New York: Free Press.

Bruno v. Codd, 47 N.Y.2d 582, 419 N.Y.S.2d 901, 393 N.E.2d 976 (1979).

Buzawa, E., & Buzawa, C. (1992). *Domestic violence: The changing criminal justice response*. Westport, CT: Auburn House.

Cahn, N. (1991). Civil images of battered women: The impact of domestic violence on child custody decisions. *Vanderbilt Law Review, 44*, 1041.

Comment. (1985). Ex parte protection orders: Is due process locked out? *Temp. L.Q., 58*, 843–872.

Corsilles, A. (1994). No-drop policies in the prosecution of domestic violence cases: Guarantee to action or dangerous solution? *Fordham Law Review, 63*, 853.

Dutton, D. (1995). *The domestic assault of women: Psychological and criminal justice perspectives*. Vancouver: UBC Press.

Finn, P., & Colson, S. (1990). *Civil protection orders: Legislation, current court practice, and enforcement*. Washington, DC: U.S. Department of Justice, Office of Justice Programs, National Institute of Justice.

Ganley, A. (1981). *Court-mandated counseling for men who batter: A three-day workshop for mental health professionals*. Washington, DC: Center for Women Policy Studies.

Goolkasian, G. (1986). *Confronting domestic violence: A guide for criminal justice agencies.* Washington, DC: U.S. Government Printing Office.

Hanna, C. (1996). No right to choose: Mandated victim participation in domestic violence prosecutions. *Harvard Law Review, 109,* 1849.

Klein, C., & Orloff, L. (1993). Providing legal protection for battered women: An analysis of state statutes and case law. *Hofstra Law Review, 21,* 801–1189.

Lerman, L. (1980). *Prosecution of spouse abuse: Innovations in criminal justice response.* Washington, DC: Center for Women Policy Studies.

Lerman, L. (1984a). A model state act: Remedies for domestic abuse. *Harvard Journal of Legislation, 21,* 61–143.

Lerman, L. (1984b). Mediation of wife abuse: The adverse impact of alternative dispute resolution on women. *Harvard Women's Law Journal, 7,* 57–113.

Note. (1982). Restraining order legislation for battered women: A reassessment. *University of San Francisco Law Review, 16,* 703–741.

Note. (1988). Mandatory arrest for domestic violence. *Harvard Women's Law Journal, 11,* 213–226.

Sherman, L., & Berk, R. (1984). The Minneapolis domestic violence experiment. *Police Foundation Reports, 1.*

Symposium on domestic violence. (1992). *Journal of Criminal Law and Criminology, 93.*

Thurman v. City of Torrington, 595 F. Supp. 1521 (D. Conn. 1984).

Tracy, K. (1997). Building a model protective order process. *American Journal of Criminal Law, 24,* 475–501.

Waits, K. (1985). The criminal justice system's response to battering: Understanding the problem, forging the solutions. *Washington Law Review, 60,* 267–329.

Watson v. Kansas City, 857 F.2d 690 (10th Cir. 1988).

Women's Legal Defense Fund. (1986). *Representing battered women in custody disputes in the District of Columbia: Litigating custody as part of a civil protection order.* Washington, DC: Author.

6

Medical Issues with Child Victims of Family Violence

Susan M. Briggs

Introduction

Trauma, either accidental or nonaccidental, is the single most common cause of death in children between 1 and 15 years of age (see Briggs, 1989). Each year, about 20 million injuries occur in children. The consequences of the permanent disability, both physical and emotional, are incalculable. Injuries caused by child abuse, either from intentional or unintentional violence against children, unfortunately constitute an increasing percentage of the trauma statistics. Our concept of child abuse must include not only the well-described "battered child syndrome" but the many children who are the innocent victims of family violence arising from domestic quarrels, drugs, or alcohol intoxication. Each day, newspapers report cases of children shot to death accidentally in drug wars, the ultimate form of child abuse.

Although the exact incidence of child abuse is not known, it is estimated that over 1 million children are maltreated in the United States each year (American Humane Association, 1984). Violence against children may take many forms, and it is important for all members of the professional community working with such situations to recognize the unique mani-

Susan M. Briggs • Massachusetts General Hospital, Harvard Medical School, Boston, Massachusetts 02114.

Case Studies in Family Violence, Second Edition, edited by Ammerman and Hersen. Kluwer Academic / Plenum Publishers, New York, 2000.

festations of injury in children from both physical and emotional abuse. Most children who die from abuse have suffered recurring episodes of battering. Early recognition of family situations at high risk for child abuse is critically important to prevent eventual death from either intentional or unintentional violence.

Violence against children, whether from emotional abuse and/or neglect or from unintentional injury to the child from violence between adults, is basically a disease of adults that finds expression in children, the innocent victims. The ultimate pathological expression of this disease is violence against children by other children seeking to emulate adult behavior for emotional or financial satisfaction. If optimal health-care resources were available to all sectors of the community, the problem of child abuse, both intentional and unintentional, could be significantly ameliorated. Until that time, the key to prevention is identifying vulnerable children and parents in high-risk family and community situations that predispose to violent behavior against children.

Identification of Victims of Child Abuse

The spectrum of child abuse can take many different forms, such as physical or mental injury, nutritional or hygienic neglect, delayed or inadequate treatment of disease, sexual abuse or verbal abuse (Green, 1975; Harris, Schwaitzberg, Seman, & Herrmann, 1989). Unfortunately, in children (especially preschool children), the spectrum of injury from accidental to nonaccidental is often quite subtle, making the diagnosis of child abuse difficult for members of the professional team dealing with such situations. Taking a careful history and physical examination of the child— together with close communication with members of the community team dealing with the family unit—is the only way to ensure that the abused child will be identified and cared for appropriately. The severely battered child or the child that is dead on arrival does not pose the diagnostic dilemma. It is the child who presents with subtle physical findings suggestive of abuse or neglect, combined with any of the warning signs of abuse, that is the most clinically demanding situation (O'Neill, Meacham, Griffen, & Sawyers, 1973).

Above all, members of the professional team must maintain a high degree of suspicion in the face of any injury to a child and remain alert to telltale signs of inappropriate behavior by family members if the true incidence of child abuse is to be appropriately identified.

Clues to the diagnosis of child abuse include the following:

History

This shows significant discrepancy between the stated history of the injury and the actual degree of physical injury observed in the child; prolonged interval between the stated time of the injury to the child and the time the child was brought to medical care; and repetitive accidents within a short period (Green, 1975).

Clinical Examination

The most common injuries to abused children are soft-tissue injuries: burns, fractures, and head trauma. The following clinical findings demonstrated by the child may alert a professional to the possibility of child abuse (see Green, 1975; Keen Lendrum, & Wolman, 1975; Sobel, 1970): poor hygiene or failure to thrive; personal injuries; odor of alcohol; fractures in children under 3 years of age; evidence of frequent injuries (scars or old, healed fractures); bizarre injuries (bites, cigarette burns, branding burns such as with iron grates, or rope marks); untreated chronic diseases; genital and perineal trauma; second- and third-degree burns, especially in anatomical distribution; subdural hematomas; skull fractures; and ruptured viscus (internal organs). If the child is dead on arrival, this too is a significant finding.

Behavioral Changes

Behavioral characteristics of the child on presentation to medical care may be important in identifying abuse. Children who cry hopelessly or cry very little under examination or treatment, those who do not look to parents or guardians for reassurance, and those who are wary of any physical contact with adults or are constantly on the alert for danger should raise suspicion that the injury may not be accidental (Caffey, 1974; Feldman & Brewer, 1978; Green, 1975).

Parental or adult behavior too may provide an important clue that the injury is a result of violence against the child. One should be suspicious of child abuse in the following instances:

- Differences in the story told by parents, guardians, and child, or changes in the story after repeated questioning.
- Failure of individuals with the child at the time of the injury to voluntarily provide information about the injury.
- Failure to demonstrate concern about the injury, treatment, or prognosis. Parents or guardians who respond inappropriately or do not

comply with medical advice—for example, refusing to admit the child to the hospital for observation if medically indicated—should alert one to the possibility of abuse.
- Lack of physical or emotional support to the child, lack of physical contact with the injured child.
- Inappropriate or no response to the crying child.

Anatomic Consideration in Injuries to Children

Size

The child's smaller size yields a smaller target to which linear forces from an injuring agent are applied. The applied energy dissipates over the smaller mass of the child, resulting in greater force to a smaller area and a high incidence of multiple organ injuries, especially internal (viscera) injuries. Children have less body fat, less elastic connective tissue, and closer proximity of multiple organs. As a result, they sustain significantly greater injuries than adults with the same applied force (American College of Surgeons, 1997).

Skeleton

The child's skeletal structure is incompletely calcified, contains multiple active growth centers, and is more resilient than the adult's. This renders the child less able to absorb significant external trauma and results in internal organ damage without overlying bony fractures; for example, rib fractures in children are unusual, but lung contusions (bruises) are common (Feldman & Brewer, 1978; Garcia, Gotschall, Eichelberger, & Bowman, 1990).

Surface Area

The ratio between a child's surface and body volume is highest at birth and decreases throughout infancy and childhood. Loss of body heat thus becomes an important factor in a young child's sustaining trauma. Hypothermia (low body temperature) can be life threatening in an injured child, especially a very young child.

Psychological Status

Caring for the injured child, especially the abused child, presents a specific challenge. The stress and pain of a traumatic injury frequently lead to marked emotional ability in the child and regressive psychologically behavior. The child's ability to interact or communicate with unfamiliar individuals in strange environments is usually severely limited in violence-related injuries, especially if the child is experiencing pain. Thus, history taking and therapeutic manipulations may be extremely difficult.

Long-Term Effects

A major consideration for all members of the professional team dealing with injured children is the effect the injury may have on subsequent growth and development. Unlike the adult who has completed the growth and development processes, the child must not only recover from the traumatic event but continue the normal growth and development processes. The physiological effects of injury on this process are significant. Children with even minor injuries may have prolonged cerebral function disabilities, psychological adjustments, or organ system deformities and disabilities.

Specific Injuries in Child Victims of Violence

All types of penetrating and blunt traumatic injuries have been demonstrated in victims of child abuse, whether intentional or unintentional. Recognition of patterns of injury suspicious for child abuse as well as characteristics of injury specific to children will alert professionals to the spectrum of child abuse.

Cutaneous Injuries

Cutaneous injuries represent one of the most common manifestations of child abuse (American College of Surgeons, 1997; Caffey, 1974; McLaughlin & Crawford, 1985). The location of the injury, the pattern of the injury, the presence of multiple lesions of different ages, and the failure of new lesions to appear after the child is hospitalized or removed from the home environment help to distinguish accidental from nonaccidental injuries.

Bruises constitute the majority of intentional cutaneous injuries. Lacerations are more commonly associated with accidental injury. The most common areas of inflicted injuries in children are the upper arms and legs, trunk, sides of the face, neck, ears, genitalia, and buttocks. Bruises (especially facial and buttock bruises) seen in infants should be considered suspicious for child abuse until proven otherwise.

The injuring instrument, whether it be animate (e.g., human hand, foot, or teeth) or inanimate (e.g., shoe, belt, electric cord, knife), will often leave a telltale mark, much like the steering wheel imprint on the chest wall of a victim who sustains a motor vehicle accident and is not wearing a seat belt. Thus, the pattern of the cutaneous injury may identify the inflicting instrument and the possible individual responsible for the violence against the child.

The typical lesion left by an electric cord is elliptical (Briggs, 1989); a belt or buckle leaves a bruise conforming to that shape. Injuries inflicted by the human hand often leave characteristic parallel linear marks representing the spaces between the fingers. Rope burns may leave circular marks around the neck, suggesting strangulation. Human bite marks are characteristic lesions, and the size of the bites helps identify the age of the biting person. Oval pressure marks in the arms or trunk suggest hard pressure from human hands.

Multiple bruises or other cutaneous lesions in varying stages of healing are indicative of repeated intentional injury. No new lesions appearing in the protective hospital environment or foster setting, combined with laboratory confirmation of normal bleeding studies, a history that suggests child abuse, and cutaneous lesions indicative of inflicted injury raise the spectrum of intentional injury to the child in the family environment.

Burns

Burn injuries are a leading cause of accidental death in the pediatric population and the source of incalculable morbidity and long-term disability. Flame burns account for approximately 15% of pediatric thermal injuries and scald burns for approximately 85%. The most disturbing cause of burns that has dramatically increased over the past decade is child abuse and neglect. Children are frequently abused with cigarettes as well as a variety of hot implements (grills, radiators, curling irons, flatirons, matches). As with all other types of child abuse, the location and pattern of the burn as well as the association of other social, psychological, and physical signs of child abuse are useful guides to the diagnosis of accidental versus nonaccidental thermal injury. Immersion burns are characterized by symmetrical anatomic region involvement (see Figure 1), such as the stocking or glove distribution pattern of burn injury in which both feet are uniformly burned secondary to forceful immersion of a child in hot water.

Most accidental, minor scald burns are characterized by a scatter distribution of thermal injury, as opposed to sharply demarcated edges, because the child will attempt to escape the burning agent unless forcibly restrained. Genital and perineal burns are suspicious areas for child abuse

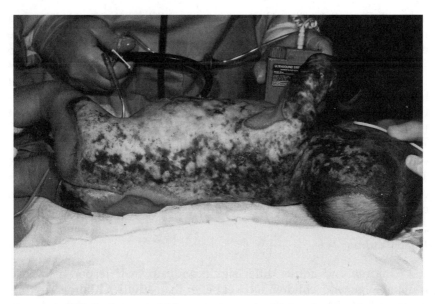

Figure 1. Full-thickness scald burn in 2-month-old female secondary to intentional immersion in hot water.

since these are unusual areas for accidental injury unless the child falls in a bathtub (American College of Surgeons, 1997).

The following characteristics will help the examiner estimate the extent of burn. In general, in children under 5 years of age scalding often inflicts third-degree burns because of the thin skin. Burns may be caused by heat from various sources, chemicals, electricity, and radiation. Extreme cold can also produce an injury similar to a burn. Burn depth significantly affects most subsequent pathophysiologic changes in the body.

A *first-degree* burn involves only the epidermis and is characteristic by cutaneous erythema and mild pain. Tissue damage is minimal, and protective functions of the skin, located in the dermis, remain intact. The chief symptom, pain, usually resolves in 48 to 72 hours. In 5 to 10 days, the damaged epithelium peels off, leaving no residual scarring. The most common causes of first-degree burns are overexposure to sunlight or brief scalding by hot liquids.

A *second-degree* burn involves injury to the entire epidermis and variable portions of the dermal layer. Vesicle (blister) formation is characteristic of second-degree burns. A superficial second-degree burn is extremely painful because a large number of remaining viable nerve endings are exposed. Superficial second-degree burns will heal in 7 to 14 days as a result of regeneration of epithelium by the epithelium cells that line the hair follicles, sweat glands, and other skin appendages. A mid to deep second-degree burn will heal spontaneously, but reepithelialization is extremely slow. Pain is present but to a lesser degree than in more superficial burns because fewer intact nerve endings remain. Fluid losses and metabolic effects of deep dermal burns are essentially the same as those of third-degree burns.

A full-thickness or *third-degree* burn involves destruction of the entire epidermis and dermis, leaving no residual epidermal cells to regenerate. The wound will not epithelialize and can heal only by wound contraction or skin grafting. The lack of painful sensation in a third-degree burn is due to heat destruction of nerve endings.

Head Trauma

Children and adults differ significantly in their response to head trauma. In general, children recover better than adults. Children less than 3 years of age have the worst prognosis from severe head injury. Head injury in abused children is often compounded by secondary brain injury from hypovolemia from associated internal injuries or hypoxemia (lack of oxygen) due to delay in appropriate treatment, especially institution of an adequate airway and ventilatory support. The young child with an open fontanel and mobile sutures is more tolerant of an expanding intracranial mass from head trauma. Vomiting is common in children after head injury and does not necessarily indicate significant increased intracranial pressure (Swischuk, Swischuk, & Johns, 1993).

Seizures occur frequently in children following head trauma and are usually self-limiting. Elevated intracranial pressure without focal intracranial masses following head trauma is more common in children than in adults. A lucid interval prior to delayed neurological deterioration is sometimes seen in children with head injuries (American College of Surgeons, 1997).

Findings on clinical examination that may suggest child abuse and dictate more extensive investigation include multiple subdural hematomas, especially without a fresh skull fracture, retinal hemorrhages, and old skull fractures on X-ray examination (Friedman & Morse, 1974). Hair pulling, a maneuver used for discipline as well as intentional injury, may cause alopecia (loss of hair) as well as scalp hematomas. Subdural hematomas are almost always traumatic in children. The signs and symptoms of head injury may be nonspecific, such as irritability, lethargy, or lack of desire to eat. More specific signs of head injury are signs of elevated intracranial pressure (e.g., vomiting, seizures, stupor, coma). The finding of retinal hemorrhages are suggestive of whiplash origin of injury. Subdural hematoma associated with a skull fracture usually leaves external marks and is more easily diagnosed.

Chest Trauma

The child's chest wall is very compliant and allows energy to transfer to the intrathoracic structures more easily than in the adult (Green, 1975). Thus, children may sustain significant internal chest injuries without evidence of external trauma. Penetrating injuries to the chest in children are usually the result of unintentional injury sustained in the physical setting of violent conflict between adults. Blunt trauma to the chest in abused children often leaves telltale cutaneous marks from inflicting agents, such as a hand mark or a belt mark.

Abdominal Trauma

Abdominal examination of the child is extremely difficult, especially in abused children. Cutaneous manifestations of injury may be present. Most infants and children who are stressed and crying will swallow large amounts of air, which may mimic the findings of abdominal injury. Ability to elicit a history of abdominal pain is probably the most reliable sign of this injury in the neurologically intact child and requires extreme patience and good communication skills on the part of the examiner.

Visceral (internal injuries) are second only to head trauma as the most common cause of death from child abuse. Nonaccidental internal injuries usually involve structures below the diaphragm, and significant blood loss may be present without external signs of trauma. Many cases of significant intraabdominal injury from child abuse, unfortunately, are first diagnosed at autopsy examination.

Extremity Trauma

History is of vital importance in the diagnosis of nonaccidental extremity trauma in children. X-ray diagnosis of fractures and dislocations around joints is difficult in younger children because of the lack of mineralization of the bone and presence of a growth plate (physis). Bone in children grows in length as new bone is laid down by the growth plate near the end of the bone. Because of the nature of the immature bones, children may sustain a fracture of only one side (cortex) of the bone, called the *greenstick fracture*. Fractures in children under 3 years of age are unusual and raise the possibility of child abuse, as does the presence of old fractures in multiple sites seen on X-ray examination.

Summary

The question, "Could this injury be the result of intentional or unintentional violence to the child?" should come to mind in all cases of traumatic injury to children.

No pattern of injury and no particular psychological or socioeconomic background of the family unit will conclusively prove an instance of child abuse. A high degree of suspicion on the part of the professional team caring for the injured child, as well as close cooperation between community and medical resources involved in the care of the child, provides the best opportunity for early detection of child abuse and prevention of the ultimate complication of child abuse: death of the child.

References

American College of Surgeons. (1997). *Advanced trauma life support provider manual.* Chicago: First Impression Publishing.

American Humane Association. (1984). *Highlights of official child neglect and abuse reporting 1982.* Denver, CO: Author.

Briggs, S. E. (1989). First aid, transportation, and immediate acute care of the burned patient. In J. A. J. Martyn (Ed.), *Anesthesia and critical care of the burned patient* (pp. 1–12). New York: Grune & Stratton.

Caffey, J. (1974). The whiplash shaken infant syndrome. *Pediatrics, 54,* 396–403.

Feldman, K. W., & Brewer, D. K. (1978). Child abuse, cardiopulmonary resuscitation and rib fractures. *Pediatrics, 62,* 1–7.

Friedman, S., & Morse, C. (1974). Child abuse: A five year follow-up of early case finding in the emergency department. *Pediatrics, 54,* 404–410.

Garcia V. F., Gotschall, C. S., Eichelberger, M. R., & Bowman, L. M. (1990). Rib fractures in children: A marker of severe trauma. *Journal of Trauma, 30,* 695–700.

Green, F. C. (1975). Child abuse and neglect: A priority problem for the private physician. *Pediatric Clinics of North America, 22.*

Harris, B. H., Schwaitzberg, S. D., Seman, T. M., & Herrmann, C. (1989). The hidden morbidity of pediatric trauma. *Journal of Pediatric Surgery, 24,* 103–106.

Keen, J. H., Lendrum, J., & Wolman, B. (1975). Inflicted burns and scalds in children. *British Medical Journal, 4,* 268–269.

McLaughlin, F., & Crawford, J. D. (1985, February). Types of burn injuries. *Pediatric Clinics of North America.*

O'Neill, J. A. Jr., Meacham, W. F., Griffen, P. O., & Sawyers, J. L. (1973). Patterns of injury in the battered children syndrome. *Journal of Trauma, 13,* 332.

Sobel, R. (1970). The psychological implications of accidental poisoning in childhood. *Pediatric Clinics of North America, 17,* 653–685.

Swischuk L. E., Swischuk P. N., & John, S. D. (1993). Wedging of C-3 in infants and children: Usually a normal finding and not a fracture. *Radiology, 188,* 523–526.

7

Medical Issues with Adult Victims of Family Violence

Richard L. Judd

Introduction

Interhuman violence is generally estimated to affect millions of persons in the United States. Violence in the context of this chapter refers to physical force that contravenes societal norms or penal codes. Abuse can generally be categorized as verbal abuse, battering, mobility restriction, communication restriction, or economic exploitation. A more inclusive categorization of abuse involves physical abuse (e.g., infliction of pain or injury), sexual abuse (e.g., rape, sexually transmitted diseases), emotional abuse (e.g., derogation, humiliation), neglect (e.g., abandonment, deliberate denial of food, medications), or financial exploitation (e.g., illegal or improper use of funds).

Violence has come to affect all echelons of our society within the adult population. While estimated figures vary widely from source to source, the number of reported abused persons is estimated to be in 4 to 5 million range (Hamburger, Saunders, & Hovey, 1992; National Coalition Against Domestic Violence, 1988; National Safety Council, 1994; "Physicians Alerted," 1985; Plotkin, 1988). Trauma as a result of domestic violence is the leading cause of death in women 15 to 44 years of age. It is estimated that 50% of

Richard L. Judd • Office of the President, Central Connecticut State University, New Britain, Connecticut 06050; and New Britain General Hospital, New Britain, Connecticut 06050.

Case Studies in Family Violence, Second Edition, edited by Ammerman and Hersen. Kluwer Academic / Plenum Publishers, New York, 2000.

women experience some form of violence from their partners each year: one-third are battered repeatedly. Visits by women to hospital emergency departments as a result of ongoing domestic violence accounts for 22% to 33% of patient numbers (American College of Surgeons, 1997).

The wide variation in estimates of individuals who have suffered violence, particularly at the hands of family members or significant others, is thought to be related to several factors. These factors include (1) fear of reporting the problem; (2) shame of having to acknowledge the person responsible for inflicting the abuse or violence; (3) unprecedented growth in the number of those over 65 years of age; and (4) lack of statutory provisions and definitive reporting systems.

It is estimated that 1 of 25 elderly women is a victim of physical abuse annually (American College of Surgeons, 1997). The physical and emotional signs of abuse—rape, spouse beating, or nutritional deprivation in the elderly—are often overlooked, or perhaps, not accurately identified. Women in particular rarely report incidents of sexual assault to law enforcement agencies. It sometimes takes years for victims to work through their apparent loss of self-respect in order to confront the feelings of fear, grief, and rage. In the elderly population, sensory deficits, senility, and other forms of altered mental status (for example, drug-induced depression) may make it impossible or extremely arduous for them to report the maltreatment.

While the categories of emotional abuse and financial exploitation are of concern to clinicians in all health-related fields, physical abuse and neglect pose the greatest concern from the medical standpoint. Sometimes during periods of acute medical illness or trauma resulting from abuse, an individual may see a health-care provider outside of the ordinary medical services system, and these providers may conduct an initial assessment. If the setting is one without medical services (e.g., a shelter for abused women), and victims access such a facility prior to receiving prehospital or definitive medical care, the facility personnel should be competent in the assessment and recognition of life-threatening problems. They should also be prepared to provide basic life support as well as referral to an appropriate medical care facility.

Initial Assessment of Abuse

Initial assessment of a patient involves evaluating those life-support processes which, if not examined during a traumatic event or acute illness, may result in serious disability or death. These initial factors have been generally referred to as the ABCs: airway, breathing, and circulation. It is not the intent, nor is it within the scope of this chapter, to provide training in the supportive or resuscitative measures required in such circumstances. Rather, major assessment regimens that are considered a standard in emergency medicine today will be presented. Indeed, any practitioner of the healing or helping medical arts who is involved with victims of adult violence should be competent in emergency medical care to a level appropriate to the environment in which the practitioner works. Human violence often involves trauma, and therefore, life-saving considerations must be part of any assessment.

The American College of Surgeons has developed a well-conceived protocol for assessing significant trauma in accident cases. These protocols are found in the College's Advanced Trauma Life Support program (American College of Surgeons, 1997) and consist of a five-step process. The steps presented in Table 1 are frequently accomplished simultaneously. For example, the response to the question, "What happened?" can provide immediate information about patient's airway, breathing, and neurologic status. Simultaneously, the examiner can assess the patient's pulse, skin color, and capillary refilling time in 30 seconds of patient contact. The Glasgow Coma Scale (GCS) is a more detailed neurologic evaluation that is also quick, simple, and predictive of patient outcome (Teasdale & Jennett, 1974). The GCS involves three determinants: eye opening, verbal response, and motor response, all of which are evaluated independently according to a rank order. A sample GCS chart is shown in Table 2. The GCS may be used to categorize patients and quantify neurologic findings. A patient in coma is defined as having no eye opening, no ability to obey commands and no word expressions. Patients with a GCS score of 8 or less are generally considered to be in coma. Patients with a GCS score of 9 to 13 are considered to be in moderate coma and those with a GCS score of 14 to 15 are considered to be in mild coma.

Characteristics of Abused Adults

Adult victims of violence most frequently are female, although males are victims as well. Likely victims are young pregnant women who are unable to resist the abuser (Goldberg & Carey, 1982). Women who have two or more children and few friends or relatives also fall into the risk category (Geis, 1982). Those adults who are unhappy with their current existence, whose spouses (particularly husbands) have job security problems (are out of work or have part-time or periodic employment), or who have a family violence history are potential victims of abuse. Families living in environments that are not conducive to normal, ordinary living or

Table 1.   Initial Assessment: ABCDE[a]

A.   Airway maintenance with cervical spine protection

Is the airway patent, i.e., open and accessible?

Patency may be accomplished by using the chin-lift or jaw-thrust maneuver.

Suction blood, secretions, remove foreign debris.

Insert an oral or nasal airway (BLS); intubation (ALS)

Remember: Assume cervical spine fracture in multisystem trauma, especially blunt injury above clavicle. Avoid hyperextension/hyperflexion.

B.   Breathing and ventilation

Expose the chest: Is there adequate ventilatory exchange?

There are generally three major problems in the trauma case that impair adequate exchange of air; these are (1) tension pneumothorax, (2) flail chest with pulmonary contusion, (3) massive hemothorax, (4) open pneumothorax.

Determine rate and depth of respirations.

Inspect and palpate the chest for unilateral and bilateral chest movements.

Auscultate the chest bilaterally.

Ascertain the respiratory rate. A respiratory rate of greater than 20 per minute or less than 8 per minute indicate respiratory compromise.

C.   Circulation

Hemorrhage is the predominant cause of postinjury deaths. What is the blood volume and cardiac output?

What is the patient's state of consciousness?

When circulating blood volume is reduced by half or more, cerebral perfusion is critically impaired, and unconsciousness results. Conversely, a conscious patient can be presumed to have at least enough blood volume to maintain cerebral perfusion.

Skin color: A patient with pink skin (or mucosa in darked-skinned persons), especially in the face and extremities, is rarely hypovolemic following injury. Conversely, the ashen, gray skin of the face and the white skin of blood-drained extremities are ominous signs of hypovolemia. These latter signs usually indicate a blood volume loss of at least 30% if hypovolemia is the cause.

Pulse: What is its quality, rate, and regularity? Full, slow, regular peripheral pulses are welcome signs in the injured patient. Check an easily accessible central pulse initially: femoral or carotid pulses signify coordinated cardiac action and at least 50% of the residual blood volume. Rapid, thready pulses are early signs of hypovolemia but may have other causes as well. An irregular pulse is usually a warning of cardiac impairment. Absent central pulses at more than one site, without local injuries or other factors, which preclude accurate palpation of pulses, signify the need for immediate resuscitative actions.

---

social customs (e.g., military camps) may also be at high risk for maltreatment. Addiction to drugs, alcohol, or other substances is a major consideration of violence potential.

Accordingly, the medical history should seek to determine information in medical records of previous injuries or illnesses that may be related to violence incidents.

Table 1. (*Continued*)[a]

C. Circulation (*cont.*)

Bleeding: Initial step in managing shock is to recognize its presence. The majority of patients in shock are hypovolemic; cardiogenic shock may be the cause and must be considered in patients with specific injuries above the diaphragm. For all practical purposes, shock does not result from isolated head injuries. A significant number of patients in hypovolemia shock will require surgical intervention. Remember that compensatory mechanisms may have precluded a measurable fall in systolic pressure until the patient has lost 30% of blood volume. Direct attention to pulse rate, respiratory rate skin circulation, and pulse pressure. A narrowed pulse pressure suggests significant blood loss. Earliest signs are tachycardia and cutaneous vasoconstriction. In adults, tachycardia is indicated with pulse rates of greater than 100. Healthy elderly patients have a limited ability to increase their heart rate in response to blood loss, obscuring one of the early signs of volume depletion, tachycardia. This is due to limited cardiac response to catecholamine stimulation or certain medications such as propanolol. Blood pressure has little correlation with cardiac output in the older patient group. Children, at the other extreme, usually have abundant physiologic reserve. When deterioration occurs, it is often precipitous and catastrophic.

D. Disability (neurologic evaluation)

Rapid neurologic evaluation using the pneumonic AVPU, which translates to:

A = Alert

V = Responds to vocal stimuli

P = Responds to painful stimuli

U = Unresponsive

E. Exposure/environmental control

Undress patient to facilitate thorough examination and assessment. The degree of undressing a patient must depend on the circumstances in which the patient is found and the current situation. If the patient is conscious and can competently advise on the nature of injuries, a full unclothing may be necessary. In a sexual assault situation, undressing the patient may be contraindicated until appropriate personnel are available. And in some circumstances, undressing the patient may not be appropriate due to psychological factors. Emergency medical personnel have appropriate backgrounds to assist in this determination, as necessary. In the hospital emergency department setting, full exposure of the patient is require to conduct a competent assessment of injuries.

[a]Adapted from American College of Surgeons (1997).

Characteristics that may assist the practitioner in identifying adult abuse include (1) repeated visits to the office, emergency department, or clinic; (2) a history of being "accident-prone"; (3) soft tissue injuries (see detail below); (4) implausible explanation of injuries; (5) simplistic, often vague explanation of injuries; (6) psychosomatic complaints; (7) pain, especially chronic pain; (8) self-destructive behavior; (9) eating and sleep

Table 2.   Glasgow Coma Scale (GCS)[a]

Eye opening response (E)		Verbal response (V)		Motor response (M)	
Spontaneous	4	Oriented	5	Obeys command	6
To voice	3	Confused conversation	4	Localizes pain	5
To pain	2	Inappropriate words	3	Withdraws (pain)	4
None	1	Incomprehensible sounds	2	Flexion (pain)	3
		None	1	Extension (pain)	2
				None	1

[a]Adapted from Teasdale & Jennett (1974).
Note. GCS score (E + V + M): best possible = 15; worst possible = 3.

disorders; (10) lack of energy; (11) depression; (12) substance abuse; and (13) sexual abuse (Goldberg, 1982). In addition, should the medical practitioner, on observant physical examination, find the following, more intensive investigation is warranted (American College of Surgeons, 1997):

- Multiple subdural hematomas
- Retinal hemorrhage
- Periorbital hemorrhage
- Ruptured internal viscera, without antecedent blunt trauma
- Evidence of frequent injuries
- Bizarre injuries such as bites, cigarette burns, bruising of breast (in women), perianal and genital injuries

Medical Issues

The medical team should undertake specific examination and inspection for bruises, burns, head injuries, abdominal injuries, fractures, and failure to thrive. It is important here that all personnel involved in violence cases, from prehospital (e.g., first responders, emergency medical technicians) to definitive care staff (e.g., nurses, physicians), perform exacting surveys and examination of the patient.

In the overall assessment of abuse, a key factor is pursuing the adequacy of explanation of the presenting incident. The astute clinician will look for those indicators that either conceal or avoid frank answers to questions that attempt to discover causation of the injury.

Often caregivers, caretakers, parents, guardians, and others charged with the well-being of the patient may not give accurate or truthful responses to the clinician as to the etiology of the presenting condition. Answers that are implausible or doubtful from anyone other than the patient, who has sustained alleged abuse, the possible inflictor, or significant witnesses, require aggressive investigation. Questions raised by the examiner—such as, "Exactly where did this happen?" "What was she (the victim) doing, exactly?" "What time did it happen?"—may provide valuable clues to the existence of maltreatment. A sense of clinical suspicion should develop when a practitioner reviews a medical history that raises such questions as: Does this make sense? Do I really believe this story? When one sees burns, especially cigarette burns (one of the stigmata of abuse), or physical marks indicative that certain portions of the body systematically have been scalded, suspicion must be raised that abuse may be the cause. It is important to remember that many patients suffering abuse are terrorized into making false statements for fear of retribution. In the case of elder abuse by family members, fear of removal from the home environment may be the cause of lying about the origin of the abuse. In other cases of elder abuse, sensory deprivation or dementia may preclude adequate explanation (Judd, 1988, 1991a,b,c; Kinsey, Tarbox, & Bragg, 1981; Schwartz, Bosker, & Grigsby, 1984).

The significance of these assessments is important in uncovering pathology as well as identifying abuse that often is not reported by the patient for fear of reprisal, embarrassment, or incapability of reporting. Some of these assessments will involve definitive diagnostic procedures by the physician, such as roentgenographic or magnetic resonance imagery. Other symptoms such as malnutrition can be observed by visual examination. Still others can be determined by palpation, as with the swelling of extremity.

In addition to the implicit life-saving care that must be administered during the assessment, one of the very significant concomitants of a thorough examination involves reducing further trauma from abuse through its very identification. It is well known that, in child abuse, the cycle of repeat abuse has a high mortality (McNeese & Hebeler, 1977). It can be inferred from the data on child abuse that one of the preventative measures in reducing additional maltreatment of adults is the knowledge of its occurrence by medical practitioners. This may allow for referral and protective services of human, social, and public safety agencies.

In the United States, health service professionals (e.g., physicians, nurses, emergency medical service personnel), teachers, social workers, and many others are obliged by law to report incidences of abuse to state human protection agencies or law enforcement officials, even if the abuse is only suspected. The statutes that require such reporting generally protect the reporter from legal liability for identifying confirmed or even suspicious cases of abuse. The sad fact is that underreporting such suspicions significantly raises the potential for increased abuse and mortality.

Clinical Signs of Physical Abuse or Neglect

The signs of physical abuse or neglect may be quite obvious (e.g., the imprint left by an item such as fireplace poker) or subtle (e.g., undernutrition in the fragile elderly). A comprehensive and thorough physical examination, in which findings are recorded and documented, is mandatory in the clinical setting. Indeed, the medicolegal implications for not doing so are enormous. In general, the physical factors to be looked for, particularly when there is inadequate explanation, are (1) inflicted bruises, (2) burns, (3) head injuries, (4) chest injuries, (5) abdominal injuries, (6) bone injuries, (7) failure to thrive, and (8) sexual abuse injuries. These will each be discussed further in turn.

Inflicted Bruises

Typical sites of inflicted bruises are the buttocks and lower back, genitals and inner thighs, cheek (slap marks) or ear lobe (pinch marks), upper lip and frenulum (from forced feeding of the elderly patient), and neck (choke marks). Pressure bruises, frequently the result of human hand marks, may be identified by oval grab marks (fingertips), pinch marks, hand print (e.g., on the face, buttocks), linear marks (fingers), or trunk encirclement bruises. Human bite marks are typically inflicted on the limbs and more likely involve the upper extremity. In addition to the trauma (lacerations, crushing) of the human bite, infection must also be a major medical concern since many diseases are transmitted from organisms located in the oral cavity.

Strap marks from belts, whips, and other similar devices may present as linear bruises and will carry characteristic marks indicative of the particular injuring agent. Loop marks from a doubled over electric cord, rope, wire, or string may leave characteristic signs as well. Many of these may have resulted from ligatures used to restrain the patient. This is especially applicable to the elderly, who, for purposes of restricting movement, may have been tied in bed. Indeed, the author has been involved in one such case in which a demented elderly patient was tied to her bed and neglected to the point where the springs of the mattress physically invaded her skin. There are other reportable cases, where in order to prevent somnambulism, falling out of bed, or behavioral problems, elders are similarly restrained. In the nongeriatric adult population, restraint can be used to control aggressive behavior in retarded individuals or for other purposes of abuse (e.g., sexual).

Bizarre marks that are not easily identifiable may be the result of unusual causation. The specific instrument may leave telltale markings of blunt trauma (e.g., hammers, pliers, and fireplace pokers). Tattoos, fork mark punctures, screwdriver indentations (Phillips head) are also highly indicative of inflicted abuse.

Multiple bruises in various states of healing also require investigation. Some bruising may be normative (e.g., those resulting from physical activity involved in playing sports, or banging into a kitchen counter). Again, careful questioning of the patient and a review of that individual's activities of daily living (ADL) are evaluative factors.

Serologic tests that include a bleeding disorder screen should be ordered in any unexplained bruising. Moreover, dating of bruising may also be helpful. Table 3 presents guidelines for judging the relative age of the bruising (Sussman, 1968).

Burns

Approximately 100,000 patients with burns require hospitalization each year; of these, 12,000 will die as a result of their injuries. It is estimated that a quarter of a million individuals sustain minor burns (e.g., second-degree burns of less than 15% of the body surface area) that are managed on an outpatient basis (Bunkis & Walton, 1986). Many burns considered less critical are not treated in any medical facility. Burns are a common form of maltreatment and it is more than likely that most of the burns inflicted are not seen in any medical setting. For many reasons the elderly, including those not able to care for themselves, can suffer from this cate-

Table 3. Coloration of Bruises According to Time[a]

Age[b]	Color
24 hours	Swollen, tender; reddish with some blue or purple discoloration
1–5 days	Blue to bluish brown
5–7 days	Greenish coloration
7–10 days	Yellowish coloration
10–14 days	Brown
2–4 weeks	Clear

[a]Adapted from Sussman (1968).
[b]Adult values of these color changes are within these parameters.

gory of physical insult. Typical abuse from burns includes those caused by (1) cigarettes; (2) match tip or incense; (3) dry contact from forced contact with heating devices (e.g., heating grates, electric hot plate, radiators, irons); (4) branding by heated metals of various types; (5) scalds from forced immersion or direct pouring of hot liquids on body surfaces; (6) chemical burns caused by acids or alkalis; and (7) electrical power sources. In the initial assessment of burns, medical personnel must direct attention to any burns that may produce airway distress. Clinical indications include facial burns, carbonaceous sputum, singeing of eyebrows, nasal, and other facial hair, and impaired mentation.

As in all abuse cases, obtaining a history of the presenting problem is imperative, but this is especially so in burn cases. The sequelae of burns and their attendant high mortality require vigorous attention to life-support measures. The history given by the patient and others needs to be considered in terms of the plausibility of the injury.

Body parts should be inspected for festering burn blisters (especially from cigarettes), excavation marks from fresh burns (with particular attention to frequently traumatized areas such as the palms, soles, and buttocks). Imprints of items such as a hot poker or household-ironing device may be indicative of abuse. In managing circumferential burns of extremity, removal of bracelets, watches, rings, and other such items is important to prevent constriction of parts distal to the circumferential item. Burns, particularly those classified as critical, are not well tolerated by the elderly for a number of complex reasons (Judd, 1991a,b,c). In fact, a 70-year-old person with burns of 30% of the body surface area has a predicted mortality of 70% (Bunkis & Walton, 1986).

Head Injuries

Head injury in abuse cases is a serious concern from a traumatic standpoint. Injuries to the head inflicted by direct blows are generally a high cause of mortality in abuse cases. Overall, trauma as a mechanism of injury to the head causes more deaths and disability than any other neurologic cause in patients under age 50 (American College of Surgeons, 1989, 1997). The latter finding is related not only to abuse but to other types of injury (e.g., motor vehicle accidents, shootings). The following general injuries may occur from direct blows: (1) skull fractures; (2) scalp swelling and bruises; (3) retinal hemorrhage; (4) subdural hematomas; (5) subarachnoid hemorrhage; (6) subgaleal hematoma and traumatic alopecia; and (7) black eyes.

In examining the head, the entire scalp and head should be examined for lacerations, contusions, and evidence of fractures. It is vitally important, due to the high mortality of head injury and its sequelae, that a physician see patients who have suffered such violent abuse in a proper medical facility capable of initial assessment and management. This requires appropriate triage, and in the initial medical management of the patient, attention to ventilation and hypovolemia. Thus is the potential for secondary brain damage obviated. Assuming that adequate and prudent initial stabilization of an abused head-injured patient has occurred, the matter of neurosurgical consultation may then be determined. At any rate, from the medical standpoint, the physician must determine what appropriate diagnostic studies (e.g., computed tomography [CT] and skull roentgenograms) are needed. CT is considered a diagnostic procedure of choice for patients suspected of having sustained serious head injury. Other tests should be left to the discretion of the neurosurgeon.

Specific Head Injuries

The scalp is one of the areas more often affected in abuse cases. Injury can result from direct blows, lacerations, and pulling of the hair. Hemorrhage is not uncommon, and due to the scalp's abundant blood supply, major blood loss is possible. The galea aponeurotica, one of the five layers of tissue covering the bone of the top of the skull, is separated by loose areolar tissue from the pericranium. It is in this area that hemorrhage can occur resulting in subgaleal hematoma. Traumatic alopecia, or baldness, can occur from vigorous pulling of the hair, as well as its removal by force. The skull is another vulnerable source of potential injury in abused adults. The skull anatomically is composed of the calvarium or cranial vault and the base. The cranial vault is particularly thin in the temporal regions. Injuries inflicted to this area of the abused patient must be regarded with great concern.

Clinically, there are four major categories of skull fracture. These are classified as (1) linear, nondepressed; (2) depressed; (3) open; and (4) basal. Skull fractures are common in violent abuse cases, but do not by themselves cause neurologic disability. Severe injury to the brain can occur without a fracture; the force alone transmitted by a blunt object to the skull can lead to damage. The significance of skull fractures from the trauma standpoint is that there is a high probability of intracranial hematoma. A victim of abuse who has sustained head injury should be admitted to a hospital for observation. Likewise, any abuse victim with a skull fracture should be seen by a neurosurgeon.

Blunt trauma, impalement injuries, and bullet wounds are the usual cause of intracranial hemorrhage. These may be classified as acute epidural hemorrhage, acute subdural hematoma, or subarachnoid hemorrhage. Acute subdural hematoma and subarachnoid hemorrhage require immediate surgical intervention because they are life-threatening. A hallmark of acute subdural hematoma is a fixed pupil on the same side as the impact area. Although alert, a patient with this type of injury typically complains of severe headache and is sleepy. It should be remembered in assessing head trauma that in cases of violent abuse, subdural hematomas are never spontaneous: someone has caused the condition! Any neurologic deficit in an abuse case involving the head should be considered critical. Alteration of consciousness is the hallmark of brain injury.

Nasal hemorrhaging, wounds or burns of the lips and tongue, missing or loose teeth, displaced nasal cartilages, fractures of the mandible, and bruises to the corners of the mouth should be evaluated in the context of the presenting patient's situation and history. Maxillofacial trauma, particularly that involving midfacial fractures, may indicate more serious skull fractures (e.g., cribiform plate).

Of particular concern for head injured abused adults is damage to the eyes. General questions to consider in ocular trauma are:

- Was there blunt trauma (e.g., fist insult)?
- Was there penetrating trauma (e.g., sharp object like a knife or pencil)?
- Were chemicals, particularly caustic, involved?

The eyes should also be evaluated for pupillary size. Commonly encountered injuries consist of periorbital ecchymoses, subconjunctival hemorrhage, dislocated lens, detached retina, retinal hemorrhage, penetrating injuries, and traumatic cataracts.

Finally, the ears should be inspected for indications of (1) twisting, pulling, or pinching; (2) ruptured eardrums caused by blows to the head; (3) "cauliflower" ear caused by frequent blows to the pinna (projected part of the exterior ear); and (4) blood behind the tympanic membrane, a possible indicator of basilar skull fracture.

Chest

Blunt or penetrating trauma is the usual mechanism of injury to the chest (e.g., hitting the chest with a baseball bat, or stabbing with an ice pick). The chest should be inspected for deformity and limitations of motion due to rib fractures. Blunt trauma from hitting with the fist or by object is a usual mechanism of injury. While marks from knuckles are sometimes discernible, often the perpetrator will use a hard bar of soap wrapped in a towel to hide telltale marks. Penetrating trauma from sharp instruments (e.g., knives and screwdrivers) must also be looked for in the examination. Observe the chest for contusions and hematomas that may be indicative of more occult or inexplicable trauma.

Careful assessment of the chest must be undertaken since the chest is often an area of assault for abuse victims. In females the breasts are often a location for infliction of nonaccidental trauma (e.g., bites, lacerations, penetrating wounds, burns, and marks of disfigurement). In the elderly, restricting their movement by restraining them with various tie-devices may result in rib fractures or more serious internal damage to the thoracic cage organs. Any impairment of respiratory effort must immediately be addressed. Definitive assessment of hemothorax, pneumothorax, and subcutaneous emphysema must be undertaken. Evaluation of the internal structures is necessary by stethoscope for auscultatory purposes followed by roentgenograms.

The elderly do not withstand even minor chest injuries very well; they advance to acute respiratory insufficiency rapidly, and support must be anticipated before respiratory collapse occurs.

Children who sustain injury to the intrathoracic structures often will not have evidence of thoracic skeletal fractures (e.g., ribs). A high index of suspicion of abuse is important.

Abdomen

Abdominal injury has the potential for grave life threat, since there is the possibility of serious hemorrhage from the many visceral organs and vessels contained in the abdominal cavity. Abdominal injuries must be identified and aggressively treated. Blunt and penetrating trauma are the usual mechanisms, although other causes such as poisoning and forced ingestion of caustic substances may be involved. The internal organs can be damaged from blows inflicted to the back by the fist; lacerations to abdominal organs such as the small intestine sometimes occur from this mechanism.

The organs and tissues contained in the peritoneum, retroperitoneum, and pelvis may be involved. Injury to the retroperitoneal organs may be difficult to determine, even with computed tomography. Knowledge of the injury mechanism is important and when an accidental nature is not well identified must raise high level of suspicion to abuse as the cause. Most frequently injured are the (1) liver and spleen, (2) intestines, (3) the duodenum or proximal jejunum, (4) major blood vessels (the vena cava and aorta), (5) pancreas, and (6) kidneys.

The liver, spleen, and kidneys are the organs preponderantly involved in blunt trauma, typically from blows administered by fists. The liver,

spleen, and major vessels are prone to ruptures, the intestines to perforation, and the duodenum to hematoma from blunt trauma.

Penetrating injuries from sharp objects (e.g., knives) and gunshot
wounds result in varied exact organ or structural damage dependent upon
the mechanism of injury. The circuitous trajectory of the bullet will determine that course; stab wounds depending on the length, width, and
mechanism of entrance will similarly determine which organs are involved.

An accurate physical examination diagnosis, diagnostic peritoneal
lavage, and other adjunctive tests such as computerized tomography (CT)
are the hallmarks of competent assessment by the physician of abdominal
trauma inflicted on abused patients. Unrecognized abdominal injury can
lead to death. Note that although genitourinary injuries fall within the
anatomical boundaries of the abdomen, they are included in the following
section on sexual abuse.

Fractures

Visual examination should be made of the extremities for contusions
or deformity. An assessment of the neurovascular integrity should be
undertaken as well. Definitive diagnosis of the existence of fractures,
which are often concealed by other injuries, must be made by roentgeno-
gram. A high index of suspicion of violent abuse must be maintained when
repeated fractures to the same site are observed.

Ordinarily, fractures do not represent a grave threat to life in the adult
patient; however, multiple fractures to major boney structures such as the
femur or pelvis can lead to greater hemodynamic instability and therefore
may pose a life threat to the patient presenting with these injuries. A sense
of urgency must accompany management of these injuries.

Failure to Thrive

In the adult abuse victim, failure to thrive (FTT) may not be as easily
discernible as in children. The frail elderly patient who may already have
reduced body volume and size is difficult to compare with others. Yet there
are factors that may be considered in identifying FTT. Some of the diagnostic criteria and other factors are

- Weight: Is the weight comparable to others in the age cohort? Is
  there undernutrition?
- Weight gain: Is there a failure to gain weight in the current environ-
  ment? Does this change when the environment is changed?
- Is there a ravenous appetite?
- Is the FTT due to withholding of medications?

- Is the FTT due to withholding of the economic capability to purchase necessary food, medicine, and other biologic needs?
- Are there signs of neglect, such as evidence of uncleanliness of body and personal clothing, unkempt hair, lack of shaving in males, poor dental hygiene, lack or deficiencies in cleanliness, temperature regulation, and reasonable amenities in the place of abode?

Sexual Abuse

Injuries to the genital, perianal areas, or rectum without direct evidence of antecedent trauma must always be regarded as suspicious in any age group. In the elderly where dementia, senility, or other causes of altered mental status (e.g., overmedication producing "chemical straightjacketing") are often observed, the abused party may never report sexual abuse. In women, as previously noted, the shame and pressure to forget are common reactions and therefore many cases go unreported for years. Because of the difficulties many sexually abused persons have in reporting the violence, it is important that inadequate or implausible explanations be carefully scrutinized and reviewed.

Urogenital Injuries

Blunt trauma from direct blows to the flank or back that result in contusions, hematomas, or ecchymosis ate the hallmarks of renal injury. A hematoma in the perianal area is indicative of bladder or urethral injury. Blood at the urethral meatus or inability to urinate are signs of urethral injury.

Penetrating trauma from sharp instruments, and particularly from gunshot wounds, produce a number of internal injuries, including perforation of the ureter and bladder.

Lacerations, bruises, or injuries to the external or internal genitalia, poor sphincter tone, and evidence of sexually transmitted disease (STD) or other infection must raise question in the practitioner's mind as to cause. Finally, roentgenographic studies, including excretory urography utilizing intravenous pyelography, cystography, and CT scan, should be undertaken for definitive assessment of the genitourinary tract in violent abuse cases.

Summary

Abuse of any person presents the diagnostician with many challenges, not the least of which may be assessment and maintenance of basic life-support functions. The clinical signs of abuse are often missed because the particular and usual mechanisms of trauma are not considered. It is abundantly and often distressingly clear, though, that the progress of the pathophysiologic insult is the same: high mortality and morbidity.

In developing the history of abuse the following key factors should be kept in mind:

- Eyewitnesses: What was seen, who is accused, and who confesses?
- In children, the following findings during the physical examination suggest abuse and require more intensive and thorough scrutiny: multiple subdural hematomas, especially without fresh skull fracture and retinal hemorrhage.
- Unexplained injuries are suspect first and ruled out only after careful analysis of all the evidence gathered, both personal and clinical.
- Implausible histories need thorough investigation before being accepted as valid.
- Alleged self-inflicted injuries must be carefully analyzed as to their origin; psychologic screening may be necessary to diagnose self-destructive behavior.
- Delay in seeking medical care in the adult, except when altered mental status exists, is always questionable.

The management of abuse that results in physical violence is always fraught with many concerns. Detection of its existence by astute practitioners may be the single most important factor in its reduction by providing the proper medical care, referral, and protection afforded by social, human welfare, and public safety agencies. The high mortality involved when the vicious abuse circle closes is all too well known.

References

American College of Surgeons, Committee on Trauma. (1989). *Advanced trauma life support for doctors*. Chicago: Author.

American College of Surgeons, Committee on Trauma. (1997). *Advanced trauma life support for doctors*. Chicago: Author.

Bunkis, J., & Walton, R. L. (1986). Burns. In D. D. Trunkey & F. R. Lewis (Eds.), *Current therapy of trauma* (pp. 367–373). Philadelphia: Decker.

Geis, G. (1982). The framework of violence. *Topics in Emergency Medicine, 3*, 2–3.

Goldberg, W. G. (1982). Behavioral assessment of the physically abused. In C. G. Warner & G. R. Braen (Eds.), *Management of the physically and emotionally abused* (pp. 111–125). Norwalk, CT: Appleton-Century-Crofts.

Goldberg, W. G., & Carey, A. L. (1982). Domestic violence victims in the emergency setting. *Topics in Emergency Medicine, 3*, 65–67.

Hamburger, K. L., Saunders, D. G., & Hovey, M. (1992). Prevalence of domestic violence in community practice and rate of physician inquiry. *Family Medicine, 23,* 283–287.

Judd, R. L. (1988). Child, spousal, and elderly abuse: An overview. *Journal of Emergency Medical Services, 17,* 43–45.

Judd, R. L. (1991a). Abuse from infancy to the grave. *Key lectures in EMS.* Akron, OH: Emergency Training Institute.

Judd, R. L. (1991b). Altered mental states. *Journal of Emergency Care and Transportation, 20,* 39–48.

Judd, R. L. (1991c). EMS strategies and the elderly. *Journal of Emergency Services, 23,* 29–31.

Kinsey, L. R., Tarbox, A. R., & Bragg, D. (1981). Abuse of the elderly—The hidden agenda: The caretakers and categories of abuse. *Journal of the American Geriatrics Society, 29,* 465–472.

McNeese, M. C., & Hebeler, J. R. (1977). The abused child: A clinical approach to identification and management. *Clinical Symposia, 29,* 31–32.

National Coalition Against Domestic Violence. (1988). *NCADU statistics.* Washington, DC.

National Safety Council. (1994). *Accident facts.* Itasca, IL: Author.

Nicholson, B. E. (1995). Family violence. *The Journal of the South Carolina Medical Association, 91,* 409–446.

Physicians alerted to risk of abuse. (1985, May 23). *The New York Times,* p. A15.

Plotkin, M. R. (1988). *A time for dignity: Police and domestic abuse of the elderly* (p. 8). Washington, DC: American Association of Retired Persons.

Schwartz, G., Bosker, G., & Grigsby, J. W. (Eds.). (1984). *Geriatric emergencies.* Bowie, MD: Brady.

Sussman, S. J. (1968). Skin manifestations of battered child syndrome. *Journal of Pediatrics, 72,* 99.

Teasdale, G., & Jennett, B. (1974). Assessment of coma and impaired consciousness: A practical scale. *Lancet, 2,* 81–84.

II

Violence toward Children

8

Child Physical Abuse

R. Kim Oates, Michael G. Ryan, and Suzette M. Booth

Description of the Problem

Historical Background

Although child abuse did not become widely recognized by the medical and other professions until the late 1960s and early 1970s, the abuse of children has been a feature of most societies for many centuries. The Punch and Judy puppet play, which originated in the mid-17th century (Opie & Opie, 1951), tells how Judy gave Mr. Punch her baby. Despite being gently rocked by Mr. Punch, the baby begins to cry. This makes Mr. Punch rock the baby harder, becoming violent. Finally, when the crying persists Mr. Punch loses control, hits the baby, and kills him. A popular English nursery rhyme dating from the 18th century (Opie & Opie, 1951) describes "an old woman who lived in a shoe" who, because of her frustration at having to care for so many of her children, "whipped them all soundly and put them to bed." Even before this time, many cultures had used infanticide as an accepted method of family planning, it also being accepted practice to dispose of weak, premature, or deformed infants (Bakan, 1971).

One of the first medical descriptions of child abuse came from France, when Ambrose Tardieu (1868), a forensic pathologist, published a medi-

R. Kim Oates, Michael G. Ryan, and Suzette M. Booth • Royal Alexandra Hospital for Children, Westmead, New South Wales, Australia 2145.

Case Studies in Family Violence, Second Edition, edited by Ammerman and Hersen. Kluwer Academic / Plenum Publishers, New York, 2000.

colegal study of 32 children who had been battered to death. Little further was published about the condition until 1946 when an American radiologist, John Caffey, reported a new syndrome. Caffey (1946) reported 6 children with subdural hematomas who also had multiple fractures of the long bones. He noted other injuries, including bruising and retinal hemorrhages, and reported that some of these children were poorly nourished and delayed in their development. Caffey concluded that, in the absence of underlying skeletal disease, the fractures were most likely to be caused by trauma. He felt that negligence may have been a factor, but he was unable to obtain any history of trauma from the parents. Others recognized this condition, which became known as "Caffey's syndrome," but the true cause of these injuries was not clear to most practitioners. Such was the level of denial that parents could actually inflict serious injury on their own children. An important contribution to understanding these injuries was made in 1955 when Woolley and Evans took a fresh look at children with Caffey's syndrome. They emphasized the traumatic nature of these injuries and pointed out that the environments of these infants were often hazardous and undesirable.

The period of awareness of child abuse was ushered in by the landmark paper from Kempe, Silverman, Steele, Droegemueller, and Silver in 1962. They coined the term *the battered child syndrome* as a way of directing attention to the seriousness of the problem and pointed out that physical abuse was a significant cause of death and injury to children. Since this time the extent of child abuse has become more widely recognized and an extensive literature has developed.

Incidence

As most physical abuse occurs within the privacy of the child's home, often to infants and preverbal children, and as most abusers give a false explanation for abusive injuries that come to medical attention, the reported incidence of abuse is an underestimate. There are also occasional reports of physical abuse that are not genuine, while others may be genuine but are unable to be substantiated. Thus there is considerable underreporting of real cases as well as some degree of overreporting. The reported incidence of substantiated physical abuse in the United States in 1993 was 254,000 (Daro & McCurdy, 1993) or four substantiated cases per 1,000 children. Although most cases go unreported or unsubstantiated, child physical abuse is a relatively common problem. It is one that has a mortality and a significant morbidity and it can have long-term adverse effects on personality development (Oates, Peacock, & Forrest, 1984). It is more common than many of the well-recognized serious disorders of childhood—for example, cystic fibrosis (1 in 2,500 births), acute leukemia (annual incidence 1 in 30,000), and juvenile diabetes (1 in every 1,000 school-aged children).

Types of Injuries

The clinical spectrum in physical abuse ranges from relatively mild trauma causing bruising through to florid cases with organ and skeletal damage. While bruises, head injuries, burns, and fractures are common, lacerations occur less often. While not as common as bruising and fractures, poisoning is a recognized form of abuse (Bays, 1990), sometimes being surreptitiously used by the parent as a way of having prolonged hospitalization and investigation to find a cause for the child's unusual symptoms (Rosenberg, 1987)—a type of Munchausen syndrome by proxy (Meadow, 1977; Schnaps, Frond, Rand, & Tirosh, 1981), now called Factitious disorder by proxy, with the mother sometimes having a history of fictitious illness (Bools, Neale, & Meadow, 1994).

The junction of the cartilage with the shaft of the long bone is one of the weakest areas in the skeleton of the growing child. These areas are very vulnerable to the torsion forces that occur when a child is pulled and shaken, so that epiphyseal separation and metaphyseal fractures are common injuries in abuse and unusual injuries in normal play or accidents. Spiral fractures of long bones also are unusual in childhood accidents and occur as a result of the twisting, shearing forces that an adult applies when violently twisting a child's arm or leg.

When an infant is shaken, the repeated acceleration-deceleration and rotation forces that are produced as the infant's head bounces back and forth can cause damage to the brain by direct contusion from the brain's hitting against the inside of the skull or by rupture of blood vessels within and around the brain. Shaking can also cause retinal injuries, so that a complete ophthalmic examination should always be included as part of the assessment of the abused child.

Burns are a relatively common manifestation of child abuse, making up approximately 10% of cases. For example, a parent may dunk a child's buttocks into boiling water as a punishment for soiling. This leaves a distinctive scald involving the buttocks and perineum with no other part of the body scalded. Other typical burns are marks caused by lighted cigarettes and glove and stocking burns of hands or feet, suggesting that the child's limbs may have been forcibly held in hot water.

Other less usual injuries include (a) drowning, suggesting that abuse should be considered in the diagnosis of atypical immersion incidents in infants, although neglect is a more common cause (Feldman, 1993); (b) subgaleal hematomas caused by hair pulling; (c) genital injuries; (d) tears to the floor and roof of the mouth caused by trauma at feeding; and (e) liver contusion or rupture, traumatic cysts of the pancreas, and intramural hematoma of the bowel caused by a direct blow to the abdomen, the latter leading to symptoms and signs of intestinal obstruction. Sometimes skin lesions take the shape of a recognizable object, such as a belt buckle, or a mark in the shape of a loop caused by a loop of rope or electric cord. When a child has multiple injuries of different ages, physical abuse should be considered as a cause of these injuries.

Why Child Physical Abuse Is Important

The answer to the question "Why is child physical abuse important?" may seem obvious, but there is more to this condition than the immediate physical injuries. It is true that child abuse is a major problem resulting in many deaths and a far greater number of injuries, many of them serious, each year. Perhaps just as important is that, with the majority of abuse being caused by the child's parent or caretaker, the actions that lead to the abuse deprive children of some of their basic needs. These are the need for love and security, for new experiences, for praise and recognition, and for the development of personal responsibility. These basic needs for security, recognition of one's worth, and praise are not met in children who see their parents as people likely to injure them and who feel they have to live in fear of a parental outburst. Some adults who were abused as children go on to abuse their own children (approximately 30%; see Kaufman & Zigler, 1987). Many physically abused children have ongoing problems with poor self-esteem, inability to make adequate friendships, lack of trust, and continuing behavior problems (Oates, 1986), with evidence of problems of poor intellectual performance and reading difficulties continuing into adult life (Perez & Widom, 1994). This makes it very difficult for many of these children to develop satisfactory adult relationships and even more difficult for them to cope with the normal stresses associated with child rearing. Thus, child abuse is a condition that can be transmitted from one generation to the next. Breaking this cycle is important, both for the abused child and for that child's own future children.

Case 1: Laura
Laura was the first child of Margaret and Danny, a young couple living in an inner-city suburb. The pregnancy that produced Laura was unplanned, and Margaret, age 20, who had been a clerical assistant in a school, had given up her job in the last trimester, remaining at home after the birth to care for Laura. Danny, age 18, was a plumber and in regular employment.

Laura was born at term weighing 3,450 grams, the pregnancy being uneventful and the delivery accompanied by a lift-out forceps procedure. She was in good condition at birth, no resuscitation being necessary, and she was breast-fed.

Margaret had a regular Monday evening activity with friends from her old place of employment, and on these occasions Laura was left at home in Danny's care. When Laura was 3 weeks old, Margaret went back to her usual Monday evening outing, being away for just under 3 hours. Later that evening Laura was noted to be restless and crying in her sleep. During the small hours of the morning Margaret went to check on Laura and found her to be very pale and breathing irregularly. The parents then took Laura to the children's hospital, where her condition was serious enough to warrant immediate admission to the intensive care unit.

The medical findings when Laura was brought to the hospital were very serious. She was gasping irregularly and was unable to be roused, although she was responsive to pain. The anterior fontanelle was raised and tense, a sign of increased intracranial pressure. Her right pupil was dilated and unresponsive to light. Examination of the eyes showed extensive retinal hemorrhages. There were no bruises anywhere on the body.

Laura's condition continued to deteriorate quickly so that she was unable to breathe spontaneously and had to be artificially ventilated. An MRI scan of the brain showed marked swelling in the right side of the brain and signs of bleeding within the brain substance. A radionuclide scan of the brain showed poor and delayed blood flow to the right side of the brain, thought to be a result of the marked swelling in this area. There was no skull fracture. These findings were consistent with an acute brain injury. A radiological survey of all Laura's other bones did not show any recent or old fractures.

The seriousness of Laura's condition was discussed with Danny and Margaret. They reported that Laura had always been an easy baby to care for, one who was fairly placid, slept well and fed readily. On this evening, Laura was said to have settled down well after her usual 6:00 p.m. feeding, and when Margaret left her an hour later she was asleep. Danny said that while Margaret was out Laura had awakened crying and could not be comforted. He tried cuddling and feeding her but with little success. However, by the time Margaret returned home Laura appeared to be sleeping peacefully. Later that evening Laura woke crying and was very irritable, taking some time to settle. Much later that night she was noted to be pale and gasping, at which time her parents rushed her to the hospital. Both parents could offer no explanation for Laura's condition, Danny very early saying, "I didn't hit her or anything like that."

After the initial interview, which was conducted without any accusations, the parents said that they were planning to visit Laura again in 2 days' time, an unusual behavior in view of the seriousness of Laura's condition and the hospital's policy of encouraging parents to live in and visit as much as possible. Margaret and Danny were told of the hospital's responsibility to report injuries that had no explanation and where child abuse could be a possibility. In a later interview with the police, Danny said that he had placed Laura in a playpen that evening when she was crying and that he had then accidentally kicked the corner of the playpen, perhaps bumping Laura as well.

The medical opinion was that Laura had sustained an acute brain injury on the evening of her admission to the hospital and that in the absence of any significant external head trauma, violent shaking was thought to be the most likely cause. Because Laura had been with only her parents during this time, it was felt that the injury must have been caused by one of the parents, the more likely one being Laura's father during the time Margaret was out of the house. It was felt that Laura probably did wake crying and that in his frustration at not being able to settle her, Danny had shaken her, not realizing the serious damage that violent shaking can cause to a young infant.

A children's court order was obtained that placed Laura in her mother's care under supervision from the Department of Child Welfare, a condition of the placement being that Danny should live out of the home and not have access to Laura. In addition to the children's court order, criminal charges were placed against Danny by the police and a number of court cases were heard over the subsequent 3 years. Despite the children's court order, there was very little in the way of welfare department supervision, and after the first few months Danny moved back into the family home. A second, healthy child was born to Danny and Margaret 14 months after Laura's injury. This child developed normally and is not known to have had any injuries. The paternal and maternal grandparents have been very supportive of the family.

At the end of 3 years the final court hearing was held, the police aiming for a conviction of Danny for attempted manslaughter. The defense case was based on the possibility that the forceps delivery may have been responsible for the injury, and this, coupled with some degree of conflict in opinion by the various hospital specialists who had seen the child, was enough for the prosecution's case to be lost.

Laura's condition remained unstable and critical for the first few days of her admission to the hospital. She was eventually able to come off the ventilator but was left with permanent, severe cerebral damage. She has been followed regularly over several years and is extremely handicapped. She is severely intellectually retarded, has spastic quadriplegia, is blind, and is very irritable. She developed infantile spasms and now has epilepsy, which is difficult to control. She has been linked with a variety of community resources, which include physiotherapy, respite care, and the state blind society's infant stimulation program, and she receives special schooling. Margaret has coped admirably with her, always keeping appointments and being fully involved in her various therapies.

Case 2: Jacinta

Jacinta is the only child of Sally and Peter, who live in a small rural town. At an antenatal clinic visit to the local hospital at 7 months of the pregnancy,

Sally was physically assaulted by Peter in front of the hospital staff. The police were called and as a result an Apprehended Violence Order was taken out by the police.

Five weeks before the expected date of birth, Peter brought Sally to a large metropolitan teaching hospital saying that they were dissatisfied with the quality of care provided in the rural hospital. At that time Sally was noted to have a black eye, which she ascribed to a recent motor vehicle accident.

Sally went into early labor and Jacinta was born at 36 weeks of gestation. She was slow to feed and spent the first 2 weeks of her life in the special care nursery requiring nasogastric feeding. During this period a social worker was involved with Sally and Peter as a result of Peter's aggressive attitude to staff.

At the hospital Sally was found to be illiterate and was thought to be mildly intellectually disabled. The social worker arranged for a community nurse in the rural town to make a home visit when Sally and Jacinta were discharged. An appointment was also made for Jacinta to be followed up by a local pediatrician. The nurse visited the family on two occasions. On each occasion there was no response, although the nurse felt that there was someone inside the house. The appointment with the pediatrician was not kept.

At 5 weeks of age, Jacinta was admitted to the local hospital with multiple unexplained injuries. She had a torn frenulum with lacerated and infected gums, a fractured nose and maxilla, and burns on her buttocks and her left upper thigh. A full skeletal X ray was done to look for other injuries, possibly of different ages. This showed a fracture in one of the bones of the forearm, the X ray appearance suggesting that the fracture had occurred approximately 2 weeks earlier.

Sally's explanation for the burns on Jacinta's buttocks was that her 17-year-old niece had allowed Jacinta to roll over and come in contact with an electric heater after she had given her a bath. The burn on the thigh was explained as having occurred when Peter accidentally spilled hot milk on Jacinta. The explanation given for the facial injuries was that when Sally was carrying Jacinta on her shoulder, she tripped over the family dog and fell backwards so that Jacinta's face hit the floor. Sally claimed that the fractured wrist must have been caused by hospital staff holding her tightly when blood was collected for pathology tests.

Sally described her relationship with Peter as happy and denied any suggestion of domestic violence. When asked about an obvious bruise to her own left cheek, she said that it was a birthmark that had always been on her face.

Following an interview by the joint investigation team (a child welfare–police interview team), Sally was told that Jacinta would be placed in foster care and that papers had been filed in the children's court for her to be made a ward of the state. Sally then divulged a long history of physical assault by Peter on her and indicated that Jacinta's facial injuries had really occurred when she had been punched by Peter.

Further inquiries found that Sally had attended a special class at high school for slow learners. She had stopped going to school at the age of 16. She described school as an unhappy experience, saying that she was teased and bullied. She had known Peter, an unemployed truck driver, for 2 years prior to their marriage 12 months earlier. Peter had a long and violent criminal history. He had been removed from his parents' care as a child and as a teenager spent a number of years in juvenile corrective institutions.

Sally's parents were fearful of Peter, as they had directly experienced threats of violence from him. Peter would never let Sally's parents visit and had threatened to cut her father's throat if he interfered in their relationship.

During Jacinta's stay in hospital, nursing staff became very concerned about the level of Sally's parenting skills. Despite encouragement from the nursing staff for Sally to care for Jacinta, she tended to leave the child's care to the nursing staff, particularly when Jacinta was crying and need comforting.

On discharge from hospital, Jacinta was placed in foster care. The child psychiatrist who assessed Sally's interactions with Jacinta while they were in hospital felt her deficits in parenting were not reversible and was concerned that she did not have the independence of mind to resist approaches from violent and exploitative men. He was concerned that Sally was unable to protect Jacinta from Peter's physical assaults and felt that Jacinta would be better cared for by foster parents.

Peter was charged by the police with violent assault and is awaiting trial.

Medical Issues

Establishing the Diagnosis

As child physical abuse is common, it should be considered a possibility, even if only to be dismissed, in any child who presents with an injury, particularly if that injury is not adequately explained. It is important for those working in emergency rooms to gain expertise in child abuse detection and management and to have an appropriate level of suspicion when seeing children with injuries. A good question to ask after examining the child is, "Is the explanation for the injuries consistent with the findings?" In Laura's case, the explanation that she had bumped against the playpen when it was kicked was inadequate. Short falls and bumps are extremely unlikely to produce serious injuries. A review of 207 cases where children fell from beds found only one simple skull fracture and no serious or multiple injuries (Lyons & Oates, 1993). Similarly, when an infant is brought unconscious to an intensive care unit, child abuse, particularly from a shaking injury, should be considered along with the other diagnostic possibilities.

The danger of shaking infants was pointed out by Caffey in 1974 when attention was drawn to the high vulnerability of the infant head, brain, and eyes to the stress of shaking. It is likely that many of the so-called spontaneous subdural hematomas of infancy described in older pediatric texts were actually cases of child abuse resulting from violent shaking. The older pediatric textbooks discussed the spontaneous subdural hematoma of infancy—a not-uncommon diagnosis in the past—but did not mention child abuse. Now pediatric texts discuss child abuse, but the so-called spontaneous subdural hematoma of infancy is no longer mentioned.

A violent shaking injury usually causes the child to become rapidly unconscious, although sometimes clinical signs may take several hours to appear. This is particularly likely when the bridging veins within the skull are torn. Bridging veins cross the potential surface between the dura, a tough, thick membrane that is the outer membrane covering the brain, and the arachnoid, a much thinner membrane lying beneath the dura. Bleeding from these veins is under low pressure and symptoms may not appear until a significant volume of blood starts to expand and accumulate in the space between the dura and the arachnoid. An ophthalmologic examination is an essential part of the assessment of children with head trauma, particularly because of the high incidence of retinal hemorrhages in children with nonaccidental head injuries (Duhaime et al., 1992).

One problem in a child with skull fracture is deciding the likelihood of it being nonaccidental. The diagnosis is based largely on the presence of any associated injuries and on the "fit" between the parents' story and the physical findings. In children under 2 years, accidents are more likely to result in single, narrow, linear fractures, usually involving the parietal bone with no associated intracranial injury. In contrast, fractures associated with abuse are more likely to be multiple, complex, depressed, or wide, to involve areas other than the parietal bone, to involve more than one bone and to be associated with intracranial injury (Hobbs, 1984, 1993).

Imaging techniques can help the diagnosis of intracranial injury (Frank, Zimmerman, & Leeds, 1985). The CT findings can include contusion and hemorrhages in single or multiple sites in the brain substance as well as evidence of bleeding between the brain and the skull. In severe cases, the CT scan later shows hypodense areas as much of the damaged brain tissue becomes resorbed, leaving markedly enlarged ventricles and atrophy of brain substance. Magnetic resonance imaging is superior to CT scanning in detecting brain injury, particularly subdural hematomas (Alexander, Schor, & Smith, 1986).

What few studies there are on the outcome of children who sustain severe head injuries suggest that, as in the case of Laura, there are usually permanent handicaps (Dykes, 1986) with a high incidence of death, vision loss, seizures, and developmental delay.

The diagnosis of physical abuse is not based solely on the injuries. It is also based on the history, particularly if the explanation is inadequate or inappropriate. Other features that may raise the level of suspicion include inconsistent explanations for the injury given by each parent, a long delay between the injury and presenting the child for treatment, and inappropriate affect on the part of the parents. Other physical findings in favor of this diagnosis include unusual patterns of bruising, especially "grab marks" in the shape of finger marks where the limbs of the child may have been forcefully gripped, bruises suggesting the pattern of an object, bruises in areas usually not injured accidentally, two black eyes, unusual fractures such a spiral fractures in long bones or chip fractures at metaphyseal regions suggesting a twisting injury, and evidence of old and recent fractures showing different stages of healing on the skeletal survey. The diagnosis of abuse is sometimes clear-cut, but often there are gray areas where clinical experience, careful family assessment, and consultation with more experienced colleagues will all help in establishing the diagnosis.

Rather than trying to reach a "whodunit" diagnosis in every case, it is far more fruitful to look at the strengths and weaknesses in the family where abuse is suspected and to take steps to relieve some of the stresses by providing realistic support services. What is most important is the future protection and mental health of the child. Most families have the same concern for the child as the child protection worker—that is, for their child to grow up well and healthy. Many families do not have the skills to achieve this, reverting to violence in the face of stress and frustration. Supporting these families in parenting and recognizing that there must be a long-term commitment to them is for most families a more realistic approach than seeing detection and prosecution as the beginning and end of involvement with the family.

One problem in making the diagnosis of child abuse may be the professional's own denial about being faced with this condition. In the past, many medical professionals have been poorly trained to deal with child abuse. They often are reluctant to become involved in court action and may be uncomfortable working cooperatively with other professionals. There is then the danger of accepting at face value a most unlikely explanation for the injury rather than seeking its real cause (Oates, 1979). With widespread acceptance that child abuse is a major problem and the availability of child protection teams in many child health centers, these difficulties in reporting have become less, although the individual practitioner still needs to be aware of the unconscious tendency to overlook this diagnosis.

Laura's injury was a typical shaking injury—the baby crying, the parent losing control and shaking the baby violently, followed by the baby appearing to go to sleep and later being found to be seriously ill. In Jacinta's case, the explanations for the injuries as given by Sally lack credibility. At 4 weeks of age an infant is incapable of rolling over, thus the burns on the buttocks could not have been caused in the manner described. Such burns are usually the result of dunking an infant's buttocks in boiling water (Hobson, Evans, & Stewart, 1994). The burns to Jacinta's thigh, if caused by hot milk, suggest either that there was inadequate parenting, to have made the milk so hot that it could burn Jacinta's skin, or else that this was not the cause of the burn.

The credibility of the explanation is further questioned by Sally's claim that Jacinta's fractured wrist must have been the result of rough handling by hospital staff, made even less likely by the X ray features showing the fracture to be 2 weeks old.

A ruptured frenulum is an uncommon accidental injury in an infant. The associated finding of a maxillary fracture and fractures to the nasal bones is highly suggestive of a blow to the face. Adding to the concern about the cause of Jacinta's injuries is the significant delay by Sally in seeking medical attention.

The Child Protection Team

The management of child abuse usually requires a team approach. However, child protection teams don't just happen. A team of individuals who work in parallel without mutual trust and respect for each other and without close cooperation is a team in name only. Considerable effort has to go into creating a child protection team with complementary skills where the members can work comfortably with each other. In Laura's case, the initial interview with Danny and Margaret was conducted jointly by the social worker and the pediatrician. Some of the subsequent interviews were held jointly or separately but always with discussion between the social worker and the pediatrician at their conclusion. The case conference is an important process in creating a management plan. In Laura's case, there was an early case conference attended by the pediatrician and the social worker, the child welfare agency (which has the statutory authority for child protection), the intensive care ward staff, and the police.

In Jacinta's case, the hospital child protection team adopted a supportive role with Sally in that it did not confront her with the inconsistencies in her history of events leading up to Jacinta's admission. In addition, the team explored with Sally and her parents Sally's strengths and weaknesses in relation to her ability to care for Jacinta.

The confrontation—when stating that Sally's explanations did not fit the known facts—was left to the joint investigative team, where police and child welfare officers work and interview together. Following their decision to initiate care proceedings for Jacinta in the children's court and to seek out Peter for further questioning, Sally began to disclose the violence that both she and Jacinta had been subjected to by Peter.

Supporting the assessment of Sally's parenting skills were the observations of the nursing staff and the consultant psychiatrist. The expansion of the hospital child protection team of pediatrician and social worker, to include the nursing staff caring for Jacinta and the psychiatrist assessing Sally, helped to develop a comprehensive picture of Sally's ability to care for her daughter.

At the case conference, minutes are taken and a management plan is made. It is essential that the recommendations made at the case conference be realistic and able to be carried out with named members of the team being recorded as responsible for particular aspects of the management. If the management plans have to be varied, subsequent case conferences or reviews are needed to ensure that any altered circumstances are taken into account and that the management plan remains viable.

It is also important for the child protection team to be involved early. Asking the team to see a child for the first time when the child is about to be discharged after 2 weeks in the hospital devalues the role of the team and makes working with the family extremely difficult. With Laura, the child protection team was notified within an hour of Laura's arrival at the hospital so that early involvement was possible. This early, initial interview often is very helpful in establishing a relationship with the parents. Child protection teams based in hospitals should try to have a high profile in terms of teaching and offering a high-quality, quickly responding 24-hour-per-day service. This credibility will encourage early consultation.

The members of the team have to be careful not to confuse their responsibility to the family with their responsibility to the child. They need to be aware of a natural tendency not to want to become involved in some cases and also of the temptation that sometimes occurs to empathize so closely with the parents that the child's needs are overlooked. While they are able to have some sympathy with and understanding for the parents' problems, it is important for them to look closely at the needs and rights of the child. This includes the provision of a treatment program made specifically for the child's needs. This is particularly important in view of the follow-up studies showing a high incidence of developmental delay in these children (Wodarski, Kurtz, Gaudin, & Howing, 1990; Perez & Widom, 1994).

Those involved in child protection often experience anger and frustration. Each team member needs to try to help the others in the team as well as those involved in the hospital, such as nursing staff on the child's ward, to contain this anger or to express it constructively. Many members often find it helpful to look beyond the team for personal support and many teams find it helpful to have an adviser not directly involved with the family with whom they can discuss the problems of the child abuse as well as their own feelings about it.

Legal Issues

In Laura's case, the legal issues were taken on two fronts. The child welfare department's interest was to protect Laura. They had her case heard in the children's court, where decisions were made "on the balance of probability," a much less stringent criterion than that of "beyond reasonable doubt," which is used in the criminal court. (Of course, legal procedures will vary from country to country and by jurisdiction.) The children's court readily accepted the need to offer Laura protection, and since the maternal grandparents were nearby and supportive and since it seemed that the injury was caused when Margaret was out of the house, a decision was made for Laura to be placed in Margaret's custody but with Danny being required to live apart from them. Supervision was not adequate, and before long Danny and Margaret were together again.

In retrospect it can be seen that no harm came to Laura from the breakdown of supervision, but this case does point out the need for court orders to be realistic and for supervision to be provided in a specified way, rather than for court orders to be made without any formal review process to ensure that they are actually happening. As it turned out, a variety of supporting services were provided for Margaret and Laura, and Margaret cooperated fully in all of these arrangements. However, if the hospital team had not worked to obtain long-term hospital and community-based support for this family, this support might not have been forthcoming. A more realistic court order might have been for Laura to live away from her parents while the assessment of their strengths and weaknesses continued, and then, if Laura was returned either to her mother or to her grandparents, or put in foster care, for an audit to be made to ensure continuing treatment for her.

The other legal avenue used was the criminal court. Because Laura was close to death, the police proceeded with an attempted manslaughter charge. Delays in the justice system, with frequent deferrals of the case and frequent adjournments, meant that it was 3 years before the case was concluded. By this time, memories were hazy, although fortunately careful documentation of the injuries and treatment had been made at the time, an essential procedure in all child protection cases.

The child protection team was convinced that the injury was not accidental, although there was a real possibility that Danny was unaware of the extent of the injury he would cause by violently shaking Laura. The evidence presented by the hospital could have been more carefully prepared. The neurosurgeon, a key witness, was very reluctant to appear in court, and as a result of several emergency neurosurgical procedures that coincided with the court hearings did not give evidence apart from a written statement describing the injuries but failing to express an opinion as to the cause.

The neurologist who had been involved in Laura's care gave evidence but was reluctant to be definite about the cause of the injury, and under pressure from cross-examination for the defense conceded that it was possible for trauma occurring at the time of the forceps delivery to be responsible for Laura's sudden illness and present condition. The child protection team had made an error in not ensuring that the neurologist was fully conversant with the obstetric details before giving evidence. The record from the obstetric hospital and discussion with the obstetrician soon after Laura's initial presentation showed that the birth was uncomplicated, that forceps were applied only lightly at the "lift-out" stage of the delivery, and that Laura was in good condition at birth. The cross-examination of the neurologist by the defense had not revealed this, the implication being that the delivery was far more hazardous than it actually was.

Another difficulty was that the neurologist was unfamiliar with child abuse literature, including studies on head injuries, and so was not able to be definite in his conclusions and was persuaded that birth trauma could have been a possible cause. This evidence was in conflict with that of the pediatrician from the child protection team, who stated that the injuries were consistent with violent shaking and not at all consistent with birth trauma. However, the conflict in evidence meant that there was "reasonable doubt," and so the prosecution's case was lost.

It can be seen now that things have probably worked out better from Laura's point of view as a result of this decision. Danny and Margaret matured considerably over the 3 years between the injury and the final court case. Danny has been able to remain in employment, and the family has been materially much better off than if he had been in prison. There has been good support from the grandparents on both sides, with little in the way of recrimination, allowing continuing support from both sides of the family. Hospital and community support have also been provided. Danny and Margaret have a continuing tragedy in their lives—having to care for a child born potentially normal but now with severe intellectual impairments and major physical disabilities. However, in other cases the result might have been different; the results in this case do not diminish the need for those involved in this area to develop expertise in preparing cases for court and in teaching other professionals who may be involved about some of the techniques needed to present effectively in court.

In Jacinta's case, there was considerable benefit in involving a joint investigative team made up of police and child welfare officers who were trained to conduct interviews together and cooperatively. The police officer concentrated on the criminal assault by Peter, while the child welfare staff looked at the need to ensure the safety of Jacinta. An interim Apprehended Violence Order was taken out by the police against Peter, which restricted his contact with Jacinta and Sally, while proceedings in the children's court placed Jacinta in foster care.

Some useful papers have been written on giving evidence in court and developing courtroom skills (Carson, 1984). It is essential for the expert witness to prepare for the case and to have a careful mastery of the facts. Doctors should not retreat into the security of complex technical jargon. This makes their evidence incomprehensible to a jury and may leave it open to misinterpretation. There is no substitute for plain, everyday language. Thus, "two black eyes" is a much more understandable term than "bilateral periorbital hematomas."

Attention to other techniques, such as dressing appropriately in a conservative manner, avoiding constantly shuffling papers, using eye contact when answering questions, and avoiding fidgeting, will all help the expert witness's credibility. It is often very helpful for those starting work in a child protection team to have several visits to court to observe more experienced members of the team giving evidence in preparation for the time when they too will be called.

It is important to remain calm and controlled. Becoming angry or sarcastic does nothing to enhance the expert witness's credibility. It also is important to be impartial and honest. Being honest may mean acknowledging when a question is outside one's area of expertise. The expert witness should never be tempted to step beyond the bounds of his or her own skill and competence. Doing so may cause embarrassment to the witness if his lack of expertise in the area into which he has strayed is revealed. It also lessens the credibility of the evidence given in an area of expertise.

Finally, the testimony of the expert witness should be regarded as a scholarly endeavor (Brent, 1982). The expert witness is there to help arrive at a decision about the truth, not to try to win a case for one side or the other. It is essential to be well informed, to be nonpartisan, and not to step beyond the bounds of one's own expertise, tempting as that may be (Oates, 1993).

Social and Family Issues

Laura's Case

Margaret

This family had a number of positive features. Margaret was of good intelligence, had a stable background, and had a good relationship with her own parents, who lived nearby. She had made firm friends in her work as a clerical assistant and also maintained contact with some of her old school friends. She was able to seek help when needed and was able to telephone her family doctor or her pediatrician whenever problems relating to Laura, such as seizures, occurred. She participated in the physiotherapy and infant stimulation programs and did all that was asked of her with regard to Laura's care, which was complex and at times stressful.

She could not be described as an "open" person, appearing calmly efficient on the outside but unwilling to discuss positive or negative features of her family life. She readily responded to all practical suggestions to assist Laura but was unable to be engaged by the social worker in any therapeutic work. This raises the question of how much one should probe or try to become involved in deeper family issues when doing so is resisted. In this case, it was decided to be available but not to exert any pressure that might have hindered cooperation with the various community support and medical treatments in which Laura and Margaret were involved.

Danny

Danny was only 18 when Laura was born. He was a large young man who had been involved in junior wrestling. He had undertaken a successful apprenticeship as a plumber and had remained in full employment during a time when unemployment was high. His parents also lived nearby and were supportive of him, Margaret, and the marriage. He had a close relationship with his mother, frequently telephoning her for advice on a wide variety of subjects, including child rearing. He was reported to have a quick temper and had been known to have been involved in fights with minimal provocation. He was proud of his physical strength.

Although his parents were supportive and readily available, the early years of his childhood had been unhappy. There had been a great deal of stress between his parents, often resulting in his father being violent toward his mother. He was unable to recall any abuse to himself, but his memory of his father, who separated from his mother when Danny was

6 years of age, was generally negative. His mother remarried when he was 11. He had no contact with his natural father but had formed a cordial but not affectionate relationship with his stepfather.

The Community

Margaret and Danny were fortunate to live in a suburb with strong community supports. While not being aware of any need for these supports before Laura's injury, the ready availability of an extremely supportive and understanding family doctor and a visiting community nurse and easy access to physiotherapy and other services for Laura were all important factors in reducing some of the stresses on the parents after the injury and in allowing a realistic management plan to be implemented.

The Future

This family had a long way to go. Laura would become an increasing physical and financial burden when older and heavier. She would never be independently mobile and continue to require almost constant supervision. Their second child had remained well and free from injury, the community support services being involved to ensure that her needs were not overlooked. Although involvement by the same professional group had continued with this family for over 4 years, many more years would be required. This is one of the major challenges in child protection work, where in many families the problems and stresses remain much longer than the involvement of any particular worker. It is important that when professionals move on to other positions they carefully prepare the family for this loss and adequately hand the case over to their successors.

Jacinta's Case

Sally

Sally's parents were extremely supportive of their daughter. However, they had retired from employment and were not in the best of health. Sally's parents lived on an isolated farm 20 miles from Sally and were unable to supply much practical support.

Sally was a headstrong young woman who in the past could not be prevented from forming a relationship with a violent partner. The inability of Sally's parents at their stage in life to provide long-term care and support for Jacinta and Sally was a major problem, particularly as the hospital's assessment was that Sally lacked the necessary skills to provide a safe and nurturing environment for Jacinta.

Peter

Peter had a long history of violence, but his mother refused to believe that he was anything but a victim of circumstances. Although she offered to have Sally and Jacinta move into her home, her ability to protect Sally and Jacinta from her son's violence was thought to be questionable. With neither Sally's nor Peter's parents judged able to meet Jacinta's needs, the child was put into foster care.

The Future

Jacinta began to thrive in the care of her foster parents. Her attachment to her foster parents increased as the placement continued. The hospital team advocating for Jacinta felt that it was in Sally's best interests to remain in foster care.

Assessment of Psychopathology

Laura's Case

Neither Danny nor Margaret had a formal psychiatric assessment. Margaret was cooperative but self-contained, a concrete thinker, and possibly not readily available for a therapeutic approach involving introspection. It was felt most appropriate to continue at a practical level, providing ready access and supportive services. On the surface this appears to have been effective, her management of Laura having been exemplary and her second child developing normally and free from abuse.

Danny appeared to be somewhat less intelligent than Margaret. He enjoyed physical activity and the company of other males, and he had a hot temper. He did not communicate easily with professionals and had had an unhappy childhood, witnessing violence toward his mother, to whom he was closely attached, but not suffering physical abuse himself. As a result of the early example of his natural father, he felt that most conflicts could be resolved by force and he demonstrated this by getting into occasional physical fights. Having married at 17 years of age, he had missed out on some aspects of normal adolescent development. It has never been established exactly what happened to Laura, but it appears likely that Danny did lose control with her, probably during Margaret's absence, resulting in the violent shaking that did far more harm than he probably intended.

Jacinta's Case

While Peter did not have a formal psychiatric assessment it was felt that he had all of the characteristics of a sociopathic personality. He had been abused as a child, had been in state care, and had moved onto juvenile justice and then corrective services institutions as he became older, committing crimes with violence. He had violently assaulted Sally during and after her pregnancy with Jacinta, and the assaults on his daughter had escalated from burns to a punch in the face.

Sally was thought to be functioning in the mild to borderline range of intellectual disability. She found it difficult to follow instructions on how to prepare Jacinta's formula, which accounted for the child's poor weight gain. Although Sally showed affection for Jacinta, it was felt that she treated her more like a doll than an infant dependent on a nurturing and stimulating environment. Sally found it difficult to resist Peter's influence, agreeing to see him and give him money while Jacinta was in hospital after having told the social worker shortly before that about the violent assaults he had made on her and Jacinta and her intention to break off the relationship.

Many abusive parents do not have clear-cut psychiatric disorders, but they do display psychopathology, with borderline personality disorder being a feature of many. Factors that are often found in child-abusing parents include arrested emotional development, poor self-image, emotional isolation, poor mental health, depressive loneliness, and poorly suppressed anger (Belsky & Vondra, 1989; Prodgers, 1984). These features were not found in Margaret, but Danny could be considered to have arrested emotional development, poor self-image, and poorly suppressed anger.

Treatment Options

Laura's Case

The management options in this case included the following:

1. *Psychotherapy.* This approach was not chosen.
2. *A practical approach providing supportive services and regular contact with the family.* This was the option chosen, although if supportive services had not been so readily available, this would have been a difficult option to organize successfully.

3. *Removal of Laura to foster care on either a short-term or a long-term basis.* This was one option available to the children's court, although the decision was made for Laura to remain with her mother.
4. *Group work with the parents.* This can be an effective form of treatment, but it requires some motivation on the part of the parents and was not chosen in this case.

Jacinta's Case

The two main management options were either to allow Sally to return to live with her parents, who would be granted custody of Jacinta, or to arrange for the removal of Jacinta to foster care on a medium- to long-term basis.

It was felt that Sally lacked the necessary skills to respond to Jacinta's needs. Although she had supportive parents, their health was in question and their ability to monitor Sally's future relationships was thought to be poor. Thus foster care was considered the better option, with Sally maintaining regular contact with Jacinta.

The evaluation of the effectiveness of treatment programs for physically abused children is difficult and there is much more written about how to treat these children than about results of treatment, suggesting that there are many problems in providing effective treatment. A literature review (Oates & Bross, 1995) on the treatment of physically abused children and the treatment of physically abusive adults found that only 25 papers published in the last 10 years had met minimal criteria for research methodology. Treatment periods ranged from 4 weeks to 2 years. Most programs showed some improvement with treatment, but the majority had no follow-up to see if improvement was sustained once treatment ceased.

Prerequisites for optimal long-term management include a comprehensive diagnostic assessment of the family; a multidisciplinary team to make decisions and to plan treatment; and most importantly, the availability of diversified treatment options for periodic assessment of treatment plans. Those involved in child abuse treatment should be clearly aware of their short- and long-term responsibilities to the families. Because the situation is complex, it is essential to have a treatment plan that is flexible, is reviewed periodically, and is realistic and practical. The multidisciplinary team that produces an ideal but totally unrealistic plan does little for these children.

The advantages of nonprofessional volunteers, who can give abusive parents some of the parenting they missed in their own childhood and thus prevent them from depending on the child for their emotional needs, have been described by Gray and Kaplan (1980). However, putting nonprofessional volunteers into direct contact with abusive families is a formidable task for the volunteer. A more effective form of home visitation is to use visiting nurses with high-risk families before the abuse occurs, something that has been shown to be effective in reducing a number of parenting problems (Olds *et al.*, 1997).

The form of treatment offered to parents depends on the degree of problem found in the family. While some parents will respond to relatively simple and supportive measures, these are less likely to work for a hard core of parents—variously estimated at between 20% and 40% of cases—who have serious personality disturbances. These parents will require intense skilled and sustained intervention, and serious consideration should be given to alternative care for the child in some of these cases.

Where there is severe family pathology it may be in the child's best interests to be removed from the parents and placed in foster care. It would be naive, however, to believe that this solves the problem. A review of over 5,000 children in foster care (Bolton, Laner, & Gai, 1981) showed that the risk of maltreatment at the hands of a foster parent was over three times greater than in a natural family. Being placed in foster care is a confusing and unsettling experience for a child. Children need to be prepared for this sort of separation and should have a specific treatment program provided for them during the period of fostering. Without this, the adverse emotional sequelae for the children may be even more harmful.

In some cases, short- to medium-term fostering with eventual return to the parents may be less in the child's interest than permanent placement. A 4-year follow-up of 50 abused children from Liverpool (Hensey, Williams, & Rosenbloom, 1983) found that those children for whom an early decision had been made to sever all family contacts fared significantly better than those who were returned to their parents.

Since most abused children remain in their homes, it is in this context that most treatment should be planned. Treatment starts with a complete evaluation of the child's strengths and weaknesses, as well as the strengths and weaknesses of the family. Preschool children often respond to a therapeutic day care center, which also involves a program for the parents to learn to relate to and care for their child (Oates, Gray, Schweitzer, Kempe, & Harmon, 1995).

Summary

As in many child abuse cases, the cause of Laura's injury was never completely determined, although it is virtually certain that it was caused by an adult, Danny being the most obvious perpetrator. The family was not known to any agencies prior to this episode and apart from Danny's youth, there was nothing to single this family out from any other. It is possible that a home visiting program commencing before birth (Olds, Henderson, & Kitzman, 1994) may have provided the family support and skills that could have prevented this injury.

In Jacinta's case, the cause of the injuries became obvious following Sally's description of her husband's behavior. Could the injuries to both of these children have been prevented?

Helfer (1987) has described a number of preventive measures aimed at parents and children at different stages of their lives that, taken together, are thought likely to prevent many cases of child abuse. The concepts are still valid today:

- Parental coaching to provide new parents with the skills necessary to communicate with their new child.
- Home care assistance, where parents are provided with visitors to help them with practical child-care problems and to improve their communication skills with their infants.
- Expanded baby care.
- Teaching preschool and primary school age children interpersonal and cognitive problem-solving skills to help them resolve everyday problems.
- Teaching interpersonal skills to high school age children, with emphasis on how to get on with people of all ages and at all levels in society.
- A crash course in "childhood" for adults and some young adults who need a second chance to learn skills that should have been learned during their childhood.
- A preparent refresher course for "soon-to-be" parents to revise previously taught concepts of appropriate ways to interact with their partners and children.

In Laura's case, supportive and preventive services could be provided only after the injury. This family has a continuing tragedy caused by Laura's severe handicap, but they seem to be managing well with a supportive approach. A long-term commitment to this family needs to be maintained, as it does to the majority of families in which physical child abuse has occurred.

References

Alexander, R. C., Schor, D. P., & Smith, W. L. (1986). Magnetic resonance imaging of intracranial injuries from child abuse. *Journal of Pediatrics, 109,* 975–979.

Bakan, D. (1971). *Slaughter of the innocents: A study of the battered child phenomenon*. San Francisco: Jossey-Bass.

Bays, J. (1990). Substance abuse and child abuse. *Pediatric Clinics of North America, 37*, 881–904.

Belsky, J., & Vondra, J. (1989). Lessons from child abuse: The determinants of parenting. In D. Cicchetti & V. Carlson (Eds.), *Child maltreatment: Research and theory on the consequences of abuse and neglect* (pp. 153–202). New York: Cambridge University Press.

Bolton, F. G., Laner, R. H., & Gai, D. S. (1981). For better or worse? Foster parents and foster children in an officially reported child maltreatment population. *Children and Youth Services Review, 13*, 127–129.

Bools, C., Neale, B., & Meadow, R. (1994). Munchausen syndrome by proxy: A study of psychopathology. *Child Abuse and Neglect, 18*, 773–778.

Brent, R. C. (1982). The irresponsible expert witness. *Pediatrics, 70*, 754–762.

Caffey, J. (1946). Multiple fractures in the long bones of infants suffering from chronic subdural hematoma. *American Journal of Roentgenology, 56*, 163–173.

Caffey, J. (1974). The whiplash shaken infant syndrome. *Pediatrics, 54*, 396–403.

Carson, D. (1984). Developing courtroom skills. *Journal of Social Welfare Law, 110*, 29–38.

Daro, D., & McCurdy, K. (1993). *Current trends in child abuse reporting and fatalities: The results of the 1993 annual fifty state survey*. Chicago: National Committee for the Prevention of Child Abuse and Neglect.

Duhaime, A. C., Alario, A. J., Lewander, W. J., Schut L., Sutton, L. N., Seidl, T. S., Nudelman, S., Budenz, D., Hertle, R., Tsiaris, W., & Loporchio, S. (1972). Head injury in very young children. *Pediatrics, 90*, 179–185.

Dykes, L. J. (1986). The whiplash shaken infant syndrome: What has been learned? *Child Abuse and Neglect, 10*, 211–221.

Feldman, K. W. (1993). When is childhood drowning neglect? *Child Abuse and Neglect, 17*, 329–336.

Frank, Y., Zimmerman, R., & Leeds, N. M. D. (1985). Neurological manifestations in abused children who have been shaken. *Developmental Medicine and Child Neurology, 27*, 312–316.

Gray, J. D., & Kaplan, B. (1980). The lay health visitor programme: An eighteen-month experience. In C. H. Kempe & R. E. Helfer (Eds.), *The battered child* (3rd ed.). Chicago: University of Chicago Press.

Helfer, R. E. (1987). An overview of prevention. In R. E. Helfer & C. H. Kempe (Eds.), *The battered child* (4th ed., pp. 425–433). Chicago: University of Chicago Press.

Hensey, O. J., Williams, J. K., & Rosenbloom, L. (1983). Intervention in child abuse: Experience in Liverpool. *Developmental Medicine and Child Neurology, 25*, 606–611.

Hobbs, C. J. (1984). Skull fracture and the diagnosis of abuse. *Archives of Disease in Childhood, 59*, 246–252.

Hobbs, C. J. (1993). Fractures. In R. Meadow (Ed.), *ABC of child abuse* (pp. 9–14). London: British Medical Journal.

Hobson, M., Evans, J., & Stewart, P. (1994). An audit of nonaccidental injury in burned children. *Burns, 20*, 442–445.

Kaufman, J., & Zigler, E. (1987). Do abused children become abusive parents? *American Journal of Orthopsychiatry, 57*, 186.

Kempe, C. H., Silverman, F. N., Steele, B. F., Droegemueller, P. W., & Silver, H.K. (1962). The battered child syndrome. *Journal of the American Medical Association, 181*, 17–24.

Lyons, T. J., & Oates, R. K. (1993). Falling out of bed: A relatively benign occurrence. *Pediatrics, 92*, 125–127.

Meadow, R. (1977). Munchausen syndrome by proxy: The hinterland of child abuse. *Lancet, 2*, 343–345.

Oates, R. K. (1979). Battered children and their families. *New Doctor, 14*, 15–18.

Oates, R. K. (1986). *Child abuse and neglect: What happens eventually?* New York: Brunner/Mazel.

Oates, R. K. (1993). Three do's and three don'ts for expert witnesses. *Child Abuse and Neglect,* *17,* 571–572.

Oates, R. K., & Bross, D. L. (1995). What have we learned about treating child physical abuse: A literature review of the last decade. *Child Abuse and Neglect, 119,* 463–473.

Oates, R. K., Peacock, A., & Forrest, D. (1984). The development of abused children. *Developmental Medicine and Child Neurology, 26,* 649–656.

Oates, R. K., Gray, J., Schweitzer, L., Kempe, R. S., & Harmon, R. J. (1995). A therapeutic preschool for abused children: The keepsafe project. *Child Abuse and Neglect, 19,* 1379–1386.

Olds, D. L., Henderson, C. R., & Kitzman, H. (1994). Does prenatal and infancy home nurse visitation have ensuring effects on qualities of parental care giving and child health at 25 to 50 months of life? *Pediatrics, 93,* 89–98.

Olds, D. L., Eckenrode, J., Henderson, C. R., Kitzman, H., Powers, J., Cole, R., Sidora, J., Morris, P., Pettit, L. M., & Luckey, D. (1997). Long-term effects of home visitation on maternal life course and child abuse and neglect: Fifteen year follow-up of a randomized trial. *Journal of the American Medical Association, 278,* 637–643.

Opie, I., & Opie, P. (1951). *The Oxford dictionary of nursery rhymes.* London: Oxford University Press.

Perez, C., & Widom, C. S. (1994). Childhood victimization and long-term intellectual and academic outcomes. *Child Abuse and Neglect, 18,* 617–633.

Prodgers, A. (1984). Psychopathology of the physically abusing parent: A comparison with the borderline syndrome. *Child Abuse and Neglect, 8,* 411–424.

Schnaps, Y., Frond, M., Rand, Y., & Tirosh, M. (1981). The chemically abused child. *Pediatrics, 68,* 119–121.

Rosenberg, D. (1987). Web of deceit: A literature review of Munchausen syndrome by proxy. *Child Abuse and Neglect, 11,* 547–563.

Tardieu, A. (1868). Etude medico-legale sur l'infanticide. Paris: J.B. Bailliere et Fils.

Woolley, P. V., & Evans, W. A. (1955). Significance of skeletal lesions in infants resembling those of traumatic origin. *Journal of the American Medical Association, 158,* 539–543.

Wodarski, J., Kurtz, P., Gaudin, J., & Howing, P. (1990). Maltreatment and the school-age child: Major academic, socioemotional, and adaptive outcome. *Social Work, 35,* 506–513.

9

Child Neglect

Arthur H. Green[†]

Description of the Problem

Neglect is by far the most common form of maltreatment. Children reported to have been neglected outnumbered those who were physically
abused by 15 to 1 in New York City in 1996. Despite the fact that neglect is
so much more prevalent than physical abuse in our country, it has received
much less attention from child-care professionals, child psychiatrists and
psychologists, researchers, and social agencies. Neglect is often less obvious than physical or sexual abuse, and it is more difficult to measure and
define. According to the New York State Child Protective Services Act of
1973, neglect is legally defined as the failure of the parent or guardian to
supply the child with adequate food, clothing, shelter, medical care, and
supervision (see the following section on legal issues).

In many cases, neglect appears to be unintentional and closely associated with substandard living conditions in impoverished inner-city areas.
Polansky, Hally, and Polansky (1975) defined child neglect as "a condition
in which a caretaker responsible for the child either deliberately or by
extraordinary inattentiveness permits the child to experience avoidable
present suffering and/or fails to provide one or more of the ingredients
generally deemed essential for developing a person's physical, intellec-

†Deceased.

Arthur H. Green • Department of Psychiatry, Columbia University College of Physicians
and Surgeons, Presbyterian Hospital, New York, New York 10032.

Case Studies in Family Violence, Second Edition, edited by Ammerman and Hersen. Kluwer
Academic / Plenum Publishers, New York, 2000.

tual, and emotional capacities." In broader terms, neglect might refer to the failure to provide the child with adequate parenting to ensure the realization of his potential for normal physical and psychological growth and development. Neglectful practices might include inadequate parenting, interrupting of maternal care, affective and social deprivation, inappropriate or premature expectations of the child, parental detachment, indifference, overstimulation, and failure to anticipate or respond to the child's needs at specific changes of development (Green, 1980). Neglect frequently involves "sins of omission," whereas abuse entails "sins of commission." It is clear that neglect, more than physical abuse, is subject to wide interpretation and is more influenced by community standards of child care. According to the New York State Central Registry for Child Abuse, 51,695 reports of neglect were made in 1996, compared with 3,807 reports of physical abuse. In 1978, almost two decades earlier, there were 19,865 reports of neglect and 6,442 reports of physical abuse. The increase in neglect during this period is striking and might reflect better reporting and heightened public awareness of child maltreatment. However, there is an apparent real increase in neglect in New York City because of larger numbers of homeless families and those living in substandard welfare hotels. At the same time, the volume of neglect reporting has been swelled by increasing numbers of mothers testing positive for drugs at the time of childbirth. These women are deemed neglectful because their infants are often addicted in utero and their substance abuse places them at risk for the maltreatment of the children.

This increase in the reporting of maltreatment has also been documented on the national level. The National Center on Child Abuse and Neglect (1997) documented 2 million reports alleging the maltreatment of 3 million children in 1995, while 1,726,649 children were reported as maltreated in 1984. Approximately 55% of the cases reported in 1995 involved neglect, 25% involved physical abuse, 13% involved sexual abuse, and 10% involved emotional maltreatment.

Yuan and Struckman-Johnson (1991), using American Public Welfare Association 1988 statistics, reported that nearly two-thirds of all children placed in substitute care because of maltreatment are neglected, with a further 16% placed for reasons of parental incapacity.

Characteristics of Neglecting Parents

A wide variety of psychological and social deviancy has been attributed to neglecting parents. Pavenstedt (1967) described typical personality characteristics of neglecting parents encountered in disorganized lower-class families during a community intervention project. Many of these parents were psychotic, alcoholic, or antisocial. Most of them had a previous history of deprivation and neglect during their own childhood, and they tended to repeat those patterns of deprivation in their own families. They were often too overwhelmed to recognize the needs of their children, and they were unable to provide them with adequate adult role models. These parents displayed poor object relationships, owing to a basic mistrust of others, and exhibited an impaired self-concept. They were also limited in language development and abstract thinking and were, therefore, action-oriented and impulsive. They failed to provide their children with sufficient physical and verbal stimulation and rarely played with them. They often left their children alone or with the nearest available neighbor and neglected their health care. They were frequently aggressive with their children in an unpredictable manner. Giavannoni and Billingsley (1970) studied neglecting mothers in a poverty-level population, using a control group of adequate mothers. The neglecting mothers had more children, were less often married, experienced greater stress, had poorer relationships with their extended families, and were poorer than their adequate counterparts. Polanski, DeSaiz, Wing, and Patton (1968) studied child neglect in a rural setting. They described five types of neglecting mothers: the apathetic–futile, the impulse-ridden, the mentally retarded, the reactively depressed, and the psychotic. Polansky, Chambers, Buttenweiser, and Williams (1981) replicated these findings in a subsequent study of neglect in an urban setting. Most of the neglecting mothers fit into the "apathy–futility syndrome" characterized by a pervasive feeling of futility, emotional numbness, clinging, and loneliness in interpersonal relationships, incompetence in many areas of living, passive-aggressive personality traits, stubborn negativism, verbal inaccessibility, and the tendency to generate the same sense of futility in others. Green (1976) compared neglecting, abusing, and normal control mothers from a similar poverty background on the basis of their responses to a structured interview. The neglecting mothers reported the highest incidence of unplanned pregnancies and the absence of a husband or boyfriend at home. They also demonstrated the highest rates of alcoholism, psychosis, and chronic physical illness. Similar findings were reported by Bath and Haapala (1993), who found that neglectful families, in contrast to abusive ones, were poorer, more reliant on public income, more likely to be headed by a single parent, and more likely to have medical, mental health, and substance abuse problems.

Ethier, Lacharite, and Couture (1995) reported that neglecting mothers exhibited higher levels of parental stress and depression than non-neglecting mothers. The neglecting mothers also experienced more frequent out-of-home placements and physical and sexual abuse.

Galdston (1968) differentiated two types of neglecting parents on the basis of their defensive organization. The first type uses projection as a major defense and perceives the child as a symbol of their own undesirable attributes. This type is similar to child abusers, who also use projection, but instead of striking out at the children, they withdraw or delegate the care of the child to someone else. The second type uses denial as the preferred defense, and they do not bond with their children and are unable to empathize with them. They have great difficulty in caring for and feeding the children.

In summary, neglect is associated with prominent psychiatric, physical, social, and cognitive impairment in the parents, which often are embedded in poverty and substandard living conditions. It is likely that neglect is the end result of a combination of these interacting factors, which interfere with the normal processes of parenting. Family disorganization and the lack of material resources further undermine parental functioning by diminishing the availability of child rearing support systems.

Characteristics of Neglected Children

The harmful sequelae of neglect and maternal deprivation in infants and young children living in institutions has been described in the pioneering studies of Bowlby (1951), Goldfarb (1945), Spitz (1945), and many others. These children exhibited physical and developmental retardation and cognitive impairment, especially in the area of speech and language. They were also impaired in their ability to form human attachments. The unavailability of a consistent caretaker in the institutional setting was felt to be the cause of these symptoms.

Subsequent studies by Coleman and Provence (1957) and Prugh and Harlow (1962) demonstrated that similar types of deprivation leading to impaired development might be encountered as a result of inadequate maternal care in children living at home. The most common sequelae of neglect in these children, as described by Marans and Lourie (1967), Malone (1967), Rutter (1972) and Green (1980) are pathological object relationships and difficulties in attachments. These result from maternal unavailability and multiple substitute caretakers, diminished initiative and enjoyment in play due to a lack of maternal support and of play materials, speech and language delays caused by inadequate verbal stimulation, poor self-care, and accident proneness due to physical neglect, depression, apathy, and withdrawal. McCrone, Egeland, Kalkoske, and Carlson (1994) proposed that maltreated and neglected children acquire internal working models of themselves as unworthy and of others as unavailable, which interfere with subsequent relationships. Many neglected children exhibit poor impulse control and conduct disorders, which may ultimately lead to delinquency and antisocial behavior (Polansky *et al.*, 1981; Manly, Cicchetti, & Barnett, 1994). Shields, Cicchetti, and Ryan (1994) reported that neglected and abused children were deficient in behavioral and emotional self-regulation, which had a negative impact on their social competence.

Numerous studies have documented intellectual impairment in neglected youngsters. Polansky *et al.* (1981) reported significantly lower IQ scores in neglected children compared with normal controls. The IQs of these children were positively correlated with the mother's Childhood Level of Living Scale (CLL), which measures the quality of child care in the family. Kendall-Tackett and Eckenrode (1996) described greater impairment in academic performance and more suspensions and disciplinary problems in neglected children than in nonneglected controls. Sandgrund, Gaines, and Green (1974) found that the mean IQs of neglected children (79.97) were 11 points below the normal controls and were not significantly different from those of a comparison group of abused children. Twenty percent of the neglected children were retarded, with IQs below 70.

Green, Voeller, Gaines, and Kubie (1981) reported significant neurological impairment in these same neglected children on the basis of pediatric neurological examination, including EEGs and perceptual motor testing designed to elicit soft signs of CNS impairment. The neurological deficits were attributed to poor prenatal and infant care, abnormal (insufficient or excessive) sensory stimulation, poor nutrition, and inadequate medical care. Neglected children, like their parents, are physically and cognitively comprised and exhibit developmental and neurological impairment. These deficits may be attributed to insufficient or inappropriate parenting during the critical periods of infancy and early childhood.

Case Description

Alan B., currently 13 years old, was referred to the Family Center (a treatment program for maltreated children and their families) when he was 5 years 10 months old and in the first grade. The school guidance counselor, who made the referral, noted Alan was disruptive in the classroom and bothered other children. He stole from these children and appeared to be restless and hyperactive. His physical appearance was often dirty and unkempt. Alan would not follow the classroom routines and rarely did schoolwork. Most striking was Alan's tendency to eat garbage and nonedible substances. Alan's mother, Miss Mary B., noticed that the child was often accident-prone (e.g., he stepped on nails in the house and he was often bruised when returning from play). He once hit himself on the head while playing with a broomstick. Mary informed the social worker that her refrigerator had not been working for the past 4 months and she kept some food on the windowsill, but Alan had to go to his grandparents' apartment for such items as milk and juice.

Mary was abandoned by Alan's father 1 week before he was born. They had known each other for a year and a half. Mary said that she wanted to have a baby, but when her boyfriend deserted she had thought about giving Alan up for adoption but then had changed her mind and decided to keep him. Alan was born after an uncomplicated pregnancy and delivery. The gestation was 36 weeks and he weighed 6 pounds, 6 ounces at birth. He developed pneumonia shortly after birth and remained in the hospital for 2 weeks. Mary was 34 years old when Alan was born. She described Alan as an active baby who sat up at 5 months and walked at 13 months. He spoke his first words at 15 months and began to use sentences when he was between 18 and 24 months. He was toilet-trained at 2 1/2 years.

When Alan was 2, he was hospitalized for 3 days with asthma. After his discharge from the hospital, Mary was provided with homemaking services because her difficulties in caring for Alan and managing the household became obvious. Alan was hospitalized once again for asthma at age 4. Following acceptance into the program, Alan was seen on a weekly basis for play therapy, and Mary was provided with child guidance sessions and psychotherapy. During this intervention, Alan frequently ran away from his mother. After a year, treatment was discontinued because Mary failed to keep her appointments and did not bring Alan for his therapy sessions.

Two years later, when Alan was 8 1/2 years old, Mary returned to the program to get help for Alan and herself. The presenting problems included Alan's leaving the house without permission and staying out late, his refusal to eat food cooked by his mother, oppositional behavior at home, and Mary's perception that she had little or no control over the child. Alan was also stealing money from his mother.

Alan was attending a class for emotionally disturbed children at this time. The guidance counselor noted problems with lateness and absenteeism, as well as Alan's arriving at school dirty and without his homework. Alan's oppositional behavior intensified to the point where he would talk back to his mother, curse her, even hit her when he did not get his way. He often ran away from his mother when they were walking on the street together, and he would roam the streets at night. Additional problems surfaced, such as frequent nightmares depicting violence, sporadic nighttime enuresis, anxiety around sexual issues, poor grooming, and academic and behavioral difficulties in school, where Alan was noted to be very distractible. Alan also experimented with lighting matches but denied any fire setting. Attendance at the program improved, although Mary was still chronically late for her appointments.

Mary B. is the third oldest of five children and was 39 years old when she was referred to our program for the first time. Her parents are still living. Her father (age 80) is a retired bookkeeper, and her mother (age 71) sells cosmetics on a part-time basis. Mary and Alan live in an apartment in the same building as her parents, who often help care for Alan. Mary's sister Janet is 4 years her senior. She is married with two children and lives in the neighborhood. Mary's brother Don is 2 years older and is a successful accountant. He is married with four children, and Alan often stays with him on holidays. Another brother, Bill, is married with one child and lives nearby, and the youngest brother died in Vietnam. Despite their proximity, Mary has little contact with her siblings.

Mary presents as an anxious, highly disorganized person who often speaks in a tangential, confusing manner, so that it is often difficult to follow her train of thought. She had been a quiet, rather timid young woman who had lived with her parents and was employed as a secretary until she was 24. At that time she began to exhibit some psychiatric difficulties, which appeared to be associated with breaking up with a boyfriend because her parents disapproved of him. She developed delusional ideas concerning people reading her thoughts and trying to influence her. She threatened to kill her father and talked about suicide. She was admitted to a psychiatric hospital at that time and was given the diagnosis of acute paranoid schizophrenia. Following this hospitalization, she had a series of part-time jobs, but her primary source of income was public assistance. Mary has taken part-time housecleaning and laundry jobs while having trouble managing these tasks in her own home. Mary's social contacts are very limited. She relates primarily to Alan and her elderly parents. She does not socialize with men, and she has few female acquaintances.

Mary demonstrates love and concern toward Alan, as well as a desire to improve her parenting skills; however, she has had chronic difficulty with understanding his needs and relating to him in an appropriate manner. She has been both neglectful and overly intrusive, and her expectations are often so high that she has difficulty rewarding Alan's progress and good behaviors without simultaneously criticizing other behaviors. Mary needs constant guidance in setting limits with Alan, reinforcing and praising good behaviors, meeting his basic needs, and keeping appropriate boundaries. For years, Alan and Mary slept in the same bed or on separate floor pads next to one another, and Mary has resisted suggestions to provide Alan with his own room.

Mary has major difficulties with her finances. Her public assistance has often been suspended for unclear reasons, and she has needed constant help in having this reinstated. She also requires assistance with budgeting, home management, and negotiating with her landlord about housing problems and the constant need for repairs in her apartment. Mary tends to be chronically late for her appointments and frequently misses them completely. Her attendance improves when she experiences crises or unusual stresses.

Medical Issues

Medical issues play an important role in child neglect in that physical and psychiatric illness in the parent is often a crucial factor in the initiation and sustaining of neglecting child rearing practices, which in turn pose a danger to the child's health and normal development. Parents with chronic medical illness are often depleted in energy and are unable to assume the burdens of child care. They are likely to become depressed or self-absorbed, which makes it difficult for them to respond adequately to the needs of their children. Their failure to provide effective supervision increases the risk of accidental injury to the child, who may sustain burns or injuries due to falls. Unsupervised children are also prone to ingesting household poisons and medications. Children who are inadequately clothed or fed are at risk for illness and impaired physical development. Neglected children who become ill are unlikely to receive prompt medical attention, or the recommended medical treatment is not likely to be implemented. Neglectful parents also fail to provide routine pediatric care for their children and rely on emergency rooms in case of illness. Neglected children often fail to obtain the required immunizations. Some neglected children who are not adequately nourished may develop the nonorganic failure-to-thrive syndrome. It is therefore imperative that all family members in a neglectful household receive medical examinations if these were not recently obtained. The adults and children should be provided with their own internist and pediatrician, respectively.

Medical services were provided to the B. family immediately after their acceptance in our treatment program. Alan was referred to the pediatric outpatient clinic at Presbyterian Hospital, in which the Family Center is located. We were initially concerned with Alan's ingestion of nonedible substances, such as garbage and crayons, which placed him at risk for lead poisoning. The B.s' apartment was inspected for evidence of toxic substances, such as lead, which might have been ingested by Alan. Lead levels in Alan's blood were determined and found to be within normal limits. Alan's pica subsided rapidly after he and his mother entered the program, and he was assigned to a pediatrician who would follow him regularly. Alan was provided with an inhaler and medication for his asthma. Mary was referred to an internist, who acted as her family physician. Even more important for Mary was the regular monitoring of her psychiatric status by the clinical director of the Family Center, who is a psychiatrist. This was the first time that Alan and Mary had had regular medical care. During his participation in the program, Alan was treated for such conditions as impetigo, shingles, poison ivy, strabismus, and an abscessed tooth, which had to be extracted.

Legal Issues

According to the New York State Child Protective Services Act of 1973, the legal definition of child neglect is the following: A "neglected" child is a child under 18 years of age, impaired as a result of failure of his parent or other person legally responsible for his care to exercise a minimum degree of care (1) in supplying the child with adequate food, clothing, shelter, education, medical or surgical care, though financially able to do so or offered financial or other reasonable means to do so; (2) in providing the child with proper supervision or guardianship; (3) by reasonably inflicting or allowing to be inflected harm or a substantial risk thereof, including the infliction of excessive corporal punishment; (4) by using a drug or drugs; (5) by using alcoholic beverages to the extent that he loses self-control of his actions; or (6) by any other acts of a similarly serious nature requiring the aid of the family court. A child is also to be considered maltreated when, under 18 years of age, he has been abandoned by his parents (or whoever else is legally responsible for his care).

Reporting Child Neglect

From 1964 to 1968, all 50 states, the District of Columbia, the Virgin Islands, and Guam enacted child maltreatment reporting laws. Physicians are specifically designated as mandated reporters in most states, along with other professionals, such as osteopaths, dentists, chiropractors, nurses, hospital administrators, psychologists, social workers, pharmacists, and religious healers. All reporting laws provide immunity from criminal and civil liability for mandated reporters. Most states have laws that include penalties for nonreporting. Friends, relatives, and neighbors are also encouraged to report suspected cases of maltreatment, but these nonmandated reporters are not required to identify themselves.

Most states have reporting systems that use one toll-free number for reports from anywhere in the state. These reports are then transmitted to the local child protective agency, which is obligated to initiate investigation within 24 hours.

The psychiatrist or mental health professional treating a member of a family in which physical abuse or neglect takes place is required by law to report such maltreatment, as is any other professional. Recurrence of abuse or neglect by parents who are receiving help for previous maltreatment must also be reported by a therapist. The reporting laws take precedence over the privileged doctor–patient relationship so that confidentiality cannot be maintained. When maltreatment takes place, the legal rights of the child take precedence over those of the parents. The potential negative impact of the reporting laws on the therapeutic relationship can be minimized if the therapist discusses his obligation to report maltreatment at the beginning of any intervention with abusing or neglecting parents.

Investigation

The child protection agency, usually located in the county or state department of social services, is authorized by law to investigate reported cases of abuse or neglect to determine the validity of allegations. The protective services caseworker carries out an intake procedure in order to obtain information about the suspected maltreatment. The worker checks the central registry for previous reports of abuse or neglect involving the child and his family. The worker may also interview neighbors, relatives, schools, and other agencies to gather relevant information about the family.

If the presence of maltreatment is confirmed by the investigation, the child may be protected in one of several ways. Depending on the severity of the case, the child may be hospitalized, may remain at home under the supervision of the child protective agency, which may provide the family with supportive services, or can be placed in a shelter or foster home on an emergency basis. If the report of maltreatment cannot be validated, the case is closed and the report is expunged from the central registry.

Legal Rights of the Child

The allegedly maltreated child is entitled to representation in all legal proceedings. Many states require that a special guardian, or guardian *ad litem*, be appointed by the court to protect the child's interest. He acts as the child's advocate and ensures that the court receives all relevant data. He also gathers relevant information concerning the causes, nature, and extent of the maltreatment, and ensures that the child's interests are protected by law.

Legal Rights of the Parents

The parents or any other alleged perpetrator of maltreatment against a child must be informed of their legal rights by the local authority. These include the right to receive written notice of one's record in the child abuse registry and of court orders and petitions filed, the right to a court hearing prior to removal of the child, the right to appeal child protective case determinations, and the right to refuse agency services unless mandated by a court. The files in the central registry pertaining to the alleged maltreatment should be kept in strictest confidence to prevent unauthorized disclosure of identifying information concerning the parents.

The Judicial Process in the Juvenile or Family Court

A pretrial conference may be held prior to any hearing in order to decide which reports and evidence will be admissible. The judge and the attorneys for all parties participate in this conference, which is usually successful in settling the majority of cases by some form of consent decree, in which the parent agrees to cooperate with the child protective agency.

If the pretrial conference is unsuccessful in settling a case, an adjudicatory or "fact-finding" hearing takes place. This is the "trial" stage of the proceedings, in which the allegations of abuse and neglect are examined and argued. The judge makes his final decision about whether allegations are confirmed. If the allegations are proven, the judge makes a finding of abuse or neglect.

A dispositional hearing follows the adjudication. At this hearing, the child protective agency managing the case presents a plan of intervention to the courts and the parents, outlining the conditions and arrangements designed to protect the child and a time schedule within which the plan is to be implemented. The dispositional order may require counseling, psychiatric treatment, or provision of social services for the parents. In case of placement of the child outside of the home, a visitation schedule should be included in the case plan. Once the plan is agreed upon, the court should ensure parental compliance by periodically reviewing their participation in the rehabilitative process.

Social and Family Issues

Poverty

The concrete aspects of poverty (i.e., lack of money, substandard and overcrowded living conditions, high crime rate, family disorganization) exert a stressful impact on families and parental functioning. While they might trigger the onset of abuse, it is likely that a background of poverty is more intimately related to neglect. Many of the substandard living conditions encountered in our decaying inner cities are considered neglectful by middle-class standards and might be used by child protection caseworkers to confirm otherwise equivocal allegations of neglect. When these impoverished parents are unable to provide adequate food, clothing, and shelter for their children, it might not be under their voluntary control. Many of these "involuntary" neglectful families are headed by overwhelmed and depleted single mothers without adequate support systems. They cannot rely on spouses or family members for child rearing assistance or emotional support. Homeless families and families living in shelters are also exposing their children to neglectful and noxious environments through no fault of their own.

Substance Abuse

The current epidemic of drug addition in the inner cities is more directly related to neglect of children. Kelleher, Chaffin, Hollenberg, and Fischer (1994), using a community-based sample of over 11,000 parents, found that 51% of parents who neglected their children had a DSM-III diagnosis of a substance abuse disorder. Chaffin, Kelleher, and Hollenberg (1996), in a prospective, longitudinal study, reported the impact of various psychiatric disorders on the onset of maltreatment. A psychiatric diagnosis of substance abuse was the most powerfully associated with the new cases of abuse and neglect appearing in a 1-year period.

Substance-abusing parents are not likely to consistently recognize and respond to the needs of their children. In addition, the children are at risk for exposure to other drug-taking adults. Women who abuse substances during pregnancy inflect medical damage on the fetus. In some states, they are automatically charged with neglect if they test positive for drugs at the time of childbirth. Infants born to these addicted mothers become addicted themselves in utero and may be born with withdrawal symptoms. Similarly, an actively alcoholic mother may give birth to a child with fetal alcohol syndrome.

Infants exposed to drugs in utero frequently suffer from prematurity, low birth weight, hypersensitivity, hypertonicity, and abnormal sleep patterns and they are often difficult to soothe or handle. These behaviors make them vulnerable to maltreatment (Kelley, Walsh, & Thompson, 1991). These difficult-to-rear children create high levels of stress in their mothers or caretakers. Kelley (1992) reported that 40% of drug-exposed infants were placed in foster care due to maternal neglect or abuse.

Assessment of Psychopathology

Since a high incidence of psychopathology and cognitive impairment has been demonstrated in neglecting families, the children and their parents should receive in-depth psychiatric evaluations designed to assess their psychopathology and document the presence of a psychiatric disorder. Exploration of the child's play, fantasy life, conflicts, and defenses will provide information about psychodynamic issues and behavioral symptoms that will assist in designing an intervention strategy for the child. Careful assessment of the parent's psychopathology, coping skills and parenting ability will provide clues for treating and supporting the parent. The psychiatric evaluation of the neglected child should be supplemented by psychological testing, which will yield additional information about how the child perceives himself, his family, and the environment and will identify the extent of any cognitive impairment.

Assessment of Alan

Psychiatric Evaluation

Alan is an appealing, "waiflike" 5-year-11-month-old boy with a dirty face and unkempt appearance. He is fully oriented and makes good contact with the examiner. Speech is coherent and goal-oriented but is somewhat pressured. There is no evidence of a thinking disorder, delusions, or hallucinations. Alan is very distractible and frequently breaks off contact as the interview progresses in order to explore the various games and toys in the examiner's office. He requires periodic refocusing during evaluation. When asked about school, where he is a first grader, he reports that the teacher says that he is a "bad boy" because he talks too much and gets out of his seat. He admits to punching kids in the classroom "if they get rough with me." Alan reluctantly acknowledges eating crayons and food from the garbage can in school because "I'm hungry and there isn't enough food at home." When asked about running away from home, Alan states that he wants to play with a friend in the neighborhood and runs off to see the boy because his mother won't let him out of the house. Alan realizes that this makes his mother "sad," and this makes him feel like a "bad boy." When he is away from home for a long time, he thinks of his mother looking for him; then he is afraid to return home because he might get a "spanking." Alan is unable to sustain interest in any of the play materials for more than a few minutes. He puts the family dolls on the roof of the playhouse, leaves them there, and is apparently unable to engage in symbolic play. His figure drawings are primitive undifferentiated stick figures. His mood is labile and ranges from overexcitement to boredom and moderate depression. His affect is constricted and shallow. He goes to open the door from time to time to peer out into the corridor to see if his mother is around. In the cognitive sphere, Alan is unable to read. He appears to be of at least low average to average intelligence.

DSM-III-R Diagnosis

Axis I	Attention-Deficit Hyperactivity Disorder
	Pica
	Oppositional-Defiant Disorder
Axis II	None
Axis III	Asthma
Axis IV	Psychosocial Stressors: Mother with chronic psychiatric illness.
	Disorganized and neglectful home.
Severity	4—Severe
Axis V [T]	Current GAF 65
	Highest GAF past year 70

Psychological Assessment

Alan was initially tested at the age of 6 years 2 months, shortly after being admitted to our program. On the WISC-R, his verbal IQ was 95, his performance IQ was 105, with a full scale IQ of 100. On the Wide Range Achievement Test he achieved a grade level of 1.7. In academic achievement he received a 1.9 grade equivalent in word recognition, 1.7 in spelling, and 0.9 in arithmetic. He scored less than 1.1 in accuracy, less than 1.0 in comprehension on the Gilmore Oral Reading Test, and 99 (age equivalent 6 years 1 month) on the Peabody Picture Vocabulary Test. In general, this hyperactive and distractible youngster fell within the average range of intellectual functioning.

When Alan returned to the program 2 years later at age 8½, he showed a deterioration in intellectual functioning. On the WISC-R he received a verbal IQ score of 86, a performance IQ of 84, and a full scale IQ score of 84. The WISC-R scaled scores were as follows:

Verbal Tests		Performance Tests	
Information	6	Picture Completion	13
Similarities	3	Picture Arrangement	4
Arithmetic	7	Block Design	5
Vocabulary	11	Object Assembly	8
Comprehension Span	14		
Digit Span	8		

Alan was in the low average range of intellectual functioning and his responses in different areas varied widely. He was above the norm in his ability to distinguish essential from unessential visual details, in his ability to find solutions to problematic social situations, and in his vocabulary and verbal fluency. Alan did very poorly on tasks involving factual information, verbal conceptual thinking, the sequential analysis and understanding of social events, and the analysis and synthesis of visual patterns in terms of their parts. His academic achievement was at a second-grade level, commensurate with his intellectual functioning. Reading was at a 1.9 grade level, spelling at a 2.4, and arithmetic at 2.6.

On the Bender-Gestalt Test of perceptual motor development, Alan's reproductions of designs contained numerous errors, including errors in integration and angulation, as well as rotations of designs. His human figure drawings were oversimplified and had peculiar characteristics. Overall graphomotor response was suggestive of both neurological and emotional difficulties. Alan achieved a social age equivalent of 7 years on the Vineland. Overall social adaptation fell into the borderline to low average range.

The projective material revealed a very confused, impulse-ridden, extremely anxious youngster who feels unstable, inadequate, and incapable of dealing with the world in an effective manner. Alan is preoccupied with his inner promptings and may perseverate on them, yet he lacks any insight; he is likely to misinterpret situations and respond inappropriately. He also has little understanding of interpersonal relationships, especially with his father, though he associates such relationships with bad feelings, including anger and sadness. There are also some indications of premature sexual feelings and preoccupations. Finally, Alan seems to feel both physically and emotionally deprived. His anxious, impulse-ridden behavior may stem from feelings of internal emptiness, hunger, and vulnerability.

Alan's most recent psychological testing at the age of 11 revealed an increase in his performance IQ to 98, a 14-point gain, while his verbal IQ remained virtually the same, at 85. His full scale IQ was 90. However, Alan failed to make any progress in academic skill since the previous testing. He was in the lowest percentile of the population in word recognition, spelling, and arithmetic, and he displayed multiple areas of moderate learning weakness with no compensatory strengths. He was weak in abstract thinking and acquired learning, with poor visual memory. In writing and reading he manifested rotational, directional, and sequential reversals of letters. His visual perception remained impaired and immature. Decoding was so laborious that the easiest reading comprehension passage could be accomplished only with great help. At the time of this evaluation Alan still retained the characteristics of an attention deficit disorder.

Assessment of Mary

Psychiatric Evaluation

Mary is a shabbily dressed 40-year-old woman who appears anxious and disorganized and considerably older than her stated age. She is fully oriented and relates to the examiner in a cooperative but rather distant manner. Her speech is coherent but occasionally tangential and rambling. Although there is no evidence of an organized delusional system, Mary displays paranoid ideas of reference pertaining to people on the street who do not like her or who talk about her behind her back. As a result, she usually stays by herself. Mary occasionally hears voices when no one is present; however, the content of these auditory hallucinations is benign. When asked about her work history, Mary admitted that she did not feel capable of having a regular job since her "nervous breakdown" several years ago. Since that time she obtained sporadic employment as a part-time clerical worker or housecleaner. She feels that the pressures of a full-time job would be too stressful for her. Mary has no real friends; she has a few real acquaintances but spends most of her time with her parents, who live in her building. Mary's affect is constricted but not grossly inappropriate. Her mood is moderately depressed. Her memory is intact, and her intellectual functioning appears to be in the low normal range. Her thinking is very concrete.

DSM-III-R Diagnosis

Axis I	Schizophrenic Disorder, Residual Type
Axis II	None
Axis III	None
Axis IV	Psychosocial Stressors: Problems with collecting welfare payments. Problems not handling her child.
Severity	3—Moderate
Axis V [T]	Current GAF 60
	[T] Highest GAF past year 65

Treatment Options

Intervention in cases of child neglect should be based on the psychopathology of the neglected child and his parents, on an assessment of their unfulfilled needs, and on the determination of the neglectful and pathological caretaking practices compromising the child's development.

In the case of Alan and Mary, Alan required individual counseling/psychotherapy to deal with his feelings of deprivation and damage, his symptoms of pica and hyperactivity, and his oppositional tendencies. In addition, he required psychoeducational assistance to help him cope with his numerous learning difficulties. It is clear that such intervention would be minimally effective without modifying Mary's neglectful and ineffective parenting. This, in turn, would require a combination of counseling and individual psychotherapy for Mary, vigorous casework intervention to help Mary negotiate the welfare system and improve the home environment, and parenting education to help Mary respond more effectively to Alan's physical and emotional needs. Both child and mother were also candidates for psychopharmacological intervention. Alan might have benefitted from Ritalin, but Mary would not agree to this plan. Mary did, however, consent to our recommendation that she receive a tranquilizer, Haldol, in order to stabilize her psychological functioning and to minimize the impact of her anxiety and disorganization.

Mary was able to benefit from our interventions and made some progress in managing the household and improving her parenting of Alan. However, renewed conflicts with her landlord and an abrupt termination of her Medicaid payments intensified her anxiety and disorganization. Furthermore, Alan's entering adolescence created additional stress for Mary, because it became more difficult for her to supervise him adequately and monitor his school attendance. Mary began to miss many of her therapy appointments, and Alan's tendency to wander away from home and to stay away from school increased. At this point, Alan was referred to a residential treatment center that could provide him with structure, supervision, therapy, special education, and socialization experiences. The latter, of course, was less available in his home environment. The residential setting would also provide Alan with positive adult role models. The final treatment goals with Mary were designed to help her to accept Alan's entry into residential treatment and to assist her in working through the separation from her son.

More intact neglecting families manifesting marked disturbances in family interactions might benefit from a family systems approach, with the use of family therapy.

Summary and Conclusions

Neglect is by far the most common form of maltreatment, having a more severe impact on the child's cognitive and psychological functioning than physical or sexual abuse. Neglectful parents are likely to be psychologically and physically compromised. The psychological deviancy and psychopathology associated with neglect is clearly described in the case presentation. Environmental factors may have a more profound effect on neglect than on the other forms of maltreatment.

Intervention with neglecting families should be based upon a careful assessment of environmental stressors, individual psychopathology, and the deficiencies in the family system. The intervention should be designed to strengthen the family functioning by (a) reducing the environmental stress through provision of concrete services and outreach and consolidating support systems, (b) dealing with the individual psychopathology of the parents and children by means of individual psychotherapy and psychopharmacological agents when necessary, (c) correcting deviations in the family system through a family therapy approach, and (d) strengthening parenting skills by providing parental education. While the general thrust of intervention is aimed at preserving and strengthening the family unit, in some cases temporary or permanent placement of the children might be necessary.

Acknowledgment

The author is indebted to Pat Coupe, M.S., for her valuable assistance in the preparation of the case description.

References

Bath, H. I., & Haapala, D. A. (1993). Intensive family preservation services with abused and neglected children: An examination of group differences. *Child Abuse & Neglect, 17,* 213–225.

Bowlby, J. (1951). Maternal care and mental health. *Bulletin of the World Health Organization, 31,* 355–533.

Chaffin, M., Kelleher, K., & Hollenberg, J. (1996). Onset of physical abuse and neglect: Psychiatric, substance abuse, and social risk factors from prospective community data. *Child Abuse & Neglect, 20,* 191–203.

Coleman, R., & Provence, S. A. (1957). Developmental retardation (hospitalism) in infants living in families. *Pediatrics, 19,* 285–292.

Ethier, L. S., Lacharite, C., & Couture, G. (1995). Childhood adversity, parental stress, and depression of negligent mothers. *Child Abuse & Neglect, 19,* 619–632.

Galdston, R. (1968). Dysfunctions of parenting: The battered child, the neglected child, the exploited child. In J. G. Howells (Ed.), *Modern perspectives of international child psychiatry* (pp. 571–586). Edinburgh: Oliver and Boyd.

Giovannoni, J., & Billingsley, A. (1970). Child neglect among the poor: A study of parental adequacy in families of three ethnic groups. *Child Welfare, 49,* 196–204.

Goldfarb, W. (1945). Psychological privation in infancy and subsequent adjustment. *American Journal of Orthopsychiatry, 102,* 247–255.

Green, A. H. (1980). *Child maltreatment*. New York: Jason Aronson.

Green, A. H., Voeller, K., Gaines, R., & Kubie, J. (1981). Neurological impairment in battered children. *Child Abuse & Neglect, 5*, 129–134.

Green, A. H. (1976). A psychodynamic approach to the study and treatment of child-abusing parents. *Journal of the American Academy of Child Psychiatry, 15*, 414–429.

Kelleher, K., Chaffin, M., Hollenberg, J., & Fischer, E. (1994). Alcohol and drug disorders among physically abusive and neglectful parents in a community-based sample. *American Journal of Public Health, 84*, 1586–1590.

Kelley, S. J. (1992). Parenting stress and child maltreatment in drug-exposed children. *Child Abuse & Neglect, 16*, 317–328.

Kelley, S. J., Walsh, J. H., & Thompson, K. (1991). Prenatal exposure to cocaine: Birth outcomes, health problems, and child neglect. *Pediatric Nursing, 17*, 130–135.

Kendall-Tackett, K. A., & Eckenrode, J. (1996). The effects of neglect on academic achievement and disciplinary problems: A developmental perspective. *Child Abuse & Neglect, 20*, 161–169.

Malone, C. (1967). Developmental deviations considered in the light of environmental forces. In E. Pavenstedt (Ed.), *The drifters: Children of disorganized lower-class families* (pp. 125–161). Boston: Little, Brown.

Manly, J. T., Cicchetti, D., & Barnett, D. (1994). The impact of subtype, frequency, chronicity, and severity of child maltreatment on social competence and behavior problems. *Development and Psychopathology, 6*, 121–143.

Marans, A., & Lourie, R. (1967). Hypotheses regarding the effects of child-rearing patterns on the disadvantaged child. In J. Hellmuth (Ed.), *The disadvantaged child* (pp. 19–41). New York: Brunner/Mazel.

McCrone, E. R., Egeland, B., Kalkoske, M., & Carlson, E. A. (1994). Relations between early maltreatment and mental representations of relationships assessed with projective storytelling in middle childhood. *Development and Psychopathology, 6*, 99–120.

National Center on Child Abuse and Neglect, U.S. Department of Health and Human Services (1997). *Child maltreatment 1995: Reports from the states to the national child abuse and neglect data system*. Washington, DC: U.S. Government Printing Office.

Pavenstedt, E. (Ed.). (1967). *The drifters: Children of disorganized lower-class families*. Boston: Little, Brown.

Polansky, N. A., Chambers, M., Buttenweiser, E., & Williams, D. P. (1981). *Damaged parents: An anatomy of child neglect*. Chicago: University of Chicago Press.

Polansky, N. A., De Saix, C., Wing, M. L., & Patton, J. D. (1968). Child neglect in a rural community. *Social Casework, 49*, 467–474.

Polansky, N. A., Hally, C., & Polansky, N. F. (1975). *Profile of neglect: A survey of the state of knowledge of child neglect*. Washington, DC: U.S. Department of Health, Education, and Welfare.

Prugh, D., & Harlow, R. (1962). "Masked deprivation" in infants and young children, *Deprivation of maternal care: A reassessment of its effects*. Geneva: World Health Organization.

Rutter, M. (1972). Maternal deprivation reconsidered. *Journal of Psychosomatic Research, 16*, 241–250.

Sandgrund, A., Gaines, R. W., & Green, A. H. (1974). Child abuse and mental retardation: A problem of cause and effect. *American Journal of Mental Deficiency, 79*(3), 327–330.

Shields, A. M., Cicchetti, D., & Ryan, R. M. (1994). The development of emotional and behavioral self-regulation and social competence among maltreated school-age children. *Development and Psychopathology, 6*, 57–75.

Spitz, R. (1945). Hospitalism: An inquiry into the genesis of psychiatric conditions of early childhood. *Psychoanalytic Study of the Child, 1*, 53–74.

Yuan, Y.-Y. T., & Struckman-Johnson, D. L. (1991). Placement outcomes for neglected children with prior placements in family preservation programs. In K. Wells & D. E. Biegel (Eds.), *Family preservation services: Research and evaluation* (pp. 92–118). Newbury Park, CA: Sage.

10

Child Sexual Abuse

David J. Kolko and Elissa J. Brown

Introduction

Definition and Prevalence

The sexual abuse of children and youth includes physical contact (e.g., penetration, touching) but may also reflect noncontact sexual acts (e.g., exposure to pornography). Actual legal definitions of child abuse differ by state, resulting in different criminal statutes regarding the types of offenders who are considered to be sexual abusers (e.g., caretaker or not), the age at which consent for sexual activity is legal (e.g., 14 years or 18 years), and whether the offender intended to commit a crime. For example, in its definition of sexual abuse, Pennsylvania law includes "any act or failure to act which causes nonaccidental sexual abuse or exploitation, or any recent act, failure to act, or series of such acts or failures to act which causes an imminent risk of sexual abuse or exploitation," when committed upon a child under 18 years of age by a perpetrator (Pennsylvania Department of Public Welfare, 1997; p. 5).

The incidence and prevalence of childhood sexual abuse (CSA) have been estimated in various ways. The third national incidence study reflects

Janet Stauffer contributed to the preparation of the first case. The clinical supervision and support of the Faculty at Medical University of South Carolina is appreciated.

David J. Kolko • Department of Psychiatry, University of Pittsburgh School of Medicine Western Psychiatric Institute and Clinic, Pittsburgh, Pennsylvania 15213. **Elissa J. Brown** • NYU Child Study Center, NYU School of Medicine, New York, New York 10016.

Case Studies in Family Violence, Second Edition, edited by Ammerman and Hersen. Kluwer Academic / Plenum Publishers, New York, 2000.

the number of child maltreatment cases reported to child protective services across the country in 1994 (National Center on Child Abuse and Neglect, 1996). The national incidence rate of CSA was 4.4 per 1000 children. Retrospective reports from adults reveal much higher rates. One telephone survey based on a national probability sample of adults indicated that 27% of women and 16% of men reported a contact sexual offense by age 18 (Finkelhor, Hotaling, Lewis, & Smith, 1990). The prevalence rates of CSA obtained from a mailed questionnaire to a national, stratified random sample of adults were 32% for women and 13% for men. Such rates may vary due to differences in the samples, definitions, methods, and screening questions used (Finkelhor, 1994), but in all likelihood underestimate the number of cases with a history of CSA (see Williams, 1994).

Acute and Long-Term Effects

Current empirical knowledge of the impact of CSA tells us that there is no single set of symptoms observed in all sexually abused children (see review by Kendall-Tackett, Williams, & Finkelhor, 1993). In fact, symptoms may be more closely related to other stressors (e.g., long-standing family problems) than the severity of the abuse. In addition, no set of behavior problems provides conclusive evidence of a sexual abuse experience. Interestingly, a subset of victims do not evidence any psychopathology following CSA (Conte & Schuerman, 1987; Finkelhor, 1990).

In their review, Kendall-Tackett et al. (1993) conclude that symptom patterns for CSA victims may differ across age groups. Preschoolers tend to experience general anxiety, internalizing and externalizing symptoms, inappropriate sexual behavior, nightmares, and posttraumatic stress disorder (PTSD) symptoms. Symptoms most commonly experienced by school-aged children include aggression, fear, hyperactivity, nightmares, regressive behavior, and school problems. Severity and complexity of symptoms appear to increase with age, with adolescent victims tending to experience depression, withdrawn/suicidal/self-injurious behaviors, somatic complaints, illegal acts, running away, substance abuse, and eating disturbances. Symptoms that may be common to all age groups include nightmares, depression, withdrawn behavior, aggression, regressive behavior, and school/learning difficulties.

In addition to symptom patterns, Kendall-Tackett et al. (1993) reviewed the research on symptom course. Longitudinal studies indicate that symptoms abate over time for one-third to one-half of CSA victims. In turn, 10% to 24% of victim-survivors become more symptomatic over time. Interestingly, signs of anxiety were more likely to disappear over time, whereas aggression tended to persist or worsen. Risk factors for a more severe reaction to CSA (e.g., PTSD) include penetration, a close relationship between perpetrator and victim, more frequent sexual contact over a longer duration, use of physical force, lack of maternal (nonoffender) support, and fear of being physically injured or killed.

Subsequent reviews have extended our knowledge of the developmental consequences of CSA (Knutson, 1995; Letourneau, Saunders, & Fitzpatrick, 1996; Putnam & Trickett, 1995), including its long-term effects (Widom, 1994) and relationship to the need for intervention (see Green, 1993). These problems include hypersexuality and sexual behavior problems, fear, anxiety, and depression, dysfunctional attributions, and social or interpersonal difficulties. Recently, these and other consequences have been described in Finkelhor's (1995) traumagenic model of CSA in which he emphasizes the developmental context of both the risks for and the effects of victimization.

Treatment Models and Clinical Guidelines

Based on this emerging evidence, greater attention has been paid to designing conceptual and therapeutic models that provide clinical guidelines for the treatment of CSA victims. These approaches include victim- and parent-oriented individual cognitive-behavioral treatment (Cohen & Mannarino, 1993; Deblinger & Heflin, 1996), expressive and skills-based group treatments (e.g., Lindon & Nourse, 1994; Zaidi & Gutierrez-Kovner, 1995), family therapy techniques (Greenspun, 1994; Roesler, Savin, & Grosz, 1993), inpatient programs (Steinberg & Sunkenberg, 1994), and models that integrate different approaches (Chaffin, Bonner, Worley, & Lawson, 1996; Friedrich, 1996b). Several professional organizations have also disseminated guidelines for the evaluation and treatment of CSA (see American Academy of Child and Adolescent Psychiatry, 1997; Cohen, 1998). In general, these treatments target both the common symptoms seen in CSA victims and the clinical and systemic concerns that arise during their treatment.

Treatment-Outcome Research

Much of the early research on the treatment of CSA revealed various benefits of therapy in the context of uncontrolled reports that described pre- and post-changes in targeted outcomes (see reviews by Beutler, Williams, & Zetzer, 1994; Finkelhor & Berliner, 1995). These early programs examined certain abuse-related and general treatment procedures in the context of multidisciplinary teams, family therapy, and individual therapy, but without much conceptual or empirical depth (see Kolko, 1987). Importantly, no controlled outcome studies had been reported at that time to guide the treatment of CSA victims.

More recently, treatment-outcome studies have documented the efficacy of cognitive-behavioral therapy (CBT) for abuse victims and their nonoffending caregivers (Celano, Hazzard, Webb, & McCall, 1996; Deblinger, Lippmann, & Steer, 1996), especially when CBT is compared to nondirective approaches (Celano et al., 1996; Cohen & Mannarino, 1997). Empirical support exists for group studies as well (Verleur, Hughes, & Dobkin De Rios, 1986). In contrast, minimal support has been found for the incremental benefit of multiple components over a single component (Berliner & Saunders, 1996; Hyde, Bentovin, & Monck, 1995) or an advantage of individual versus group treatment (Perez, 1988). In general, significant improvements have been demonstrated in levels of internalizing (Cohen & Mannarino, 1996) and externalizing problems (McGain & McKinzey 1995), and modest changes have been obtained in social competence and sexualized behavior (Stauffer & Deblinger, 1996), with some reports of deterioration over time (Lanktree & Briere, 1995). Of course, studies vary considerably in several parameters, including client age, developmental level, treatment content and format, and inclusion of family members. Discussion of the abuse experience, training in some type of coping skills, and attention to the child's general safety are among the more common elements in these interventions. The following two cases of CSA illustrate the variability in symptoms reported and thus, techniques with these children and their families.

Case Description 1: Early Work

Neil was a 7-year-old white male who attended second grade in a regular school. He lived with his 35-year-old mother, a 10-year-old brother, and for much of the time, the mother's 41-year-old boyfriend. He had three prior admissions to a local psychiatric hospital in the past 9 months.

Neil was referred by the hospital to which he had been admitted three times previously due to long-standing problems with impulsivity and aggressiveness. Various medications had been tried at this hospital with little improvement. Requests of hospitalization were to verify diagnosis, evaluate medication needs, and increase family involvement in inpatient and follow-up services.

In terms of sexual behavior, Neil admitted to pulling up girls' skirts and pinching their buttocks in the past, though this was not confirmed. According to his mother and her boyfriend, Neil was precocious in his discussion of sexual activities. They denied his having a history of sexual abuse by a caretaker but acknowledged his involvement the previous summer with a 9-year-old neighborhood boy who offered Neil his friendship in return for fondling his genitals.

His peer relations were described as poor. Neil seldom kept friends for any length of time and was unable to share a friend. He frequently fought both at school and in the community, which became a chronic problem resulting in a school suspension. At the same time, he appeared to compete for mother's attention at home and frequently complained of vague aches and pains in an effort to get her attention. Since his mother's car accident in February of 1987, he had been more jealous of mom's affection and voiced concerns that she might die. He also became more clingy and demanding of her attention at this time.

Mother reported hyperactivity, inattentiveness, aggressiveness, and intrusiveness at school since age 3. This corresponded to the time of Neil's father's death, at which time his mother became depressed and began to abuse solvents. He was expelled from preschool at age 4 due to inappropriate sexual acts with the girls at the school. The expulsion prompted referral to a partial hospitalization program.

Neil's first hospitalization was initiated for treatment of these chronic conduct problems and a possible attention deficit disorder. The latter disorder was adequately controlled with medication for several months until his behavior began to deteriorate, as evidenced by a loss of weight, insomnia, and frequent temper tantrums. Alternative medications only worsened his behavior, and the situation was compounded by the family's failure to comply with outpatient sessions. Readmission was sought to address Neil's increasingly destructive, agitated, and belligerent behaviors. Additional medications resulted in some symptomatic relief. However, Neil returned home occurred after his mother's separation from her boyfriend (as a result of the boyfriend's alcohol abuse) and became increasingly unmanageable, aggressive, and destructive. A third hospitalization was initiated during which he received additional medications and a recommendation for further treatment.

Prenatal history was positive for several complications (e.g., smoking, alcohol, marijuana use). Labor and delivery were uncomplicated. However, he was hospitalized four times at an early age after suffering from gastrointestinal problems and intolerance to formulas. He also had a history of asthma, which required approximately 15 hospitalizations since birth. Developmental milestones were reached within normal limits and physical growth parameters were at least average. He was Tanner I. Family history was positive for cardiovascular disease, substance abuse, seizure disorder, hypothyroidism, obesity, and leukemia.

Neil's biological father died suddenly of a heart attack in 1983 at age 36. Family psychiatric history was positive for maternal depression and substance abuse, and for paternal substance abuse and PTSD. There was also a family history of drug abuse, alcoholism, suicidal behavior, and possible bipolar disorder. In addition the patient's maternal uncle had sexually abused Neil's mother.

The mother's boyfriend attempted to serve as a parental figure for Neil, although mother frequently undermined his efforts. He was a veteran with a history of PTSD, depression, and abuse of alcohol and illicit substances, though he provided few details regarding the nature of these problems.

The patient was well-groomed and neat in appearance, and displayed appropriate and pleasant affect. He indicated that he had been hospitalized because he was "hyper," which was consistent with his behavior throughout the interview. He displayed a high activity level, fidgeted, and was distractible by irrelevant noise. His attention span was short and he needed prompting or restatement of a question when his focus shifted to an irrelevant subject or object in the room. Speech rate and rhythm were a bit pressured at times, but never unintelligible. There was no evidence of a formal thought disorder, and he denied depressive affect, sleep and appetite disturbance, anhedonia, and other mood symptoms. However, he admitted to being annoyed easily and unhappy that he lacked friends. When asked why he lacked friends, he stated, "because I fight with them," and excitedly bragged about a recent run-in with a neighborhood boy. He denied fears or phobias and other anxiety-related symptoms with a similar degree of certainty.

Neil's initial problem list included the following psychiatric and behavioral symptoms: (1) impulsivity, distractibility and other ADD/H symptoms; (2) verbal and physical aggressiveness; (3) precocious sexual play; and (4) lack of friends. Family problems included marital conflict, a weak parental coalition, and parental psychiatric problems.

It was during this final hospitalization that concerns about sexual abuse and permissiveness were raised. A brief inquiry into the possibility of sexual abuse conducted on admission was negative. Upon reviewing Neil's sexual activities and family history, however, the team became increasingly concerned about the possibility of abuse and requested an interview by a specialist in the area of CSA to further explore his sexual behavior.

At the outset of the interview, Neil willingly discussed some concerns regarding his sexual feelings toward a 13-year-old female on the unit. He acknowledged sending her notes and feeling "in love" with her, and also cautiously reported that he had thought of raping the girl. His verbal and nonverbal behavior—along with picture drawings—graphically depicted his knowledge of, and desire for, sexual activity.

Although appearing anxious when asked if anyone had touched or abused him sexually, he proceeded to describe an incident 3 years earlier when the mother had left her boyfriend and Neil in bed together one night after she had moved to the sofa downstairs. Neil alleged that the boyfriend initiated anal intercourse ("he bopped me up the butt"), but denied any subsequent occurrences. At this point, the interview was terminated because of a concern about Neil's jumping on tables and chairs in the room.

In subsequent interviews with his psychiatrist, Neil verified his allegation and addressed his anxiety around the disclosure. He was very concerned about his family's reaction and the impact of his allegation on his relationship to his mother's boyfriend, denying that the boyfriend made any threats to Neil regarding disclosure.

Medical Issues

Neil's medical status and general physical health were normal. An admission physical suggested the possibility of an inguinal hernia. There was no evidence of sexually transmitted disease, hickeys or facial bruises, or related findings that would suggest oral sex or anal penetration. Precocious sex play was reported by the mother.

Legal Issues

Involvement in the legal or judicial system is often prompted by the need to protect children, even though such involvement may elicit or exacerbate other adjustment difficulties. Although not new concerns, the family's sexual permissiveness, Neil's history of sexualized behavior, and his recent allegation of sexual abuse committed by an adult nearly 3 years ago implicated the mother's boyfriend, who had continued to live in the home. In light of the disclosure and Neil's appearance as a credible source, we responded to the legal mandate as professionals to file a SCAN (suspected child abuse or neglect) documenting the incident to the child abuse hotline for further investigation by the local child protective services agency (children and youth services; CYS). Neil's credibility was upheld on the basis of their interview findings, which included his verbal report and several sexually explicit drawings of the incident. The local CYS worker forwarded a report to Neil's home county CYS with the findings.

Our report of the incident and the discussion with mother that ensued regarding the need for a prompt investigation diverted the focus of intervention away from the family system and toward the determination of whether this man was guilty and should remain with the family. One consequence of filing the report was the family's preoccupation with understanding why Neil would make the allegation, whether he was credible, and how their family life and the boyfriend's future would be harmed if the investigating agency found the allegations to be true. We chose to discontinue our efforts at clarifying the family's boundaries and structure, Neil's sexual knowledge and acting out, existing community supports, and the impact of the mother's boyfriend's alcoholism on family life and his sexual behavior. Instead, it appeared more important to prevent Neil's involvement in further episodes of abuse, though it was equally clear that this could be accomplished only by a comprehensive intervention with the family that extended beyond his involvement in an incident that occurred 3 years ago.

Neil's mother, in particular, responded to her son's allegations with considerable apprehension. She was asked to describe any information that could aid in understanding the basis of the allegation. Reportedly, she was surprised by the allegation and denied having any such knowledge. Initially, she vacillated between being suspicious of and angry toward her boyfriend and defending the boyfriend by maintaining his innocence and attributing Neil's lack of credibility to his apparent psychological problems.

During the initial family session, she vigorously attempted to find inconsistencies in Neil's statements. Soon thereafter, she began to question him repeatedly during phone conversations, conveying in subtle but meaningful ways both her disbelief of this report and her anxiety over the implications of his statements. Sensing her disbelief and anxiety, Neil changed his story, perhaps as a way of showing his loyalty to his mother. According to his mother, Neil admitted to some confusion and reported that it had actually been his now-deceased father who had molested him. Upon recounting this information to the treatment team, his mother and the rest of the family were greatly relieved to hear this alternative allegation and to receive confirmation of the boyfriend's innocence. Because of the traveling distance, Neil's home county CYS agency waited to interview him until he was discharged from the hospital several weeks later. In the meantime, the mother's boyfriend was ordered out of the home until the SCAN could be evaluated in order to ensure Neil's safety. Eventually, Neil maintained the accuracy of his revised claim upon subsequent interview by a representative of his home county CYS agency, who then unfounded the SCAN.

Aside from this reversal in his allegation, of clinical import was the fact that Neil maintained that he had been sexually abused, though neither his family nor the children's agency seemed interested in addressing this experience. As long as there was no one to prosecute, it was as if the event had never happened. No legal recourse seemed available to initiate comprehensive family therapy or therapeutic involvement designed to address the sequelae following his victimization. In retrospect, the family's focus on our filing of the SCAN and its eventual status as unfounded may have impeded therapeutic efforts to address family issues regarding loyalty, protection, and sexual intrusiveness. The family had attended three sessions at the sexual abuse outpatient treatment center to which we had referred them, but terminated as soon as the SCAN was unfounded.

The appropriate legal response had been made by filing the SCAN and reporting Neil's allegations to CYS to assure protection. Despite the appropriateness of filing a SCAN report, however, the investigation itself may have placed him at greater risk for reabuse or family rejection, if not both (Newberger, 1985). This investigation process appeared to contribute to further family disruption as mother's boyfriend was restricted from residing in the home until the investigation was completed. Potentially, the family's anger toward Neil about the disclosure placed him at risk for emotional and psychological abuse. Furthermore, Neil's relationship with the boyfriend, who provided emotional support and structural stability in the family as a primary disciplinarian, may have been weakened. One, then, has to wonder to what extent Neil, or his family, will confide and trust in other mental-health professionals as they recall the distress associated with the investigation of these allegations.

Social and Family Issues

CSA cases require an analysis from a systems perspective because these events are often related to factors that interact to weaken the natural protective elements of the family. Understandably, abusive experiences do not occur in a vacuum but instead are abetted by dysfunction in the family and social system. As argued by Tierney and Corwin (1983), life stressors can precipitate involvement in incestuous relationships, which, in this case, reflected a vulnerability the family had experienced after a tragic death. The goal of conceptualization from a systems perspective should go beyond "blaming the victim" or the family, especially since this often increases the tendency to ignore the perpetrator's culpability. Rather, it provides the framework from which to address a continuum of issues that influence the initiation and maintenance of abusive environments, beginning with prevention, proceeding to assessment of allegations of abuse, and then designating treatment services.

There were many weakened social and familial factors in Neil's case. First, there was inappropriate sexual permissiveness in the family. The mother was unable to establish boundaries designed to protect her children from overstimulation and sexual exposure. For example, they were given access to pornographic movies and magazines. During periods of the mother's absence from the home, substitute adult caretakers exhibited sexually inappropriate behavior and used sexually provocative language in front of the children. The boys were permitted to watch pornographic movies and read explicitly sexual adult books. For 9 months following their father's death, Neil's mother and both of her sons slept together in the family living room where his cremated ashes lay in a vase. This lack of privacy may have resulted in sexual activity being displayed in front of the boys. Neil's sexually inappropriate behavior was often minimized by his mother, as evidenced by the fact that repeated contacts to the mental health system were initiated for complaints regarding related problems, such as aggression, hyperactivity, or peer conflicts.

Neil's mother was also overwhelmed by her own psychological problems as she continued to experience complicated bereavement related to her husband's death. In addition to living without a partner, she had to assume several new responsibilities for which she was unprepared. Although she had entered a drug rehabilitation program to deal with her addiction to solvents, she was unable to complete the treatment and signed herself out prematurely. She then continued to abuse drugs actively and was occasionally "high" at home. A serious motor collision left her in a condition of chronic and disabling back pain that limited her mobility to the first floor of the house. She had difficulty setting limits and disciplining the children on a consistent basis, which often seemed to relate to her own feelings of guilt and inadequacy as a parent. This apparent overprotectiveness or limited involvement shielded the boys from the structure and boundaries they needed, heightening their vulnerability to physical or sexual misconduct. Neil's mother also expressed an ambivalence regarding her relationship with her boyfriend, which was exacerbated during conflicts around discipline. During these angry incidents, his mother's successful efforts to elicit the children's loyalty against the boyfriend compromised any efforts the couple made to achieve consistency in their exercise of control strategies.

In terms of her own vulnerability, Neil's mother had been sexually abused as a child by her uncle on one occasion while he was intoxicated, although this had not been revealed prior to making this disclosure to a member of her hospital treatment team. She was unable to tell her mother because her mother was emotionally close to her uncle. Thus, Neil's mother appeared to minimize the importance of the event in her own life, saying that "we don't talk about those kinds of things." Being unable to acknowledge and confront effectively her own victimization in all likelihood contributed to her unavailability in providing support for her son at the time of his disclosure. On a more practical level, she had minimal energy to nurture and care for her sons as a consequence of her unresolved grief over the husband's death, abuse of solvents, physical disability, and relational conflicts.

Other sources of existing family stress were evident. Two other children—Neil's 12-year-old biological brother and 17-year-old adopted sister—stayed at home with the boyfriend when mother was out of the home. The 12-year-old brother was physically aggressive toward Neil. During one altercation 2 months prior to admission, his brother had forced a rope around Neil's neck and caused an asthma attack. The two boys frequently fought about minor matters. The boyfriend's alcoholism and seriousness of his medical problems also affected the family in that he was frequently unemployed and spent much of his time in the house. Because of the conflictual nature of his relationship to the mother, there were occasional fights at home and brief, but disruptive, separations.

A comprehensive assessment of family functioning would be incomplete without recognizing and validating the family's strengths. Throughout these proceedings, the family managed to maintain its many important functions. There was much genuine care and concern for each family member, despite some limitations in focusing their attention in productive ways. Neil's mother's requests for mental health services on several occasions were based, albeit circuitously, on a sincere desire to address Neil's behavioral difficulties. The boyfriend continued to reaffirm the need for added structure and more effective behavior management with the children. He and Neil had established several common recreational pursuits and hobbies, such as water sports and fishing. The family also looked to the boyfriend for emotional support and stability throughout the SCAN process. At certain times, the family appeared to share several positive experiences and several humorous moments.

Outside of the family, however, Neil was socially unable to maintain friendships, and his peer relationships often had a sexual quality to them. As noted earlier, Neil had been coerced by a neighborhood boy to engage in mutual fondling and other sexual activities during the past year, though few details were recalled regarding this relationship. In yet another incident that occurred just before admission, Neil was observed fondling a young girl in his neighborhood. The family as a whole lacked a strong support system with extended family or regular contacts with the neighborhood, church, or social community. These indigenous supports might have been helpful in altering the family's reluctance to participate in treatment at the mental health or drug and alcohol centers.

It seems quite unfortunate that family intervention was not initiated earlier in Neil's childhood. Instead of expulsion from the preschool program due to what the school perceived as sexualized behaviors toward classmates, school personnel who were better trained to identify families who are susceptive to violence and sexual exploitation could have performed a more extensive assessment or engaged the family in a preventive, community-based program. This involvement could have enhanced the family's supports in a way that might have reduced the continuation of inappropriate family routines and relationships. Of course, no such family intervention was implemented at that time. Even upon Neil's referral for mental health treatment for aggression and attention-deficit problems, the family's sexualized routines remained unexplored. Eventually, Neil was brought to our tertiary care facility for inpatient psychiatric hospitalization on the children's unit in light of these and other concerns.

Assessment of Psychopathology

The case manager and attending physician conducted a comprehensive psychiatric interview with Neil and his mother on admission. An interdisciplinary team conference that was conducted 2 weeks later evaluated the admission data (e.g., clinical findings, unit observations, academic reports, social history) and yielded an Axis I diagnostic of conduct disorder: undersocialized/aggressive and other specified family circumstances. The diagnosis of attention deficit disorder with hyperactivity had been ruled out using teacher ratings on the Connor's Teacher Questionnaire and unit observations. On the WISC-R, he obtained a verbal IQ of 105, a performance IQ of 104, and a full-scale IQ of 104. His mother's completion of the Interview for Antisocial Behavior yielded a high score on the overt behavior factor (82), and low scores on the covert behavior (19) and self-injury factors. Neil's overall score on the Matson Evaluation of Social Skills of Youngsters (−22) indicated greater involvement in inappropriate than appropriate behaviors.

The frequency with which Neil engaged in the eight symptom categories of the hospital chart review was determined in order to compare his behavior to those of sexually abused, hospitalized children (Kolko, Moser, & Weldy, 1988). Children with a history of sexual abuse have been found to exhibit a greater frequency of problems in a few of these categories (e.g., sexual behavior, fear/anxiety) than nonabused children. During his eight weeks of hospitalization, Neil exhibited 23 separate incidents of sexual behavior, primarily involving sexual gestures and play with other peers. He also appeared to be sad or depressed on 15 occasions and engaged in physical aggression five times.

In terms of family characteristics, the Family Environment Scale revealed low cohesion, high conflict, and high organization and control. On the Dyadic Adjustment Scale, the couple was rated as somewhat low in satisfaction, cohesion, and affective expression. The mother's score on the Beck Depression Inventory was 27, which suggested a moderate level of depressive symptoms. It should be recalled that Neil's mother and father, and the mother's boyfriend, all suffered from problems with depression, anxiety, and substance abuse. These problems may have resulted in the caregivers increasing their dependency on Neil and limiting their availability to both provide for his own needs and promote his interests. In addition, these problems diminished their general involvement in family activities. The relationship between these vulnerabilities and the occurrence of abuse, however, can only be roughly approximated at this point.

Treatment Options

Treatment

Brief treatment was initiated with Neil and his family during hospitalization, but was impeded due to the limitations of a short hospital stay and a driving distance of 3 hours for the family. Therefore, greater attention was paid to adequately assessing the nature of any psychiatric dysfunction and Neil's experience of victimization in order to facilitate referral for the most appropriate type of treatment in his home area. To provide a context for his experience, Neil met on an individual basis during hospitalization with his attending child psychiatrist for supportive work around his disclosure of abuse. Two additional concerns directly related to the abuse were his fear of having AIDS and being homosexual. The psychiatrist also helped him to express his anxiety following the disclosure and his apprehension about the family's reaction and impact on his mother's boyfriend.

Neil participated in a group therapy program designed to encourage the use of appropriate social skills with peers. A special behavior program was also implemented to reduce nighttime noncompliance and encourage going to bed on time and without disruption. Briefly, compliance with these expectations was reinforced with extra social time the next day or bonus points in the milieu program. Both of these therapeutic efforts resulted in improvements.

Prior to Neil's disclosure, meetings with the family attempted to address the family's permissive attitude toward the viewing of sexually explicit materials, the need for appropriate structure and boundaries for the boys, and the frequent conflicts between Neil's mother and her boyfriend. Following the disclosure, an effort was made to help the family understand Neil's experience and better respond to his needs, though this was met with minimal success. The family's own disinterest in discussing the allegation made it especially important for the treatment team to avoid perpetuating a denial of the family's sexual problems and adopting the system's idiosyncratic perception of reality.

In such cases, the development of long-term intervention plans is often suspended. A decision first must be made as to whether the family's strengths are sufficient to support a child's return home or the family's resistance to change and anger at the child are likely to complicate the child's reintegration and later adjustment. It was certainly possible that Neil might sustain greater impairment in his emotional and sexual development by continuing to reside in an environment of sexual stimulation fostered in his family and community. We were very concerned that Neil was at great risk to become a sexual perpetrator himself should he remain in his environment without receiving follow-up treatment. Out-of-home treatment in a group facility was an alternative option that would have fostered intensive individual work under controlled living circumstances. However, the goal of group home facilities is often to eventually return the client to his family. It was felt that Neil's family ties could be utilized constructively to facilitate change and maintain more appropriate interactional patterns among family members. To remove Neil permanently from the family at this point did not seem wise. He was emotionally very close to family members and such an action might simply compound the unresolved losses that had already incapacitated the family.

Steps for Reunification

A decision was made to have Neil return home to his family. Treatment was encouraged to focus on each of the weakened aspects of the family system noted previously and to ensure future protection for Neil and his siblings. A complementary strategy would also involve teaching Neil to manage better both his own and others' behavior. Of course, there was also a need for Neil to participate in counseling designed to address the sequelae of victimization and his concerns regarding sexuality and appropriate sexual expression. It was also assumed that mother would benefit from the resolution of her grief over the loss of her spouse, as well as her own childhood sexual victimization. In addition, a commitment to protecting the children by providing more consistency in the setting of boundaries and use of structure was seen as crucial. Neil's mother was encouraged to engage in more active problem-solving to mediate individual conflicts with her boyfriend and free the children from loyalty struggles that prevented them from trusting either caregiver. Finally, Neil's mother and her boyfriend needed to confront their respective problems with drug use and alcoholism. The couple's fragile relationship also was seen as a primary therapeutic target.

The reality, however, was that the family was not ready to undertake these challenges and confront these issues. We referred them to an excellent agency in their geographical area that specialized in the treatment of sexually misused and abused persons. Concerned with the possibility of sexual abuse, the agency was prepared to help Neil understand his own sexuality and express his feelings about his abuse. Agency staff expressed an additional concern about Neil's risk of becoming a sexual perpetrator should he not find more healthy expression of his sexual feelings and were willing to work toward ensuring Neil's protection within the family system. Neil participated in three sessions before the allegations against the mother's boyfriend were considered unfounded by CYS. The family promptly terminated treatment at that time. Although sexual expression issues were still of real concern, the family was reluctant to pursue this threatening topic further. Instead, the family took Neil and his brother to a former counselor with whom sexuality was not a focus of treatment. This episode of treatment also lasted only a few sessions. Because the CYS focus was limited to finding the SCAN valid or invalid, they were unable to mandate that the family continue with treatment.

Outcome

A 1-year follow-up phone call revealed that Neil was attending a specialized child behavior management class in his school district and had brought his school marks up to As and Bs. At the same time, a Child Behavior Checklist completed by the mother indicated that Neil continued to exhibit clinically significant levels of both externalizing and internalizing symptoms. Specifically, he engaged in hyperactive (e.g., "can't concentrate," "hyperactive"), aggressive ("fights," "unliked"), and delinquent ("destroys property," "steals") behaviors, was withdrawn ("poor peer relations," "teased"), and showed obsessive-compulsive (e.g., "obsessive," "can't sleep") and depressive (e.g., "lonely," "cries") symptoms. He was perceived as doing well in social activities and school performance, but was showing significant problems in social skills and peer relations. There were no difficulties reported on individual items representing sexual behavior and preferences.

The functioning of the mother and family had improved significantly. Neil's mother was now employed full-time and her health was much improved. No further episodes of abuse by the boyfriend or neighborhood children were reported. She was successful in imposing additional structure in the home for the boys and had curtailed their exposure to pornographic movies in the house. She also acknowledged her boyfriend's assistance in providing this needed structure and a more cohesive relationship with him due, in part, to the threat of his removal from the home as a result of the allegations. In turn, the boyfriend was relating more positively with Neil.

Case Description 2: Recent Work

Annie was an attractive 6-year-old Caucasian girl who had been sexually abused at the age of 5 by her biological father. She was the only child of her biological parents, with whom she resided in a small rural town. Disclosure of the abuse occurred when Annie's father, Fred, reported to medical staff during his own treatment that he had fondled his daughter. Originally, he presented the narrative as if it had been a dream but later admitted that the abuse had actually occurred. The medical staff then reported the child sexual abuse to child protective services (CPS).

Although Annie, Fred, and Annie's mother, Mary, agreed that the sexual abuse occurred, their descriptions of what the abuse entailed were inconsistent. Annie reported that Fred forced both her and her cousin, Ruth (age 6), to remain in a room in their home while he engaged in digital and lingual touching of the girls' vaginal and anal areas. He also forced the girls to manually touch his penis. According to Annie, her mother entered the room upon hearing the girls scream and told her husband that "he was wrong to do that to kids."

In contrast to Annie's report of the abuse to professionals, Mary asserted that she had not been aware of the abuse prior to Fred's disclosure. After Fred's disclosure and the initiation of CPS involvement, Mary discussed the abuse with Annie. According to Mary, Annie described three distinct abusive incidents. In the first, Annie had been "half-asleep" while her father "rubbed her down there." In the second, Annie had touched her father's genitals after he stepped out of the shower and he "allowed" it. In the third, Fred had "laid on top" of Annie and her cousin at their grandfather's house. Interestingly, when questioned about the three incidents, Fred admitted to the first two but denied that the third incident occurred.

One of the most controversial issues in the area of child sexual abuse is the nature of the assessment procedure. In most cases, children complete either a forensic evaluation *or* a clinical assessment. The goal of a forensic evaluation is to determine the veracity of the sexual abuse, specifics of the incidents, current safety of the child, risk for future abuse, and ability of the nonoffending caregiver to protect. Law enforcement, CPS, physicians, and mental health professionals typically participate in a forensic evaluation. In contrast, a clinical/psychological/psychiatric assessment is completed to examine the level of psychosocial functioning of the child (and her family) and may be conducted by a single mental health professional.

Annie was seen at a clinic designed to coordinate systems of care (i.e., legal, medical, mental health) for abused children and participated in a forensic, rather than a clinical, evaluation. This evaluation included a forensic interview, designed to obtain Annie's narrative of the abuse incidents under the observation of a CPS worker and police officer. Annie also completed a medical exam.

The majority of the psychological information was collected through interviews with Fred and Mary. First, each caregiver described the abuse incidents and impact of disclosure on Annie. Second, information was gathered on each family member regarding their medical history, mental health history (including substance use), experience with law enforcement, education, employment history, previous physical assault, sexual assault and neglect experiences, other traumas (e.g., car collisions), and family stressors (e.g., financial, marital, custody). Third, as the primary caregiver, Mary answered a series of questions about Annie's developmental history, school/day-care history, social/peer relationships, types of discipline used in the family, family privacy rules and sleeping arrangements, past exposure to sexual information, and family terms for genitals (to assist with the child's interview). Mary also provided information about Annie's psychiatric symptoms, including behavioral sequelae of abuse (e.g., aggression, sexual behaviors, posttraumatic stress disorder symptoms), mood and affect, and mental status.

Medical Issues

According to Mary's report, Annie had a history of enuresis. At the time of the evaluation, Annie experienced sporadic bouts of enuresis when she was playing outside of the home. Mary was unsure whether the bouts of enuresis were related to the sexual abuse incidents. During the forensic medical examination, the pediatrician found evidence of a urinary tract infection, but no other medical problems.

Fred's medical history was quite relevant to the family dynamic. He was borderline diabetic and began dialysis 1 year prior to the forensic evaluation as a result of blood clots in his legs, lungs, and kidneys. Dialysis occurred 3 days per week for 3 hours each day and, according to Fred, was "very stressful." Additionally, Fred had high blood pressure, poor vision (resulting in cornea transplants), and a speech impediment. Given his medical problems (and mild mental retardation), Fred was unable to maintain full-time employment.

Mary's medical history was insignificant with the exception of hypothyroidism. Interestingly, although she invested time and money in her husband's medical care, Mary received no treatment for her own medical problems. Both Fred and Mary denied having any history of substance abuse or dependence.

Annie and Mary had no prior history of mental health problems. In contrast, Fred reported having been institutionalized in a state mental hospital as a child for "depression and hyperactive fits." His depressive disorder was recurrent, with the most recent episode occurring within the year prior to the disclosure of the sexual abuse. The staff conducting Fred's dialysis had noted his symptoms of depression. When questioned, Fred reported having distress about financial and medical difficulties. Suicidal ideation was also endorsed. The medical staff referred Fred to a mental health professional, and he was hospitalized for 1 month for depression.

He was receiving no mental health care at the time of the disclosure and forensic evaluation.

Legal Issues

As mentioned, Annie participated in an interview under the observation of a CPS worker and police officer as part of the forensic evaluation. This forensic interview included a controversial procedure, the use of anatomically detailed dolls. According to an excellent review of the literature by Koocher, Goodman, White, Friedrich, Sivan, and Reynolds (1995), the hypothesized benefits of these dolls are that they may provide a memory cue and a simple, concrete means for reenactment of the abuse. However, they also may be suggestive and stimulate sexual and other fantasy.

Anatomically detailed dolls are used in a decision-making process, as props to evaluate whether or not the sexual abuse occurred. According to the American Psychological Association (1985), a psychological test is an assessment procedure that includes a set of tasks or questions intended to elicit particular types of behavior when presented under standardized conditions. The behaviors are interpreted based on standardized rules for scoring and assigning meaning to the responses. However, at this time there is no standardized procedure for the use of anatomically detailed dolls; in fact, procedures vary across setting in number of sessions, number of dolls, doll features (e.g., race, facial features, sexual features), presence or absence of clothing when presented, and presence or absence of background knowledge of the assessor regarding the abuse incidents (Koocher et al., 1995). In addition, there are no quantitative results (i.e., score) elicited from an assessment with anatomically detailed dolls.

The capacity for children to remember traumatic experiences and use these dolls as aides in their reconstruction may be limited by cognitive development. The research on developmental changes in memory indicates that, in general, children are able to give a complete and accurate report if the task is simplified and appropriate cues are available in a supportive context (Koocher et al., 1995). However, there is evidence that children younger than 4 years cannot use a prop to relate one social category (e.g., parent) to another (e.g., child).

A series of empirical studies have been conducted to evaluate normative behavior with anatomically detailed dolls (Koocher et al., 1995). The participants were samples of nonreferred children (who may have been unreported abuse cases). Sexual behavior was most often a function of the norms in the children's families. Virtually all studies found that many children inspect and touch sexual body parts; however, play showing explicit sexual activity was rare. In comparisons of referred (for sexual abuse) versus nonreferred groups of children, findings are equivocal. Unfortunately, the studies differ widely in the size and composition of samples and methodology. Koocher and colleagues concluded that these dolls do not inherently distress or overstimulate the children, can assist in identifying names for body parts, and result in more verbal productions during the interviews (with Ken and Barbie dolls doing just as well). Furthermore, the authors assert that no conclusion can be drawn as to whether the determination of child sexual abuse is more or less accurate with anatomically detailed dolls.

During Annie's forensic interview, anatomically detailed dolls were utilized in her descriptions of the sexual abuse. Dolls that varied by age, gender, and race were introduced to Annie and she was then asked to "show" the interviewer where and how her father touched her and she touched him, using "Daddy" and "daughter" dolls. While describing the abusive incidents verbally, Annie placed the father's hand on the daughter's breasts, vagina, and behind. She also placed the daughter's hand on the father's penis.

Behavior, affect, and speech tone and content were also monitored throughout the interview. Annie's speech had a "singsong quality," potentially indicative of either overwhelming anxiety with attempts at distraction or a sense of play (calling the validity of the interview into question). Nevertheless, she was consistent and accurate in reporting background information. Less open-ended questions revealed that she was suggestible and influenced by questions. However, there was no indication that Annie had been coached.

Social and Family Issues

During her interview, Mary provided the developmental history of each member of the family. According to Mary, Annie experienced deficits in her cognitive development. She evinced language delays, such as using "me" instead of "I," and spoke in a voice tone typical of a younger child. Mary also reported that Annie's scores on tests of intelligence and achievement were low and that she was "almost held back in school." Although she had completed 1 year of kindergarten at the time of the assessment, Annie did not know the alphabet and could count consecutively only from 1 to 10.

Annie's social development was also limited. She was an only child, and prior to the disclosure of the sexual abuse, spent most of her time playing alone or with her father. Also prior to the disclosure, Annie socialized with her cousin, Ruth. Ruth was Mary's sister's daughter, and Annie's age. According to Annie, Ruth had been her "best friend." At the time of the assessment, Ruth's family had moved out of state and Annie had not seen her in weeks. Ruth's mother refused to discuss the abuse and prohibited contact between the two girls. Annie reported a great deal of distress and confusion regarding the lack of contact with her cousin.

Fred was a 36-year-old Caucasian male who had been married to Mary for approximately 10 years. Like Annie, Fred experienced cognitive deficits, including mild mental retardation, illiteracy, and speech deficits. Because of his inferior intellectual functioning and serious medical problems, Fred received social security and disability payments (SSI). He had completed some high school, and although he was unemployed at the time of the evaluation, had been employed previously as a security guard for his father's business and a janitor.

Annie's mother, Mary, was a 31-year-old Caucasian woman who was also unemployed at the time of the interview and received Aid to Families with Dependent Children (AFDC). She had "dropped-out of school" during the eighth grade. When asked about employment experiences, she replied that she "[had] not worked consistently." She was the primary caregiver of Annie. When asked about her parenting style, Mary reported using the "time-out" procedure and viewed herself as having been the only disciplinarian. Fred and Mary denied having a history of childhood abuse or neglect.

At the time of the evaluation, Annie was a 6-year-old girl with possible mental retardation, who, with her cousin and best friend, had been sexually abused by her father. She was experiencing anxiety symptoms, regressive, and inappropriate sexual behaviors. Social support had decreased because she no longer had contact with her father or cousin, both of whom had been playmates. Her mother was providing some emotional support while simultaneously voicing sadness and frustration at being separated from her husband.

Annie's mother, Mary, was a 31-year-old wife and mother with cognitive limitations, experiencing emotional conflict since the disclosure of Annie's abuse. Although she was concerned about her daughter, Mary was very protective of her husband, who functioned on a childlike level. She also missed her husband, and thus attempted to convince the therapists that he was ready to return home. Mary would make these attempts in Annie's presence, conveying a lack of consistent support. In addition, she may have known about the abuse prior to Fred's disclosure and not acted to protect Annie. Mary's stress was also affected by the loss of social support (i.e., absence of her sister) and financial problems.

Assessment of Psychopathology

Results of the mental health evaluation revealed that Annie was exhibiting many of the symptoms seen typically in preschool- and school-aged sexual abuse victims, including regressive behaviors, anxiety, and inappropriate sexual behaviors. When punished by her mother, Annie would often bite herself. Mary also reported that Annie experienced bouts of enuresis when playing outdoors. Anxiety symptoms included reexperiencing the abuse ("stories in [her] head"), fears that the abuse would recur, and physiological reactions when reminded of the abuse (e.g., hypervigilance, sleep disturbance). Annie also reported affective symptoms, such as self-blame, sadness, and anger. Although she slept in her own room through most of the night, Annie would crawl into her parents' bed in the morning. She would also sit in bed with her father and watch television during the daytime. In addition, Mary believed that her daughter masturbated excessively (three to four times per day) and attempted to terminate this behavior.

After reviewing the information gathered from the three sources during the forensic evaluation, Annie was diagnosed with Adjustment Disorder with Anxious Mood (DSM-IV code of 309.24; American Psychiatric Association, 1994) and Sexual Abuse of Child (DSM-IV code of 995.5). Given the lack of formal psychoeducational testing during the forensic evaluation, mental retardation, learning disorders, and communication disorders could not be ruled out. As mentioned, the only notable medical condition was a urinary tract infection. Annie's psychosocial and environment problems included a loss of social support (due to the absence of her father and cousin), poor school performance, and a change in the family structure.

Treatment Options

The treatment approach used at the clinic had three primary components, (1) child safety; (2) treatment; and (3) clarification. Child safety was initiated immediately following the report of sexual abuse. In this particular case, child safety was accomplished by a number of steps: (1) the medical staff to whom the abuse was disclosed contacted CPS; (2) CPS removed the perpetrator from the home and organized the forensic evaluation; (3) the police observed the evaluation and formalized the complaint; and (4) the clinic's pediatrician conducting a medical exam. Based on the findings of the forensic evaluation, the charge of sexual abuse was founded. CPS and clinic staff then promoted child safety by scheduling treatment for Mary and Annie at the clinic and scheduling treatment for Fred elsewhere (with a clinician specializing in the treatment of sexual offenders). Fred was to remain out of the home until his and Annie's therapists recommended reunification.

Treatment

Annie and Mary participated in parallel individual psychotherapy for eight sessions over 2½ months, each with a different therapist. Based on empirical support (reviewed later in the chapter), cognitive-behavioral techniques were selected for Annie's treatment. Initial treatment sessions indicated that Annie was experiencing emotional and cognitive conflict about her relationship with her father. Using toys to describe her situation, Annie's conveyed that she felt unsafe with her father, yet missed him. She reported anger at his behavior, yet sadness about his (and Ruth's) absence and guilt regarding the reason for his absence. As a result of her cognitive developmental level, Annie experienced these conflicting emotions simultaneously without the vocabulary to identify them or the cognitive capacity to understand the relationship among them.

Thus, the initial phase of treatment involved psychoeducation. First, Annie was told about typical reactions to sexual abuse, with the goal of normalizing her symptoms. Second, Annie was taught to identify various emotions using pictures of faces and verbal descriptions. Once she was able to label her emotions, Annie recognized that she was experiencing "conflicting" emotions simultaneously. In-session and mother-reported anxiety decreased with the normalization of this affective pattern.

Psychoeducation was also used for affect regulation. Annie was taught the relationship between emotions, thoughts, and experiences and behavior. Emotions of sadness and guilt were associated with thoughts of self-blame about her father's absence from the home and her mother's loneliness. Cognitive restructuring techniques were used to challenge these thoughts and replace them with adaptive self-talk (e.g., "What Daddy did was not my fault").

Exposure therapy, another cognitive-behavioral technique, was used to address Annie's anxiety symptoms. She reported having "stories in her head" about being locked inside a room with her father. Thus, Annie participated in a flooding procedure in which she "relived" the situation by describing the events in the present tense while reporting her level of anxiety. In-session decreases in anxiety were evident during each of three exposure sessions. Between-session anxiety decreased across the three sessions such that the flooding procedure was discontinued after the third session.

In spite of the anxiety reduction, social support remained a problem for Annie. She had experienced the loss of Ruth and Fred as playmates and needed to learn to develop friendships with children outside the family. Thus, Mary was encouraged to schedule supervised play-dates for Annie with female peers. Although Mary viewed the responsibility as a burden at first, Annie reported enjoying the socialization, which was reinforcing for her mother.

Mary also participated in individual treatment with her own therapist. Psychoeducation was used to teach her about the typical psychosexual development of children. Her therapist also incorporated both supportive psychotherapy and cognitive restructuring to challenge Mary's belief that the goal of therapy was to have Fred return home rather than to protect and assist Annie.

Mary also attended group therapy for nonoffending mothers on a weekly basis for approximately 3 months. Using supportive psychotherapy, the group therapist encouraged participants to explore feelings, thoughts, and behaviors about the abuse and reaction of the system to the disclosure. After initial resistance, Mary took the opportunity to discuss her frustrations and loneliness with her peers in the group, rather than with Annie.

Clarification/Reunification

The clarification process began during the second month of therapy and continued through termination. There are a number of goals in the clarification process between the victim and offender: (a) acceptance of responsibility for CSA by offender; (b) presentation of an apology to the victim and family by the offender; and (c) development of a plan by the family for continued child safety and family restructuring. The nonoffending caregiver also is expected to participate in clarification, with the goals of reducing his or her own symptoms and providing support to the victim and expressing belief that the abuse occurred.

As a result, successful completion of clarification requires a systematic progression through several steps. The nonoffending parent must complete the clarification process prior to the offender doing so; the offender has to complete clarification prior to family reunification. Thus, clarification was conducted first between Mary, the nonoffending caregiver, and Annie, the victim. The need for this step was evidenced by Annie's report that Mary knew about the abuse and did not protect her and Mary's focus on Fred's (perhaps premature) return to the home rather than Annie's anxiety.

The rationale and steps for the clarification process were presented to both Mary and Annie (i.e., apology, chance for the victim to ask questions, chance for the nonoffending caregiver to answer questions, and discussion of prevention). Beginning during the sixth week of individual treatment, Mary and her therapist drafted a letter in which Mary apologized for not protecting Annie and not listening when Annie attempted to disclose the abuse. Mary and her therapist included terminology that was familiar to Annie (i.e., "coo coo" for vagina, "boobies" for breasts, and "heiny" for behind). In addition, Mary included in the letter a plan for protection against abuse in the future, encouraging Annie to report any further incidents of sexual abuse. Completion of this letter took 3 weeks. Concurrently, Annie and her individual therapist identified rules for the clarification meeting. They also developed a list of what Annie would like to say to her mother (e.g., Annie's reactions to the abuse) and questions she had for her mother (e.g., regarding the nature of Annie's future relationship with her cousin).

Clarification occurred after Mary's therapist approved of her letter and Annie completed the cognitive-behavioral treatment for symptom reduction (at week 9). Annie attempted to console her mother during Mary's reading of her apology letter. With support from therapists, Mary was able to take a parenting role and Annie was able to listen to the content of the letter without self-distraction. During subsequent sessions, Annie was encouraged to recall the content of the letter to ensure that she incorporated that her mother had apologized for not listening when Annie told about the abuse, had removed blame from Annie for the abuse, and had promised to protect her in the future.

Fred also participated in the reunification process. Contact between Annie and Fred was gradually increased, from phone conversations (under the supervision of both of their therapists) to holiday visits. Visits were initiated after Fred completed the clarification process with Annie. Specific rules regarding physical contact and discipline were established for Annie and Fred's relationship (e.g., no sleeping in the same bed). The expectation was that Mary would be responsible for enforcing these rules.

Working with Fred was especially challenging because of his cognitive rigidity and lack of understanding of consequences. Unfortunately, few studies have been conducted to evaluate treatment for sexual offenders with mental retardation. This is especially alarming given that counselors providing treatment to sexual offenders report that approximately one-fourth of their clients experience severe cognitive delays (Lundervold & Young, 1992). Contrary to popular thought, the sexual offenses committed by offenders with mental retardation are serious, including rape and oral and anal sodomy. However, research conducted on treatment efficacy has involved the evaluation of therapy for relatively benign inappropriate sexual behavior.

Outcome

Child safety, treatment, and clarification was completed in approximately 5 months. At termination, Annie evidenced little affective and cognitive conflict. She was able to describe her emotions about the abuse, including the anger toward her father and sadness about losing him and Ruth as playmates. Compared to the initial evaluation, she reported less anxiety in session, when discussing the abuse with her mother, and in her daily life. In addition there was no evidence of self-blame or fear of being reabused.

Mary also reported posttreatment improvements. She was more knowledgeable about normal psychosexual development and applied this knowledge to Annie's behavior. She recognized her role as Annie's protector and identified methods by which she could protect her daughter. There was no evidence of inappropriate sexual conversations or behaviors during the supervised interactions with her father. Group therapy provided information about and support for her marital relationship. Social support for both Annie and Mary had improved somewhat since the beginning of treatment, but further work in this area was recommended as a future goal.

Summary

The two clinical cases described here share some similarities as well as differences on key therapeutic and systemic issues. The treatment approach adopted in both cases incorporated multiple procedures, targets, and participants. This was prompted by the identification of various child, parent, and family issues raised during the assessment phase to which specific intervention techniques were applied. Certainly, clinical recommendations in recent years have highlighted the many issues and potential therapeutic obstacles that may need to be addressed during different phases of intervention, including minimizing the child's and family's denial of the abuse, protecting the child, mobilizing family support, and identifying treatment targets among the family (see Berliner & Elliot, 1996; Chaffin et al., 1996; Friedrich, 1996a).

Differences between the two cases are also worthy of discussion because they help to reflect some of the changes that have occurred over the past 10 years in both the conceptualization and treatment of CSA.

Because of significant psychiatric problems, the child in the first case was hospitalized; however, the child treated more recently was not. This difference may reflect actual clinical differences between the two cases (e.g., severity), change in hospital policy as a result of managed care, and progression in CSA treatment approaches over the past 10 years.

Clearly, whether a child should remain in the home is a major initial decision related to the capacity to protect the child and the child's treatment needs, among other characteristics (e.g., need for family stabilization). This decision may also have a significant effect on all aspects of the treatment process. Sometimes children are admitted to an inpatient setting due to the severity of the child's psychopathology or the potential risks to the child of staying in the home after disclosure. At other times, the perpetrator may be removed from the home when a child's level of maladjustment has been low and removal of the child is not seen as necessary in order to stabilize or protect the child. Because it is plausible that children's reactions to removal from the home may vary widely, it may be useful to give greater attention to the influence of removal on the child's later adjustment.

The presenting complaints of the two children also differed. Whereas in the first case the focus was on externalizing symptoms (e.g., aggression), the focus in the second case was primarily on internalizing symptoms (e.g., anxiety). This difference may be related to the difference in the gender, but it is equally important to appreciate the wide diversity in the clinical sequelae documented among abuse victims (Berliner & Elliot, 1996; Kendall-Tackett et al., 1993). Clinicians need to be prepared both to assess and to intervene with a range of psychopathology in any given case, especially given the absence of a unique profile or clinical syndrome associated with CSA (Kendall-Tackett et al., 1993). As reflected in both of these cases, child victims may show mixed clinical pictures that include both externalizing and internalizing symptoms and other unusual or socially inappropriate behaviors (e.g,. sexual behavior, dissociation, self-mutilation) that make diagnosis and treatment planning challenging and complicated.

The specific treatment approach adopted in the first case drew heavily upon various family therapy, psychiatric, and general clinical approaches. At that time there were few if any generally accepted treatment procedures for use in CSA cases. The second case, however, reflects a more contemporary approach to working with child sexual abuse. Specifically, treatment emphasized several cognitive-behavioral techniques, such as psychoeducation about the responsibility for and effects of abuse, anxiety management, cognitive restructuring, exposure treatment, and the scheduling of social activities. The judicious use of these procedures, among others, has been found effective in clinical and experimental studies (see Cohen & Mannarino, 1996, 1997; Deblinger, McLeer, & Henry, 1990; Deblinger *et al.*, 1996). It is noteworthy that such an "abuse-specific" approach to treatment has achieved greater improvements on key outcomes than more general or indirect clinical treatments (see Finkelhor & Berliner, 1995). Several sources have been disseminated that clearly describe the application of these techniques in clinical practice in cases of sexual abuse (see Berliner, 1997; Cohen & Mannarino, 1993; Deblinger & Heflin, 1996). In general, there is growing recognition of the need to encourage the exposure of child victims to traumatic material or cues through discussion or other elicitation techniques (e.g., stories, drawings, role-plays), to train them in anxiety management and coping skills, and to maximize family support for the child.

The two cases also illustrate different concerns about parental, marital, and family dysfunction and treatment cooperation. In each case, efforts were made to enhance the level of motivation and consistency shown by the offending and nonoffending adults. Certain psychological and medical problems were documented that increased marital-partner tension, and reduced the level of communication and overall effectiveness in their parental roles. The mothers' loyalty to the offenders in both cases also appeared to limit their level of cooperation. Thus, the presence of adult clinical disorders and potentially adversarial partner alliances may obstruct full parental participation in the treatment process.

The nature of the parent and family work varied somewhat between the two cases. In the first case, family work began shortly after the child's hospitalization and addressed family boundaries, conflicts, and relationships. In the second case, the offender was removed from the home, and parallel services were developed for the child and parents that paid considerable attention to developing a clarification session in which mother sought to apologize to daughter and suggest how she was to protect her in the future. The use of this clarification procedure has been discussed in a few clinical cases, but it has not been researched in its own right. Specialized procedures such as clarification may enhance the likelihood that reunification can be accomplished in an atmosphere of trust and security, rather than one characterized by a sense of betrayal and hostility. Clearly, there has been increasing attention paid to the way in which children are reintegrated into their family environments and, in some cases, reunified with their offenders (see Chaffin *et al.*, 1996). This delicate process may require considerable clinical resources and time in order to assure that the child's experience is both supportive and therapeutic.

Neither case involved any legal involvement or considerable involvement in other systems because no criminal charges were filed and no court hearings were held. Legal involvement is common in cases of child sexual abuse and has been associated with different outcomes, such as symptom improvements relative to those who have not testified (Runyan, Everson, Edelsohn, Hunter, & Coulter, 1988) and an increased likelihood of receiving services and heightened perception of intervention stress (Runyan, Hunter, Everson, Whitcomb, & De Vos, 1994). The overall impact of any legal involvement in these cases cannot be estimated. Indeed, they were withheld in part because neither nonoffending spouse opted to press charges. Determining how to minimize the adverse effects of legal involvement has been the subject of considerable empirical work (see Saywitz & Goodman, 1996).

Evidence from surveys of child victims and their parents on the effects of disclosure and intervention suggest that they are influenced by the nature of the interactions they have when evaluated and treated and that they see some benefit from the professional contacts they receive following the abuse (Berliner & Conte, 1995). These beneficial impressions are confirmed in recent clinical outcome studies showing the benefit of abuse-specific treatments for CSA victims and their parents. Further clinical reports and empirical investigations are needed to enhance the effectiveness of these interventions for the many victims who receive services in various community settings.

References

American Academy of Child and Adolescent Psychiatry. (1997). Practice parameters for the forensic evaluation of children and adolescents who may have been physically or sexually abused. *Journal of the American Academy of Child and Adolescent Psychiatry, 36,* 423–442.

American Psychiatric Association. (1994). *Diagnostic and statistical manual of mental disorders* (4th ed.). Washington, DC: Author.

American Psychological Association, Committee to Develop Standards for Testing. (1985). *Standards for educational and psychological testing.* Washington, DC: Author.

Berliner, L. (1997). Intervention with children who experience trauma. In D. Cicchetti & S. Toth (Eds.), *Developmental perspectives on trauma: Theory, research, and intervention. Rochester Symposium on Developmental Psychology* (Vol. 8, pp. 491–514). Rochester, NY: University of Rochester Press.

Berliner, L., & Conte, J. R. (1995). The effects of disclosure and intervention on sexually abused children. *Child Abuse & Neglect, 19,* 371–384.

Berliner, L., & Elliot, D. M. (1996). Sexual abuse of children. In J. Briere, L. Berliner, J. A. Bulkley, C. Jenny, & T. Reid (Eds.), *The APSAC handbook on child maltreatment* (pp. 51–71). Thousand Oaks, CA: Sage.

Berliner, L., & Saunders, B. E. (1996). Treating fear and anxiety in sexually abused children: Results of a controlled 2-year follow-up study. *Child Maltreatment, 1,* 294–309.

Beutler, L. E., Williams, R. E., & Zetzer, H. A. (1994). Efficacy of treatment for victims of child sexual abuse. *Sexual Abuse of Children, 4,* 156–175.

Celano, M., Hazzard, A., Webb, C., & McCall, C. (1996). Treatment of traumagenic beliefs among sexually abused girls and their mothers: An evaluation study. *Journal of Abnormal Child Psychology, 24*, 1–17.

Chaffin, M., Bonner, B. L., Worley, K. B., & Lawson, L. (1996). Treating abused adolescents. In J. Briere, L. Berliner, J. A. Bulkey, C. Jenny, & T. Reid (Eds.), *The APSAC handbook on child maltreatment* (pp. 119–139). Thousand Oaks, CA: Sage.

Cohen, J. A. (1998). Practice parameters for the assessment and treatment of children and adolescents with posttraumatic stress disorder. *Journal of the American Academy of Child and Adolescent Psychiatry, 37*, 45–265.

Cohen, J. A., & Mannarino, A. P. (1993). A treatment model for sexually abused preschoolers. *Journal of Interpersonal Violence, 8*, 115–131.

Cohen, J. A., & Mannarino, A. P. (1996). A treatment outcome study for sexually abused preschool children: Initial findings. *Journal of the American Academy of Child and Adolescent Psychiatry, 35*, 42–50.

Cohen, J. A., & Mannarino, A. P. (1997). A treatment study for sexually abused preschool children: Outcome during a one-year follow-up. *Journal of the American Academy of Child and Adolescent Psychiatry, 36*, 1228–1235.

Conte, J. R., & Schuerman, J. R. (1987). Factors associated with an increased impact of child sexual abuse. *Child Abuse & Neglect, 11*, 210–211.

Coppens, N. M. (1986). Cognitive characteristics as predictors of children's understanding of safety and prevention. *Journal of Pediatric Psychology, 11*, 189–195.

Deblinger, E., & Heflin, A. H. (1996). *Treating sexually abused children and their nonoffending parents: A cognitive-behavioral approach.* Thousand Oaks, CA: Sage.

Deblinger, E., McLeer, S. V., & Henry, D. (1990). Cognitive behavioral treatment for sexually abused children suffering posttraumatic stress: Preliminary findings. *Journal of the American Academy of Child and Adolescent Psychiatry, 29*, 747–752.

Deblinger, E., Lippmann, J., & Steer, R. (1996). Sexually abused children suffering posttraumatic stress symptoms: Initial treatment outcome findings. *Child Maltreatment, 1*, 310–321.

Finkelhor, D. (1990). Early and long-term effects of child sexual abuse: An update. *Professional Psychology: Research and Practice, 21*, 325–330.

Finkelhor, D. (1994a). Current information on the scope and nature of child sexual abuse. *Future of Source, 4*(2), 31–35.

Finkelhor, D. (1994b). The international epidemiology of child sexual abuse. *Child Abuse & Neglect, 18*(5), 409–417.

Finkelhor, D. (1995). The victimization of children: A developmental perspective. *American Journal of Orthopsychiatry, 65*(2), 177–193.

Finkelhor, D., & Berliner, L. (1995). Research on the treatment of sexually abused children: A review and recommendations. *Journal of the American Academy of Child and Adolescent Psychiatry, 34*, 1408–1423.

Finkelhor, D., Hotaling, G., Lewis, I. A., & Smith, C. (1990). Sexual abuse in a national survey of adult men and women: Prevalence, characteristics, and risk factors. *Child Abuse & Neglect, 14*(1), 19–28.

Friedrich, W. N. (1996a). Clinical considerations of empirical treatment studies of abused children. *Child Maltreatment, 1*, 343–347.

Friedrich, W. N. (1996b). An integrated model of psychotherapy for abused children. In J. Briere, L. Berliner, J. A. Bulkey, C. Jenny, & T. Reid (Eds.), *The APSAC handbook on child maltreatment* (pp. 104–118). Thousand Oaks, CA: Sage.

Greene, A. H. (1993). Child sexual abuse: Immediate and long-term effects and intervention. *Journal of the American Academy of Child and Adolescent Psychiatry, 32*, 890–902.

Greenspun, W. S. (1994). Internal and interpersonal: The family transition of father-daughter incest. *Journal of Child Sexual Abuse, 3*, 1–14.

Hyde, C., Bentovin, A., & Monck, E. (1995). Some clinical and methodological implications of a treatment outcome study of sexually abused children. *Child Abuse & Neglect, 19*, 1387–1399.

Kendall-Tackett, K. A., Williams, L. M., & Finkelhor, D. (1993). Impact of sexual abuse on children: A review and synthesis of recent empirical studies. *Psychological Bulletin, 113*, 164–180.

Knutson, J. F. (1995). Psychological characteristics of maltreated children: Putative risk factors and consequences. *Annual Review of Psychology, 46*, 401–431.

Kolko, D. J. (1987). Treatment of child sexual abuse: Programs, progress, and prospects. *Journal of Family Violence, 2*, 303–318.

Kolko, D. J., Moser, J. T., & Weldy, S. R. (1988). Behavioral/emotional indicators of child sexual abuse among child psychiatric inpatients: A comparison with physical abuse. *Child Abuse & Neglect, 12*, 529–541.

Koocher, G. P., Goodman, G. S., White, C. S., Friedrich, W. N., Sivan, A. B., & Reynolds, C. R. (1995). Psychological science and the use of anatomically detailed dolls in child sexual-abuse assessments. *Psychological Bulletin, 118*, 199–222.

Lanktree, C. B., & Briere, J. (1995). Outcome of therapy for sexually abused children: A repeated measures study. *Child Abuse & Neglect, 19*, 1145–1155.

Letourneau, E. J., Saunders, B. E., & Kilpatrick, D. G. (1996, January). In B. E. Saunders (Chair), *Adolescents and abuse: Results from a national survey study*. Paper presented at the annual meeting of the San Diego Conference on Responding to Child Maltreatment, San Diego, CA.

Lindon, J., & Nourse, C. A. (1994). A multidimensional model of group work for adolescent girls who have been sexually abused. *Child Abuse & Neglect, 18*, 341–348.

Lundervold, D. A., & Young, L. G. (1992). Treatment acceptability ratings for sexual offenders: Effect of diagnosis and offense. *Research in Developmental Disabilities, 13*, 229–237.

McGain, B., & McKinzey, R. K. (1995). The efficacy of group treatment in sexually abused girls. *Child Abuse & Neglect, 19*, 1157–1169.

National Center on Child Abuse and Neglect. (1996). The third national incidence study of child abuse and neglect. Washington, DC: Department of Health and Human Services.

Newberger, E. H. (1985). The helping hand strikes again: Unintended consequences of child abuse reporting. In E. H. Newberger & R. Bourne (Eds.), *Unhappy families: Clinical and research perspectives on family violence* (pp. 171–178). Littleton, MA: PSG Publishing.

Pennsylvania Department of Public Welfare. (1997). *Child abuse report '98*. Harrisburg, PA: Commonwealth of Pennsylvania.

Perez, C. L. (1988). A comparison of group play therapy and individual therapy for sexually abused children. *Dissertation Abstracts International, 48*, 3079.

Putnam, F. W., & Trickett, P. K. (1995, September). *The developmental consequences of child sexual abuse*. Paper presented at the Conference on Violence Against Children in the Family and the Community, Los Angeles.

Roesler, T. A., Savin, D., & Grozs, C. (1993). Family therapy of extrafamilial sexual abuse. *Journal of the American Academy of Child and Adolescent Psychiatry, 32*, 967–970.

Runyan, D. K., Everson, M. D., Edelsohn, G. A., Hunter, W. M., & Coulter, M. L. (1988). Impact of legal intervention on sexually abused children. *Journal of Pediatrics, 113*, 647–653.

Runyan, D. K., Hunter, W. M., Everson, M. D., Whitcomb, D., & DeVos, E. (1994). The intervention stressors inventory: A measure of the stress of intervention for sexually abused children. *Child Abuse & Neglect, 18*, 319–330.

Saywitz, K. J., & Goodman, G. S. (1996). Interviewing children in and out of court. In J. Briere,

L. Berliner, J. A. Bulkey, C. Jenny, & T. Reid (Eds.), *The APSAC handbook on child maltreatment* (pp. 104–118). Thousand Oaks, CA: Sage.

Stauffer, L. B., & Deblinger, E. (1996). Cognitive behavioral groups for nonoffending mothers and their young sexually abused children: A preliminary treatment outcome study. *Child Maltreatment, 1,* 65–76.

Steinberg, R., & Sunkenberg, M. (1994). A group intervention model for sexual abuse: Treatment and education in an inpatient child psychiatric setting. *Journal of Child and Adolescent Group Therapy, 4,* 61–73.

Tierney, K. J., & Corwin, D. L. (1983). Exploring interfamilial child sexual abuse: A systems approach. In D. Finkelhor, R. J. Gelles, G. T. Hotaling, & M. A. Straus (Eds.), *The dark side of families: Current family violence research* (pp. 102–116). Beverly Hills, CA: Sage.

Verleur, D., Hughes, R. E., & Dobkin De Rios, M. D. (1986). Enhancement of self-esteem among female adolescent incest victims: A controlled comparison. *Adolescence, 21,* 843–854.

Widom, C. (1994). Childhood victimization and adolescent problem behaviors. In R. D. Ketterlinus & M. E. Lamb (Eds.), *Adolescent problem behaviors: Issues and research* (pp. 127–164). Hillsdale, NJ: Lawrence Erlbaum.

Widom, C., & Ames, M. A. (1994). Criminal consequences of childhood sexual victimization. *Child Abuse and Neglect, 18*(4), 303–318.

Williams, L. (1994). Recall of childhood trauma: A prospective study of women's memories of child sexual abuse. *Journal of Consulting and Clinical Psychology, 62,* 1167–1176.

Zaidi, L. Y., & Gutierrez-Kovner, V. M. (1995). Group treatment of sexually abused latency-age girls. *Journal of Interpersonal Violence, 10,* 215–227.

11

Incest

Judith A. Cohen and Anthony P. Mannarino

Description of the Problem

Incest is a particular type of child sexual abuse that often has severe consequences for the child, the perpetrator, and the family as a whole. *Webster's Dictionary* defines incest as "sexual intercourse between persons too closely related to marry legally." However, in the field of child sexual abuse, it more commonly refers to any sexual activity between a child and a close relative. This obviously includes many diverse behaviors, which vary in frequency, duration, and type of contact.

There is no "typical" psychological outcome of incest. As with other forms of child sexual abuse, children exhibit a wide variety of psychological symptoms in response to incest. In two different studies, the authors found no significant group differences in symptomatology between children abused by relatives and children abused by nonfamilial perpetrators (Cohen & Mannarino, 1988; Mannarino, Cohen, & Gregor, 1989). This supports the notion that the child's relationship to the perpetrator *per se* does not determine the degree of trauma he or she experiences. However, there are several other aspects of intrafamilial sexual abuse that may make it particularly difficult for victims to recover.

The first is frequency of sexual abuse. There is some evidence to indicate that with a greater number of abusive episodes, there is a higher

Judith A. Cohen and Anthony P. Mannarino • Department of Psychiatry, Allegheny General Hospital, Pittsburgh, Pennsylvania 15212.

Case Studies in Family Violence, Second Edition, edited by Ammerman and Hersen. Kluwer Academic / Plenum Publishers, New York, 2000.

rate of self-reported symptomatology, such as depression, anxiety, and poor self-esteem, although findings in this regard are not consistent (Mannarino *et al.*, 1989). Although some cases of incest involve only one abusive episode, many incest victims have experienced ongoing sexual abuse. Some of these children have been abused for months or years on a regular basis. In these cases, frequency of abuse may result in an increase in psychological symptoms.

The incest victim may be more vulnerable than victims of extra-familial abuse to developing distorted cognitions about abuse. Intra-familial perpetrators may present the abuse to child as a "normal," loving family interaction. For example, one father said he wanted to "teach my daughter about sex rather than having her learn it from someone else who doesn't even care about her." Intrafamilial perpetrators may frame the abuse as "just a special way of showing I love you," in order to convince the child that incestuous behavior is acceptable. When such a child does not resist abusive acts, he or she may feel partly or wholly responsible for their occurrence. This type of self-blame for sexual abuse has been demonstrated to be a strong mediating factor in symptom formation in children (Mannarino & Cohen, 1996c). Children abused by a close relative may also be more likely to have ambivalent feelings toward the perpetrator than children abused by someone outside the family. This issue is discussed in more detail in the following sections.

The family's reaction to abuse and its disclosure may also be a very important determinant of the child's symptomatology. Familial support has been found to be a very important factor in the child's symptom formation and recovery (Friedrich, Leucke, Beilke, & Place, 1992; Mannarino & Cohen, 1996a). It is important to note that the stereotypical incestuous family, where the "collusive mother" knows all along about the sexual abuse of her child and tolerates or even promotes it, is not representative of the families that we have seen. Other researchers report this also (Faller, 1988). Many of these children report the first episode of abuse to their mothers, who often take immediate appropriate action to protect the child and remove the perpetrator from the home (Mannarino & Cohen, 1986). Many other mothers express a great deal of ambivalence and have difficulty in "choosing sides" but still take steps to prevent ongoing abuse. There are, unfortunately, some families that tolerate the abuse or persistently disbelieve the victim despite significant evidence that incest is occurring. (It should be noted that much variability in response to the victim occurs in extrafamilial sexual abuse cases as well; these victims' families are also not uniformly supportive, protective, or readily willing to believe the child.)

The nonoffending parent's emotional reaction to the child's sexual abuse has also been found to strongly mediate symptomatology in the child (Mannarino & Cohen, 1996a, 1996b; Cohen & Mannarino, 1998a). Children whose nonoffending parents are able to resolve their own emotional upset about abuse are less symptomatic as a group than children whose parents remain highly upset about the abuse.

Legal involvement is often more complex in an incest case than with extrafamilial sexual abuse. Frequently, the perpetrator represents the main source of family income. Pressing charges that eventuate in the perpetrator being sentenced to prison may in such cases significantly decrease the family's standard of living, resulting not only in financial hardship but also in resentment of the victim by other family members. Removal of the perpetrator (with or without criminal charges being pursued) frequently deprives other family members of an emotionally important figure in the home, which may also cause ambivalence, anger, or resentment toward the victim. Custody issues frequently have an impact not only on the abused child but on other siblings as well. In addition, public knowledge about the sexual abuse may cause significant shame or embarrassment to family members because of their relationship to the perpetrator. All of these factors may significantly add to the stress experienced by the family and the abused child.

In the case of incest, the victimized child usually has a relationship with the perpetrator that also has had positive aspects. Although the perpetrator objectively has betrayed the child's trust, the latter may not perceive it this way. The emotional attachment that the child has to the perpetrator may make it much harder for her or him to reach some resolution about the abuse because the perpetrator is still, and may always be, a member of the family. This may add complications and conflicts that a victim of extrafamilial abuse would not have to address.

The following cases demonstrate many of these issues, which are potential problems that may be encountered in incest. However, it is important to recognize that each sexual abuse case has its own characteristics, and there are no "absolute" dimensions that distinguish incest from extrafamilial child sexual abuse. Each situation must be assessed individually to determine relevant clinical, familial, and legal issues.

Case Description 1

Ann and Marie were sisters, aged 14 and 13, respectively, who were brought for an evaluation by their mother because of the girls' disclosure of sexual abuse by their natural father. The girls were living with their mother (a college-educated housewife) and their 18-year-old sister, Michele. The father, a Protestant minister, had lived with them until his arrest a few weeks prior to evaluation.

Ann had first attempted to tell her mother about the sexual abuse 2 years previously. She did this by asking her mother, "Do you know what sexual abuse is?" The mother apparently did not make anything of Ann's question and did not pursue the subject at that time. Ann let the matter drop. The following year, Marie disclosed the sexual abuse to a counselor at a church camp. Child protective services were called to investigate, but Ann was very angry at Marie for telling someone at camp (partly because it was affiliated with the father's church). Consequently, Ann refused to talk to the case-worker. In an attempt to lessen Ann's anger at her, Marie also refused to talk to the worker. Because the girls would not speak to the investigator, the report was unfounded. Apparently, the mother did not question the girls about whether they had been abused or why Marie had reported it. She did, however, confront the father, who was already in individual therapy for treatment of work-related stress. The mother went with the father to see the father's therapist, and he did admit to "inappropriate love and affection" for both girls. (It should be noted that this was the first time his therapist learned about this, after 5 years of ongoing psychotherapy.) Shortly thereafter, the father called the child into his room, and in his wife's presence, praised Marie for her disclosure and apologized for his behavior. He promised it would never happen again, and the mother assumed that it would not.

However, in the last several months, the mother had noted that Marie was frequently fighting with her father and seemed to feel a great deal of hostility toward him. For this reason, the mother brought Marie to a private therapist for individual treatment. During the evaluation by this therapist, Marie again disclosed ongoing sexual abuse by her father. Child protective services (CPS) was called and this time Marie described the abuse to the investigators. The father was arrested, and both Ann and Marie were re-ferred to our clinic for treatment.

Apparently, abuse of both girls began at about the same time, when Ann was 5 years old and Marie was 4 years old. Each girl was evaluated individu-ally. Ann presented as an attractive, well-developed, articulate adolescent. She felt very ambivalent about Marie's disclosure, expressing both relief that her father would get some help and anger that Marie had gotten him into trouble by disclosing the abuse.

Ann reported that, most commonly, her father would fondle her in the breast area and between the legs. At different stages of her life, he would perform different sexual acts on her, which she and Marie would discuss on occasion. The most extensive abuse Ann experienced was what the girls called the "full treatment." This consisted of the father's undressing her, fondling her, and lying in bed with her back to his chest. He would roll her around his genital area and touch her on her breasts and vaginal area. During the course of the interview, Ann related many incidents of this type being perpetrated against her, almost on a weekly basis during certain periods of her life. She could remember one of many trips out of town with the family, when the mother slept with Michele in one room and the father slept with Ann and Marie in another room. She stated that while they were sleeping together in the same bed, he attempted to fondle her once again. She asked him to stop and he did. He asked her if she wanted to go in with her mother and she replied yes. Ann related that she felt guilty that she went into the other room with her mother and left Marie alone with her father. She stated that she always knew that the abuse was wrong but did not know how to stop it at the time.

Abuse continued on a regular basis, with Ann stating that frequently she would see her father entering Marie's bedroom and would know the abuse was occurring. On several occasions, she attempted to stop her father from abusing Marie by entering the room and beginning a conversation. In her estimation, she was never able to ask him to stop abusing Marie or herself until the first disclosure. Ann stated that she felt in her mind that she had given her mother many hints that the abuse was occurring. When she went to her mother and asked her, "Do you know what sexual abuse is?" Ann felt that this should have been a sufficient hint for her mother, but it was not. After the first disclosure, with her father apologizing to her and Marie, she felt the abuse would no longer continue. Even when he would still attempt to enter her bedroom and give her back rubs, which resulted in his hands moving to her chest, she was able to say no, but she knew in her heart that the abuse was continuing with Marie. She was very angry at Marie for disclosing at camp and felt that it threatened the family. She was "trying to be good for mom" so as not to add any additional emotional burdens on her mother. She was unsure that her mother would be able to handle the family without her husband and felt quite guilty about having "wrecked" their marriage. She was able to state that she felt that she needed help to discuss feeling "dirty" about what had happened and what effect this would have on her future relationships with the opposite sex. She was also able to express some anger at Marie for acting out emotionally when she herself was trying to be so good and hold the family together.

Ann expressed fear that Michele would be angry at her, although Michele had expressed support for her. Ann stated that what she dreaded the most was having to go to court and face everyone and discuss what had happened to her. She stated that she felt everyone would be looking at her, thinking about the abuse that had been perpetrated against her, and that this made her feel "dirty." She was somewhat angry at father but expressed more sorrow for him, stating that he "must have problems" and that he "is a sick man." Ann denied any suicidal thoughts or ideation. She reported being sad, angry, and confused, and believed very strongly that she needed to talk to somebody about this. She felt that her mother was torn between her daughters and husband and worried about the outcome of their relationship and their marriage.

Marie was also evaluated individually. Like her sister, Marie was attractive, intelligent, and articulate. She was tearful during most of the interview. Marie described the same type of fondling as Ann (as stated earlier, the two girls occasionally discussed the abuse with each other). As Marie got older, the father would perform oral sex on her as well. In describing this, Marie became quite tearful and felt guilty and "dirty" because of this particular abuse. She wondered if it was her fault and if she should be blamed for not stopping her father sooner. She was angry at him but also said that he has lost his wife, children, and possibly his job over this disclosure. She was also fearful that he would go to jail and wondered what would become of her mother and the family. She reported an inability to concentrate in school and some sleep disturbance. She reported that it took several hours for her to fall asleep at night and frequently she would awake in the middle of the night or early in the morning. She reported constant sadness and frequent tearfulness since the disclosure as well.

Marie was extremely angry that her father continued to abuse her (and not Ann) even after he promised to stop. She said this was why she began fighting and being noncompliant with the father in the last several months. She was relieved and glad that she had at last followed through on disclosing the abuse because this would finally make it stop.

Case Description 2

Norman was an 8-year-old boy brought for an evaluation by his parents after disclosing sexual abuse by his 14-year-old brother Gerard. Norman had been caught fondling a 6-year-old boy in a school rest room. He was taken to the principal's office and the school nurse was called. When she asked where he learned this behavior, he said "on TV." When asked whether anyone at home did this kind of thing to him, he became withdrawn and refused to answer. The nurse contacted CPS, who interviewed the child at school. During the interview, Norman disclosed that Gerard had been molesting him for the past 2 months. He described that Gerard had engaged him in mutual genital fondling as well as oral–genital contact. CPS interviewed Gerard and the boys' mother. Gerard denied the allegations, and mother expressed disbelief and anger at Norman's allegations. Mother denied that Gerard could have engaged in such behavior, and suggested that the actual perpetrator was Andre, the 16-year-old son of father's paramour. Andre and his mother had been living with Norman's father since his separation from Norman's mother 3 years ago. Norman had bimonthly weekend visits at father's home and had contact with Andre during these visits.

CPS reinterviewed Norman and asked him whether Andre had engaged him in any inappropriate sexual behaviors. Norman denied sexual abuse by Andre but at this point also denied sexual abuse by Gerard, saying he was "only messing with" the CPS worker when he made the initial allegation. Because of the inconsistency of Norman's disclosures, CPS did not indicate the report and Norman and Gerard remained in their mother's care.

One month after CPS closed the case, mother came home early from work. She heard footsteps running in the hall and when she went to investigate, she found Norman running from Gerard's bedroom with his jeans unzipped. She entered Gerard's room in time to see him fastening his pants.

Mother questioned Norman privately and he admitted to mother that Gerard had been "playing the sex game" again. He described that he had been performing oral intercourse on Gerard while Gerard fondled Norman's genitals, until this activity was interrupted by mother's return home. Mother then questioned Gerard, who initially denied this behavior, but when threatened with being questioned by his father, admitted to fondling Norman. Mother called father, who agreed that CPS be informed. Mother called CPS, who referred Norman to our clinic.

Norman presented to the initial evaluation as a cheerful, cooperative youngster. He was quite verbal when describing his school, friends, and sports. However, when asked about Gerard and the sexual abuse, Norman became very agitated and distracted. He began grabbing toys off the interviewer's shelves and ignoring the interviewer's questions. When redirected, he became silly and started using "toilet" words. Norman became calmer when he was told that he could write or draw what happened with Gerard instead of having to describe it verbally. Norman drew a picture and said, "That's Gerard's dick. He had me suck his dick." When asked whose fault it was that this happened, Norman said, "His and mine. It was both of us together doing it." Norman denied being angry at Gerard, and was instead angry at his mother for telling father and CPS about the abuse. Norman denied having any symptoms of depression but did acknowledge having some posttraumatic stress disorder (PTSD) symptoms. He denied initiating sexual activity with other children and said that the episode in which he was caught with the 6-year-old in the school rest room was the younger child's idea.

Mother was interviewed individually. She stated that since she and Norman's father had separated, Norman had looked up to Gerard "like he was his substitute father." Gerard had been tolerant of Norman tagging along with him and his friends, and spent time playing sports and video games with Norman. Mother had depended on Gerard to care for Norman after school while she worked. She was tearful when she said that she never worried about Norman "because Gerard was always there with him and he wouldn't let anyone hurt his little brother." Mother said that she could not have believed that Gerard was capable of abusing Norman "until I saw it with my own two eyes." Mother was quite distraught and expressed a great deal of guilt that she had not believed Norman when he made his original allegation. She felt responsible for allowing the abuse to continue and expressed fear that Norman "will never trust me or really believe in me ever again" because of this. Mother also described that Norman's behavior had deteriorated in the past 3 months in that he had been more "hyper," mouthy, and oppositional with her. He was also having trouble falling asleep at night. Norman's teacher had also noticed that Norman was less focused and more restless in class. In fact, a few weeks before sexually inappropriate behavior was observed in the school rest room, the school had raised the possibility of Norman being evaluated for attention deficit hyperactivity disorder. Mother had wanted to wait until the end of the semester, in the hope that Norman would "settle down." Mother had also had concerns about the possibility that such an evaluation could result in a medication trial, and she was hesitant to follow up on the school's suggestion because she did not want to "drug" Norman to get him to behave.

Medical Issues

It may be helpful to digress from the case studies at this point in order to discuss general medical issues in the case of incest. (For the purpose of this discussion, the collection of medical evidence for legal proceedings will not be addressed.) The medical approach to incest is basically the same as in any other case of child sexual abuse. The type of sexual activity experienced will determine whether and what type of a medical examination is indicated. For a sexually transmitted disease to be contracted, the child generally must have had contact with the perpetrator's bodily fluids.[1] Unless one is very confident that there has been no contact with the perpetrator's body fluids or any traumatic injury (i.e., violent penetration), a physical exam is indicated. Because children often do not disclose the full extent of the sexual abuse they have experienced, physical examinations are usually routinely performed after any disclosure of sexual abuse.

In the prepubertal female child, if there is a possibility that contact with the perpetrator's bodily fluids has occurred, introitus cultures are generally obtained for chlamydial and gonococcal organisms. Blood samples are obtained for syphilis and HIV titres. (If the abuse occurred less than 3 months prior to the exam, HIV titres should be repeated at a later date, since these frequently do not become positive until 3 to 6 months following exposure.) With either a male or a female child, if there is a history or suspicion of anal penetration, anal gonococcal cultures should also be obtained.

In a prepubertal child, there will rarely be significant internal genital trauma without evidence of severe external trauma. If external injury is severe enough to require suturing, or there is significant intravaginal or intraanal bleeding, an internal exam is generally indicated. In the prepubertal child, this may need to be done under general anesthesia to minimize traumatization of the child as well as to assure an adequate exam. When this situation occurs, children are often frightened of being put to sleep and need careful explanations and reassurances about the procedures to be done.

---

[1] This may occur without ejaculation; there may be exchange of body fluids with any oral–genital, anal–genital, genital–genital, or oral–anal contact. It might also occur if, for example, the perpetrator ejaculated into his hand, then fondled the child's genitals with that hand.

For postpubertal girls, a serum pregnancy test is required in addition to the tests for sexually transmitted diseases. If possible, an internal exam should be performed. The main purpose of the internal exam in this situation is to obtain cervical cultures for gonorrhea and vaginal cultures for chlamydia, because these are more reliable than cultures from the introitus. However, the risk of further psychological trauma to the child should be carefully weighed against benefits of performing an internal exam. If the child seems to experience a significant degree of fear or psychological stress about having an internal exam, the exam can usually be deferred. It should go without saying that any medical procedures should be explained to the child in a supportive way and that no method requiring forcible restraint of the child is acceptable in this situation. If the child is fearful or resistant, the medical examination will simply victimize that child further. Generally, even very young children can cooperate with the medical procedures involved with they are explained with care and a parent or advocate is available for comfort and support during the exam.

If the child has contracted a sexually transmitted disease, appropriate antibiotic (or in the case of HIV or herpes, antiviral) therapy must be instituted. The issue of incest resulting in pregnancy is very complex, and a detailed discussion is beyond the scope of this chapter. The medical and psychological risks of bearing a child conceived from an incestuous relationship are significant. Abortion is frequently the best available option in this situation. However, such decisions are generally conflict-laden, and each situation must be evaluated individually.

With regard to the first case history, Marie had experienced oral intercourse with her father on several occasions. Ann gave no history of contact with her father's bodily fluids. However, because the abuse had gone on for so many years and it was possible that some such contact had occurred earlier (without Ann's realizing or remembering it), medical evaluations were performed on both girls at a large metropolitan children's hospital. Cultures and blood tests were obtained from the girls to detect the presence of sexually transmitted diseases. All of these were negative. Both girls continued to have regular, asymptomatic menstrual periods, and neither girl had any significant somatic complaints. With regard to the second case history, Norman had described oral intercourse as well as fondling. He received a medical examination, which revealed no abnormalities. Cultures and blood tests were negative.

Legal Issues

When incest has been disclosed, there is usually a great deal of ambivalence about pressing charges against the perpetrator. Many procedural requirements, particularly in the criminal justice system, may further traumatize the child witness (Landwirth, 1987). One group of researchers found that while testimony in juvenile court may be beneficial for the child (in the case of a juvenile perpetrator), protracted criminal proceedings may have an adverse psychological effect on the child victim (Runyan, Everson, Edelsohn, Hunter, & Coulter, 1988). The risks and benefits of the child's testifying in court should be weighed carefully in each individual situation before the decision to press charges is made. Generally, the prosecuting attorney will respect the child's wishes in this matter, although there have been a few unfortunate cases where the child incest victim has actually been held in contempt of court for refusing to testify against the perpetrator.

In case 1, the father was arrested shortly after sexual abuse was indicated by child protective services. Bail was posted by authorities in his church. Child protective services informed the parents that both girls should be removed from the parental home if the father returned. The mother and father agreed that he should move into an apartment to "keep the rest of the family together."

The family was very ambivalent about pressing legal charges against the father. (Charges included indecent assault, involuntary deviant sexual intercourse, and corruption of a minor.) The mother fretted that pressing charges would shame the family because it would be on public record that the father had done these things. She did not pressure the girls to avoid pressing charges but also did not encourage them to do so, saying that "it has to be their decision." This obviously placed the responsibility (and subsequent guilt) squarely on Ann or Marie. They did agree to press charges, at which point the father said he would plead guilty. He claimed this plea was to "spare the girls having to testify," although it clearly also spared him from having the details of his behavior come out in court.

A presentencing interview was conducted by the probation office. This involved each girl's talking with an investigator about her own preferences with regard to sentencing. Theoretically, the purpose of this interview is not only to ascertain how much harm has come to the victim but also to determine what sentence would be most beneficial to the victim (i.e., some children would be further traumatized by the perpetrator's being imprisoned).

At this interview, Ann expressed much ambivalence. She said she would feel terribly guilty if her father were sent to jail; she would feel "like I put him in prison." This seemed to be her strongest feeling. However, she was also clear that if he were not put in jail, he would have "gotten off easy, gotten away with doing that to us with no consequences." She then pointed out that he had "lost his family and his job and that's probably bad enough." (Church authorities accompanied the father to the trial to provide support. However, following the trial, he was dismissed from his job.)

Marie was much less ambivalent than Ann. She felt strongly that the father should be put in jail, no matter what it meant to the family in terms of embarrassment or loss of income. She expressed this clearly to the probation officer. However, Marie later changed her mind about this option; she indicated that her father had "made improvements" in therapy, that he now understood some of his own underlying conflicts, and that he did not need to be punished any more. (It is not clear how much of Marie's change of heart was actually due to ongoing family pressure on her.) Sentencing is still pending.

This is a case in which the legal system worked promptly and effectively in the victims' best interests. This was in part due to the fact that the girls were able, and ultimately willing, to testify against the perpetrator. Although the presentencing investigation may place too much of a burden of responsibility on the young incest victim, in general it tends to serve the victim's needs as much as possible.

The initial disclosure in this case highlights a shortcoming of the child protective system. After Marie disclosed the sexual abuse to a counselor, she experienced a great deal of pressure from Ann. This caused Marie to refuse to confirm her claims during the actual child protective services' investigation. Accordingly, the case was unfounded. The pathological enmeshment, guilt, and responsibility evident in this and many other incestuous families makes it more likely that these victimized children will not speak out against the parent–perpetrator. In such cases, unless there is other convincing evidence of abuse, protective services are legally unable to intervene. Unfortunately, there are many situations where this occurs and the incest most likely continues. When such a case is unfounded because of lack of evidence, there is no requirement for the family to enter therapy; indeed, such families probably tend to avoid treatment, in part for fear that allegations will be brought up again by the abused child. These children frequently fall through the "cracks" in the legal system and are unavailable for therapeutic or protective intervention. This was initially true in case 2. However, when Norman's mother discovered evidence of sexual abuse by Gerard, she became invested in protecting Norman from further abuse, even if it meant she would have to testify against her older son. Mother insisted, with father's support, that Gerard "own up" to what he had done. Parents both told Gerard that he could either acknowledge the full extent of the abuse and enter counseling for this behavior or he would have to go through a juvenile court hearing and risk being sent to a juvenile detention center. Gerard was initially resistant to admitting that he had engaged in oral intercourse with Norman and stated that Norman would never testify to this because "he knows it's a lie." In fact, Gerard felt confident that he could convince Norman not to testify against him at all. Mother was concerned about this possibility because of Norman's past close relationship with Gerard. Mother told Gerard that it did not matter what Norman said at the hearing because she herself would testify against Gerard if he decide not to go to court. Because mother had defended Gerard when Norman made the original allegations, Gerard was taken aback by mother's willingness to testify against him. He eventually acknowledged that oral intercourse had occurred on several occasions, and agreed to attend treatment. He pleaded guilty prior to the court hearing and was placed on probation and mandated into treatment.

CPS was initially adamant that Gerard be removed from mother's home. However, mother was proactive in suggesting several safeguards to protect Norman from further abuse by Gerard. These included locking Gerard in his bedroom at night (as his bedroom was on the ground floor, he could escape in case of fire); arranging for Gerard to enter an after-school program and taking away his house key so that he could not enter the home until mother let him in; and hiring a sitter to watch Norman after school. Mother provided constant supervision in the evenings and made sure the boys were never alone together. These arrangements and mother's position that she would testify against Gerard herself if necessary, convinced CPS to allow Gerard to remain in the home with the understanding that any inappropriate behavior by him would result in his immediate removal. Norman felt a great deal of guilt and distress about the possibility that Gerard would no longer be living at home and was very relieved to learn that Gerard would remain unless he behaved inappropriately.

Social and Family Issues

The family in case 1 illustrates many maladaptive patterns of interaction and communication, which allowed the father's abusive behavior to persist for a number of years. These patterns include an unrealistic overdependence or enmeshment in the family, to the degree that any threat to family stability was seen as a threat to each member's very survival. There were inappropriate generational boundaries and coalitions, as evidenced by a dysfunctional marital relationship and delegation of parental responsibilities to the children. Communication was characterized by ambivalent, mixed messages; the need not to hear statements that were threatening or dangerous; and placating "at all costs" rather than discussing and working out problems constructively. These problems not only contributed to onset and maintenance of the father's incestuous behavior but also interfered with the family's ability to cope with events subsequent to the disclosure. These familial problems are illustrated in detail in the following discussion.

Ann initially asked the mother about sexual abuse at a time when this was a widely publicized subject. The mother had been a schoolteacher prior to the birth of Michele and should thus have been more likely than some mothers to be sensitive to this kind of "hint." However, the mother made no attempt to pursue the question with Ann at that time. The mother revealed to us that for several years prior to that episode, the father had wanted to do "kinky" sexual things with her. She refused, and the couple had minimal sexual contact for many years. Despite this, she denied any suspicions of a problem when Ann raised the subject. Whether this was indicative of collusion (i.e., the mother knew or suspected the abuse was occurring and did nothing) or of the mother's need to deny any threatening communication is impossible to determine.

After Marie disclosed abuse the following year, mother did confront father, and to her credit, she forced the issue to be addressed by his therapist. However, she did not try to persuade either girl to speak to child protective services workers, preferring to "work it out as a family." She also did not maintain close supervision of where the father slept at night and whether the abuse had indeed stopped. She never encouraged the girls, even at the family meeting where the father promised to stop the abuse, to report any future abuse to her. Marie was clear that had she felt this kind of support and backing from her mother, she would have been more assertive about reporting or stopping the abuse.

Ann and Marie both feared that if they reported their father's sexual activities, the family would "fall apart." This inappropriate sense of responsibility for holding together a dysfunctional family seems to be a more common finding in victims of ongoing incest. It was certainly reinforced by the mother's overt and covert attitudes. Even after the trial, the mother tried to influence the girls with regard to sentencing, saying things like, "I don't know how we'll manage if your father goes to jail. I'd have to get a job and I don't know if I can find one. How will we live?" When confronted with this in therapy, she denied wanting to influence the girls. Ann and Marie both genuinely feared what would happen to their family without their father. They were unable to view that scenario realistically and reacted with global feelings of impending catastrophe if the family changed in that way.

The mother did many things to indicate her ambivalence toward family members. She told the girls she was "behind them all the way," but she also said she "couldn't take sides" by supporting the girls over her husband. Ann picked up on this and adopted many of her mother's empathic attitudes toward the father; subsequently, even Marie displayed signs of doing this. A few specific episodes are illustrative of the ambivalent message the mother gave to the father and the girls. Once when the electricity went off in the father's apartment, he called the family home and the mother brought him candles, staying with him for an hour while the lights were out. Marie was angry about this, but both the mother and Ann pointed out that "he's still our family and we should take care of him." Marie wondered why no one felt compelled to protect and take care of *her* during the years she was being abused, and why she should worry about her father when he clearly did not worry about how he was hurting her. She quickly felt guilty for having these "vicious" thoughts, however— a guilt that the mother subtly reinforced.

Another time, Michele had a college event that both the father and the mother wanted to attend. Ann and Marie at that time felt very betrayed by their father and said they would not go if he was going to be there. The mother tried to coerce them into going even though Michele said she did not care whether any of the family attended. The mother was unable to side with Ann and Marie, and instead said that if they did not want to go, she and the father would go together. The parents did go together for 3 days (Michele attended college out of town), and Ann and Marie felt their mother "chose him over us." The therapist tried to point this out to the mother, but she was unable or unwilling to consider this view. She said that Michele deserved to have both of her parents there, despite Michele's repeated statements that she did not care whether her parents were present or not. (Michele, in fact, disclosed in family therapy shortly thereafter that the father had also sexually abused her for many years, until she was in her midteens. She had never told anyone about this. She refused to press charges, saying, "It's over; I want to forget it and go on with my life.")

It is clear through all of these events that the mother was unable to take a strong position against the father in order to protect the children. They felt much lack of support and later reported that this contributed to their not taking a stronger stand against their father's behavior. They simply felt that mother accepted what he did, so they should as well. The family's religious background probably contributed to this problem. The guilt of getting a family member in trouble or hurting someone else, and the overly developed sense of responsibility these girls felt, was encouraged by their strong religious training. The fact that their father was a respected minister also probably contributed to their hesitancy to become angry at him or report his abusive behavior.

Even at the present time, the mother continues to give mixed messages to her daughters. She cloaks this in the guise of giving them "control over their lives." When Ann became resistant over coming to therapy, the mother said, "That has to be Ann's decision, not mine." The mother has been unwilling to encourage her daughters to do positive things for themselves, yet has been perfectly ready to coerce them when it is to her own or the father's benefit. The mother has been totally lacking in insight with regard to this pattern, no matter how it has been pointed out to her. No doubt this style enabled the sexual abuse to go on for as many years as it did. The only way Marie was able to break free of this pressure was by rebelling against both parents. She became angry and confrontative with her father prior to her second disclosure and has continued to be much more symptomatic than Ann, who has felt less anger and has been less assertive about reporting or pursuing the legal aspects of the abuse. Marie has received overt and covert messages because of her actions, being told she has "destroyed the family" and that she is a "troublemaker." At some points, Marie has become suicidal because of this betrayal by her family; the possibility of her being placed outside the home has been discussed recently. Marie's perception is that she has been punished for "rocking the boat" and reporting the abuse. This certainly seems accurate (particularly because after the first disclosure, the father continued to abuse only her, not Ann). Unfortunately, if the family cannot change this pattern, Marie may have to leave the home in order to maintain any degree of emotional health.

The father has been in therapy at a facility that specializes in treating sexual offenders. According to his therapist and reports from Ann and Marie, he has focused therapy on his own issues, such as conflicts with his mother when he was a child. He has yet to identify himself as a perpetrator of abuse, saying only that he "loved the children too much." He apparently has had no insight into the fact that he caused long-lasting emotional trauma to his daughters. In fact, he has expressed hurt that they do not want him to return home now that he has been in therapy. (In her typical fashion, the mother has left the responsibility for this decision on the girls' shoulders, saying, "He won't come home until you agree that he can.") Ann has felt guilty for hurting her father and would probably agree to his returning home at this point. Marie also has felt sorry that her father has lost his prestige in the community, and has felt that he has been improving in treatment. (He speaks to the family on the phone frequently and has communicated to them the issues he is addressing in therapy.) However, Marie is still angry and appropriately expects the father to have some understanding of the damage he has done to her and the family. A simple apology is not enough for Marie, she says, because he apologized before but then went right on abusing her.

In summary, the family patterns of overenmeshment, poor communication, needing to maintain the family at all costs, and inappropriate responsibility being placed on the children, along with parental abdication of responsibility, all enabled incest in this case to continue. These patterns have persisted, causing ongoing problems for the victims. In Ann's case, this has been manifested by her need to "be a perfect daughter," requiring herself to care for her mother rather than allowing herself to need nurturance. The only family member who has significantly broken the pattern is Marie. She has been able to do this only by becoming alternatively angry and depressed. She has been on the verge of being rejected from the family because of her refusal to comply with the dysfunctional "rules" of the family. Unfortunately, neither parent has shown any significant motivation to acknowledge or change the way the family operates.

In contrast, the family in case 2 demonstrated much more adaptive interactions. Although mother was initially disbelieving of Norman's allegations, and responded to them by casting blame on father's paramour's son Andre, once she became convinced that the abuse had occurred, she became very supportive of Norman and appropriately set limits on Gerard's behavior. Mother immediately included the boys' father in the decision making by informing him of what she had observed and discussing with him the importance of calling CPS. Despite father's previous anger at mother for trying to blame Andre, he was able to discuss the current circumstances calmly and without blaming mother for the recurrence of the abuse. He supported her decision to contact CPS and was also supportive of mother's insistence that Gerard acknowledge his abuse behavior and accept full responsibility for it. Many families would have faltered in this regard; despite their desire to stop the abuse, they would not have been willing to report and convict another family member. These parents were able to act appropriately because they believed this was not only the best thing for Norman's safety but also the only way that Gerard would get the kind of help he needed. The parents' ability to present a united front to Gerard was probably instrumental in his pleading guilty and cooperating with treatment. At the same time, the parents remained supportive of both children and made arrangements so that Gerard could remain at home (albeit under strict supervision and restricted activities) while assuring Norman's safety. Father transported Gerard to his after-school program and provided backup sitting for Norman when his new sitter was unavailable. Both parents participated in Norman's treatment as well as Gerard's. They praised Norman for his courage in disclosing the abuse and encouraged him to report promptly any inappropriate behavior by Gerard (or others).

Father was very helpful to mother in her attempts to resolve her own guilty feelings. Father stated that he also had had trouble believing Gerard could have abused Norman and never made recriminating remarks to mother about this. He often made supportive comments to mother in therapy, such as, "If it weren't for you, Gerard could still be abusing

Norman." Mother was able to move from guilt to positive action by providing a safe environment for Norman and thus show him that she believed him and wanted him to trust her ability to protect him. This contributed significantly to Norman's recovery, and to the gains Gerard made in treatment as well.

Assessment of Psychopathology

Ann and Marie were assessed individually. On the surface, Ann appeared to be coping fairly well. She was maintaining her honor grades in high school and continued to be involved in her usual activities. Her main symptoms were anxiety and panic attacks. These were not specifically related to the abuse but to events subsequent to the disclosure.

They occurred in relation to what would happen now that her father had left the home. She worried that the family would have to move, that her father would have a nervous breakdown, that her friends would find out about the abuse, and that her mother would "fall apart." She had panic attacks related to these concerns several times a week. Ann denied any depressive symptoms and also denied that she ever thought about her father's abusive behavior, except when police, her therapist, or other authorities brought it up. She denied dissociative features or flashback phenomena. Ann was diagnosed as having an adjustment disorder with anxious features and a panic disorder.

Marie was more symptomatic than Ann. Her grades had fallen from As to Bs and Cs. She fought with her friends more frequently. Marie had many depressive symptoms, including a significant sleep disturbance, frequent crying, and suicidal thoughts. At stressful times, she thought about cutting her wrists or overdosing to "end the pain." Marie had poor concentration and frequent fatigue. In addition to these depressive features, Marie had significant behavioral problems. She had become oppositional with her mother, and in angry outbursts she would throw objects around her bedroom or leave the house for hours at a time without saying where she was going. She was very irritable with her sister Ann, as well as with friends. This profile of anger and aggressive behavior in adolescents who have experienced long-term sexual abuse has been well described in the literature (Runtz & Briere, 1986). Often, when such behaviors occur in the context of frequent intense mood changes and suicidal behavior, the adolescent incest victim may be misdiagnosed as having a borderline personality disorder (Briere, 1989). In evaluating adolescents such as Marie, it is important to understand the etiology of the symptoms rather than focus on the symptoms themselves. Briere believes many female adolescents are misdiagnosed as "borderline" when in fact they are manifesting problems directly related to long-term sexual abuse.

In addition to these symptoms, Marie described frequent intrusive memories of her father abusing her. When she became very sad, she would occasionally experience derealization symptoms. Her diagnosis was major depressive disorder and adjustment disorder with mixed disturbance of conduct and emotion. A rule-out diagnosis of acute posttraumatic stress disorder was also made.

Norman was evaluated individually; parent and teacher reports were also solicited. Both of these informants endorsed significant ADHD symptoms, including hyperactivity, distractibility, impulsivity, and an inability to concentrate. Mother also endorsed symptoms of oppositional defiant disorder, such as Norman being "mouthy" and testing limits at home. However, a careful history revealed that most of these symptoms were fairly recent and had developed around the time when the sexual abuse began. In his individual interview, Norman displayed few ADHD symptoms until the subject of the sexual abuse was raised; at that point, these behaviors became more prominent. It therefore appeared that Norman's ADHD behaviors were in fact symptoms of anxiety, which had emerged soon after the abuse began. It has been noted that PTSD symptoms in young children may mimic ADHD ("Practice parameters," 1998). In fact, Norman's sexually inappropriate behavior with a younger peer at school probably represented posttraumatic play, a form of traumatic reexperiencing displayed by younger children. Although Norman initially denied other reexperiencing or avoidant symptoms, he eventually acknowledged that he often thought about what Gerard did to him while he was in school, and in fact, he was thinking about this when the episode in the school rest room occurred. When he was physically active, the intrusive thoughts were less likely to occur, so Norman said that he usually tried to get these thoughts out of his mind by "doing something else so I don't think at all." This may have explained why Norman became hyperactive and appeared impulsive and distractible in school. Although mother did not report hypervigilance or increased startle reactions in Norman, she did endorse that he was having trouble falling asleep. Norman reported that he also often woke up in the middle of the night with "scary" dreams; although these dreams were not specifically about the sexual abuse, they had begun within the past few months. Norman thus met most of the necessary criteria for PTSD, and this was his provisional diagnosis. (The fact that he reported only one avoidant symptom is not unusual in children and may reflect developmental differences in the manifestation of PTSD ["Practice parameters," 1998].)

Treatment Options

Most programs that specialize in treating incestuous nuclear families have very specific requirements, such as the perpetrator's admitting to his or her inappropriate sexual behavior, the nonabusive parent's providing a safe or supportive home situation, and the perpetrator's not having unsupervised access to the children until various treatment goals have been achieved (Meinig, 1989). Most such programs combine several of the following elements: group therapy for perpetrators, group treatment for spouses of perpetrators, dyadic therapy for mothers and child victims, child victims' groups, individual therapy for victims, and eventual family therapy including the victim, perpetrator, nonabusing parent, and siblings of the victim. Unfortunately, the majority of incestuous families do not meet the entrance requirements for such programs because the perpetrator denies the abuse and/or the mother is unable or unwilling to protect the children adequately from the perpetrator. With these families, therapy is frequently a long and frustrating process. It is not unusual in such circumstances for the child victim to be removed from the home. When the victim remains with family members who are ambivalent or unsupportive, he or she frequently becomes more symptomatic and may require hospitalization. This is what happened with Marie.

Ann was referred for individual and group psychotherapy, as well as family therapy (which was provided through her father's treatment center). After a few months, Ann began missing individual appointments, saying she was "over this" and just wanted to "put it all behind" her. The mother has refused to ask Ann to comply with treatment, saying, "It has to be Ann's decision whether she needs treatment or not; you or I can't decide that for her." It is unclear at this time whether Ann will resume treatment.

Marie began group and individual therapy, and established very positive relationships with the other group members. She was able to provide and accept support very constructively. Soon after the 12-week group ended, Marie became increasingly depressed, culminating in a suicidal gesture (an attempt to stab herself, which the mother stopped). Marie was hospitalized on an adolescent psychiatric unit for 3 weeks. In the hospital, she rapidly improved and stated frequently that she did not want to return home because she felt she received no support there. However, as her discharge approached, she reluctantly agreed to return home at the mother's persistent requests. She continues in individual therapy and family therapy. The possibility of placement outside the home is being seriously considered because of her recurring depressive symptoms and the difficulty her family is having in making significant changes.

Norman received individual treatment based on a cognitive-behavioral treatment model for sexually abused children and their nonoffending parents (Deblinger & Heflin, 1996). This model focuses on correcting attributional errors (i.e., self-blame for the abuse) and other cognitive distortions in the child and nonoffending parent, and includes gradual exposure techniques to decrease PTSD symptoms. This type of treatment has been empirically demonstrated to be superior to nondirective supportive therapy (Cohen & Mannarino, 1996a,b; Cohen & Mannarino, 1998b) and to standard community care (Deblinger, Lippman, & Steer, 1996) in decreasing PTSD, depression, and sexually inappropriate behaviors. Both Norman and his mother experienced a decrease in self-blame and emotional distress; Norman's PTSD and ADHD-like symptoms also responded well to this treatment. Father participated in some of these sessions and provided appropriate support to Norman and mother. Gerard was referred to an adolescent perpetrators' program, which included individual, group, and family components. Gerard was readily accepted into this program because of his willingness to admit to his abusive behaviors. He continues in treatment at this time and has made significant progress. He has apologized to Norman for his abusive behavior and has told Norman he is glad that he told about the abuse because this has helped Gerard understand himself better. There has been no known recurrence of sexually inappropriate behavior in either boy.

Summary and Conclusions

Incest has the potential for causing significant and long-lasting psychological problems for its victims. Children and adult incest survivors exhibit a wide range of psychological responses to the incest experience (Russell, Schurman, & Trocki, 1988); there is no "typical" symptomatology that characterizes most of these victims. Although it does not appear that the child's relationship to the perpetrator *per se* determines psychological outcome, there are many aspects of intrafamilial sexual abuse that may make the experience more difficult for the victim. Some of these legal, social, and familial issues have been presented in this chapter and illustrated by the case histories. As in other cases of child sexual abuse, each child and family must be carefully evaluated to determine the specific dynamics, psychological symptoms, and family issues that are relevant. Treatment should be tailored to address these specific needs. More systematic empirical research is needed to determine how treatment can most effectively aid in optimizing recovery for incest victims, perpetrators, and their families.

References

Briere J. (1989). *Treating adults molested as children: Beyond survival.* New York: Springer.

Cohen J. A., & Mannarino, A. P. (1988). Psychological symptoms in sexually abused girls. *Child Abuse and Neglect, 12,* 517–577.

Cohen, J. A., & Mannarino, A. P. (1996a). Factors that mediate treatment outcome in sexually abused preschool children. *Journal of the American Academy of Child and Adolescent Psychiatry, 35,* 1402–1410.

Cohen, J. A., & Mannarino, A. P. (1996b). A treatment outcome study for sexually abused preschool children: Initial findings. *Journal of the American Academy of Child and Adolescent Psychiatry, 35,* 42–50.

Cohen, J. A., & Mannarino, A. P. (1998a). Factors that mediate treatment outcome of sexually abused preschoolers: Six and twelve-month follow-ups. *Journal of the American Academy of Child and Adolescent Psychiatry, 37,* 44–51.

Cohen, J. A., & Mannarino, A. P. (1998b). Interventions for sexually abused children: Initial treatment findings. *Child Maltreatment, 3,* 17–26.

Deblinger, E., Heflin, A. H. (1996). *Treatment for sexually abused children and their nonoffending parents: A cognitive behavioral approach.* Thousand Oaks, CA: Sage.

Deblinger, E., Lippman, J., & Steer, R. (1996). Sexually abused children suffering PTSD symptoms: Initial treatment outcome findings. *Child Maltreatment, 1,* 310–321.

Faller, K. C. (1988). The myth of the "collusive mother." *Journal of Interpersonal Violence, 3,* 190–196.

Friedrich, W. N., Luecke, W. J., Beilke, R. L., & Place, V. (1992). Psychotherapy outcome of sexually abused boys: An agency study. *Journal of Interpersonal Violence, 7,* 396–409.

Landwirth, J. (1987). Children as witnesses in child sexual abuse trials. *Pediatrics, 80,* 585–589.

Mannarino, A. P., & Cohen, J. A. (1986). A clinical-demographic study of sexually abused children. *Child Abuse and Neglect, 10,* 17–28.

Mannarino, A. P., & Cohen, J. A. (1996a). Family related variables and psychological symptom formation in sexually abused girls. *Journal of Child Sexual Abuse, 5,* 105–119.

Mannarino, A. P., & Cohen, J. A. (1996b). A follow-up study of factors which mediate the development of psychological symptomatology in sexually abused girls. *Child Maltreatment, 1,* 246–260.

Mannarino, A. P., & Cohen, J. A. (1996c). Abuse related attributions and perceptions, general attributions, and locus of control in sexually abused girls. *Journal of Interpersonal Violence, 11,* 162–180.

Mannarino, A. P., Cohen, J. A., & Gregor, M. (1989). Emotional and behavioral difficulties in sexually abused girls. *Journal of Interpersonal Violence, 4,* 437–451.

Practice parameters for the diagnosis and treatment of PTSD in children and adolescents. (1998). *Journal of the American Academy of Child and Adolescent Psychiatry, 37*(10) Supplement, S4–S26.

Runtz, M. T., & Briere, J. (1986). Adolescent "acting out" and childhood history of sexual abuse. *Journal of Interpersonal Violence, 1,* 325–334.

Runyan, D. K., Everson, M. D., Edelsohn, G. A., Hunter, W. H., & Coulter, M. L. (1988). Impact of legal intervention on sexually abused children. *Journal of Pediatrics, 113,* 647–653.

Russell, D. E. H., Schurman, R. A., & Trocki, K. (1988). The long-term effects of incestuous abuse: A comparison of Afro-American and white American victims. In G. E. Wyatt & G. J. Powell (Eds.), *Lasting effects of child sexual abuse.* Newbury Park, CA: Sage.

12

Maltreatment of Children with Disabilities

Robert T. Ammerman, Martin J. Lubetsky, and Karen F. Stubenbort

Description of the Problem

As professional and public awareness of the problem of child maltreatment expands, increased attention is being directed toward abuse and neglect of children with disabilities. Indeed, in the initial stages of controlled empirical research on child maltreatment, several authors speculated that children with disabilities are at greater risk for abuse and neglect relative to their peers without disabilities (Helfer, 1973; Solomons, 1979). This belief was derived, in large part, from the growing literature reporting a disproportionate number of individuals with disabilities in samples of abused and neglected children (e.g., Birrell & Birrell, 1968; Lightcap, Kurland, & Burgess, 1982). Methodological shortcomings in much of this literature, however, prompted some authors to reject the link between disability and subsequent maltreatment (Starr, Dietrich, Fischhoff, Ceresnie, & Zweier, 1984). In contrast, others have acknowledged the relative paucity of and methodological limitations in much of the research con-

Robert T. Ammerman • Division of Psychology, Children's Hospital Medical Center, Cincinnati, Ohio 45229.   **Martin J. Lubetsky** • University of Pittsburgh School of Medicine, Western Psychiatric Institute and Clinic, Pittsburgh, Pennsylvania 15213.   **Karen F. Stubenbort** • Department of Psychiatry, Allegheny General Hospital, Pittsburgh, Pennsylvania 15212.

Case Studies in Family Violence, Second Edition, edited by Ammerman and Hersen. Kluwer Academic / Plenum Publishers, New York, 2000.

ducted to date, but argue that there are compelling reasons to suspect that a significant number of children with disabilities are at heightened risk for maltreatment in general, and physical abuse in particular (Ammerman, Van Hasselt, & Hersen, 1988).

Most theoretical models of child abuse and neglect include the contribution of certain child characteristics to the etiology of maltreatment (Ammerman & Galvin, 1998). In general, these factors consist of severe behavior problems (e.g., oppositionality, aggression, defiance) or variables that often elicit negative reactions from caregivers (e.g., prolonged crying). The relationship between disability and maltreatment is based upon the similarity between hypothesized "abuse-provoking" behaviors of some maltreated children (Ammerman, 1991; deLissovoy, 1979) and those often exhibited by children with disabling conditions.

Ammerman et al. (1988), describe three processes whereby children with disabilities are at heightened risk for maltreatment: (1) disruption in the formation of infant–caregiver attachment, (2) prolonged stress associated with raising some children with disabilities, and (3) increased vulnerability to certain types of maltreatment. Insecure attachment is a common finding in maltreated children and their caregivers, and is primarily thought to be a consequence of abuse and neglect (Cicchetti, 1987), although some authors have suggested that it can play a causative role in maltreatment as well (Ainsworth, 1980). A number of factors may impede the formation of secure attachment in children with disabilities, including frequent mother–infant separations secondary to illness and deficits in specific attachment-promoting behaviors (e.g., gaze, responsiveness) in physically and sensory-disabled children.

Stress is an additional risk factor in families of children with disabilities. Some of these children display difficult-to-manage behavior problems that are resistant to intervention. These consist of stereotypies, self-injurious behaviors, aggression, hyperactivity, crying, and screaming. Moreover, children with disabilities often require increased care and supervision that further adds to caregiver stress. The frustration engendered by these difficulties may contribute to subsequent abuse.

The final risk factor associated with maltreatment in children with disabilities is vulnerability. Specifically, many children with disabilities are more vulnerable to maltreatment in that cognitive or communicative deficits prevent them from revealing to others information regarding mistreatment. In addition, their greater need for care, assistance, special education, or medical support, provides unique opportunities for neglect.

Of course, the degree to which the aforementioned factors contribute to risk for maltreatment is dependent upon the type of disabling condition, its severity, the functional limitations of the child, and the course of disorder (stable versus degenerative). Furthermore, it is acknowledged that other variables (e.g., social isolation, financial hardship, substance abuse) are more influential in the etiology of maltreatment than the presence of a disability. Risk for abuse and neglect is posited to increase when a child with a disability is introduced into a family that *already* displays those characteristics that can lead to maltreatment (e.g., poor parenting skills, impulse-control deficits, unemployment, past experience of abuse).

More recent research has underscored the importance of context in the elevation of risk for maltreatment. For example, Ammerman, Hersen, Van Hasselt, Lubetsky, and Sieck (1994) identified a variety of factors that differentiated mothers of children with disabilities who used harsh physical punishment and those who used mild or no corporal punishment: mother's age, knowledge of parenting skills, social support, IQ, stress, and child behavior problems. However, use of more severe disciplinary practices was best explained by the interaction of maternal anger reactivity and child's rebellious behavior; diminished maternal social support and increased independence in the child; and child's younger age and more mature socialization. The *context* of maternal variables (anger reactivity and poor social support) and child characteristics (higher functional abilities—which, in turn, indicate less severe and less overt disabling conditions—and externalizing behaviors) were most strongly related to the use of harsh physical punishment.

The importance of context is also evident in a study of abuse potential in young children with and without disabilities (Ammerman & Patz, 1996). Using the Child Abuse Potential Inventory, Ammerman and Patz (1996) found that variability in obtained Abuse Scale scores was best accounted for by the interaction of negative child characteristics (hyperactivity, demandingness, moodiness) and diminished social support in mothers. This relationship was evident in both children with and without disabling conditions.

Some have argued that children with "less severe" disabilities are more vulnerable to physical abuse than their more functionally limited peers. Indeed, findings from the Ammerman *et al.* (1994) study support the premise that children with milder disabilities (but who exhibit significant behavior problems) are at great risk of receiving harsher physical punishment. Examples of these disabilities include mild mental retardation, attention-deficit/hyperactivity disorder, and learning disabilities. Ammerman and Boerger (1998) elucidated the process by which this increased risk might be manifested. They derived a measure of parental intent (the attribution that children misbehave for manipulative and purposeful reasons) in mothers and fathers of children with disabilities who were involved with child protective service agencies secondary to indicated or substantiated physical abuse or neglect. Parental intent was significantly correlated with child's age, child behavior problems, stress related to parenting, low frustration tolerance in parents, diminished empathy, and use of more severe disciplinary practices. Such misattributions may be more likely to occur in children with less severe and overt disabilities, thereby facilitating the expression of physical disciplinary practices in high-risk parents.

Regardless of whether or not children with disabilities are at higher risk for maltreatment, the fact remains that a significant proportion of these children are abused or neglected and are in need of intervention. For example, in a study of children involved with child protective service agencies in the United States, Crosse, Kaye, and Ratnofsky (1993) found a substantial over-representation of children with disabilities in child welfare caseloads. In comparison to maltreated children without disabilities in the sample, those with disabilities were 2.8 times more likely to be emotionally neglected, 2.1 times more likely to be physically abused, 1.8 times more likely to be sexually abused, and 1.6 times more likely to be physically neglected. In 47% of cases, caseworkers believed that characteristics associated with disability contributed to the maltreatment. Sullivan and Knutson (1998) retrospectively examined the medical charts of over 39,000 hospitalized children. Of the 15% that were identified as having been maltreated, 64% had a disability. Ammerman *et al.* (1994) prospectively interviewed caregivers of 138 children and adolescents with disabilities who were psychiatrically hospitalized. Sixty-one percent of the sample were found to have experienced a severe form of abuse or neglect at some point in their lifetime. Clearly, clinicians and other professionals involved in helping these families must be sensitive to the unique issues encountered in treating the abused or neglected child with a disability. Although there is content overlap in assessment of and intervention with families who maltreat their children with disabilities and those who abuse or neglect their nondisabled children, a number of special considerations must be taken into account when working with this population. The complexities associated with such families are illustrated in the following cases involving abuse and neglect if children with disabilities.

Case Description 1

Peter L. was a 6-year-old white male who lived at home with his mother (Ms. R., age 24) and younger brother Nick (age 3). Peter's father (Mr. L.) and mother had lived together 7 years, and then separated 1 year prior to Peter's hospitalization. Up until 5 months prior to admission, Mr. L. maintained contact with the family but had since left the state. Ms. R. received public assistance and lived in a subsidized housing project. Peter was referred by a local mental health center to the John Merck Program for Multiply Disabled Children at Western Psychiatric Institute and Clinic (Pittsburgh) for overactivity, impulsivity, and inattentiveness. Because of the severity of these problems and their resistance to prior treatment, an inpatient evaluation was recommended. This was Peter's first psychiatric hospitalization.

A comprehensive neuropsychiatric assessment revealed a variety of disruptive behavior problems and concomitant physical conditions. Peter was observed to be impulsive, oppositional, inattentive, and hyperactive. These problems were reported to occur both at school and at home. In addition, Ms. R. complained that he was aggressive, especially toward his younger brother. Ms. R. also reported weekly occurrences of nighttime enuresis. Finally, Peter exhibited self-injurious behavior (self-biting), masturbation, bolting from his mother and running away, recklessness, and a lack of awareness of danger. Examples of the latter include an incident in which he swallowed an entire bottle of aspirin, and another where he jumped into a frozen pond because "he wanted to swim."

Upon admission to the John Merck Program, Peter was receiving 10 mg of methylphenidate three times per day to treat his inattention and overactivity. Moderate improvement in attention span was noted both at home and at school, although no changes occurred in Peter's aggressiveness, defiance, and noncompliance. One year prior to admission, Peter was prescribed 100 mg of Pemoline once per day. This was discontinued because of several negative side effects, including irritability, lethargy, and increased noncompliance and aggression.

Ms. R. was distraught over her difficulties in handling Peter and managing his behavior problems. In particular, she was quite concerned about his aggression, which she described as being unpredictable and severe. Typically, she responded to his aggression with physical restraint. Upon being released, he would often continue to aggress against his younger brother. She also expressed frustration that, because of his language and cognitive limitations, she was unable to "reason" with him. Ms. R. reported frequent use of moderate to severe corporal punishment. These involved slapping Peter in the face, and spanking him on the buttocks and legs with a stick, paddle, fly swatter, or belt. Although Peter's younger brother "did not need" this form of discipline, Peter's misbehavior was "serious enough" that Ms. R. resorted to physical punishment at least once a day. In addition, on one occasion during which Peter was biting other children, she instructed the other children to "bite him back, to teach him what it is like." Ms. R. acknowledged that these methods were ineffective in managing Peter. In addition, she described two incidents, the last occurring 6 months prior to admission, in which she had "lost control" and spanked Peter until he had black-and-blue marks on his buttocks that lasted for several days.

Ms. R. was raised in an intact family with two sisters. Her father was an alcoholic, and she witnessed his physical battering of her mother that often resulted in facial marks and bruises. Ms. R. was disciplined, primarily by her father, with a belt, paddle, and hairbrush. During high school, Ms. R. used drugs (i.e., marijuana, amphetamines) and alcohol. She quit school on her own at the age of 17 because she "wanted to have children." At the age of 18, she moved in with Peter's biological father. When she was 20, Peter was born.

Peter was 6 weeks premature and weighed 5 pounds 6 ounces at birth. He had respiratory problems that required oxygen treatment. Ms. R. described Peter as a "jittery" baby who was difficult to comfort, did not like to be held, and had problems sleeping through the night during his first year of life. Shortly after Peter's birth, Mr. L. became physically abusive toward Ms. R. and Peter. He did not accept Peter's medical problems and developmental delays, and he would frequently hit Peter to "toughen him up." This abuse lasted from age 1 to 5, often resulting in welts and bruises that lasted up to 2 days. These incidents were more likely to occur when Mr. L. drank alcohol excessively. Ms. R. also was physically abused by Mr. L. approximately every 4 months, resulting in facial bruising. On one occasion, Ms. R. took Peter and hid in the woods next to their home when Mr. L. returned home drunk. Ms. R. reported that both children witnessed the physical violence directed toward her.

Also around this time, Ms. R. had a variety of odd jobs in order to support the family. While she was working, Mr. L. was responsible for care of the children. She reported that during her absences the children were neglected, and she described several accidents to underscore his lack of supervision of the children. For example, at one point, Peter cut his foot on a piece of glass while walking barefoot through some garbage near the home. On another occasion, he put his hand in a blender and was seriously cut.

Ms. R. was evaluated by a comprehensive assessment and treatment program conducted in collaboration between Western Psychiatric Institute and Clinic and the Western Pennsylvania School for Blind Children (Pittsburgh) and funded by The National Institute on Disability and Rehabilitation Research (U.S. Department of Education). Because of her serious parenting difficulties and history of abuse, she was offered treatment in conjunction with the psychiatric interventions that were implemented during Peter's hospitalization.

Case Description 2

Alicia was a 7-year-old white female who lived at home with her mother (Mrs. S.), step-father (Mr. S.), and a sister (5 years old), and a brother (2 years old). Alicia had been diagnosed with mild mental retardation and had been placed in EMR classes since the first grade. She was also diagnosed with attention-deficit/hyperactivity disorder. However, the family had failed to follow up with outpatient treatment, and Alicia was not prescribed stimulant medications. Alicia and her family were referred to the Child Assessment and Management Project (CAMP), a treatment evaluation study conducted at the Western Pennsylvania School for Blind Children and funded by the National Institute on Disabilities and Rehabilitation Research (U.S. Department of Education). The referral was made by a local child protective service agency. The incident that led to their involvement had occurred several months prior to their involvement with CAMP. Alicia's parents had taken her to the hospital after she broke her arm. They claimed that Alicia's cousin had caused the arm to be broken during rough play, although hospital staff suspected that Alicia had been abused by her parents, and they contacted the child protective service agency. The family had been involved with a child protective service agency in an adjacent county a year before. At that time, Alicia had a bruise on her face that was noticed by her teacher. According to her parents, she had fallen on a cement floor as a result of "clumsiness." Alicia was sent to the hospital at that point, staff were suspicious about inconsistencies in parental reports about the injury, and the child protective service agency was brought in. Regarding the most recent incident, the child protective service agency found *indicated* abuse, stating that they could not directly prove that her parents had perpetrated the injury. Prior to their referral to CAMP, the family had been involved with several caseworkers and had undergone a number of evaluations and participated in various interventions. All of these had resulted in little positive change. Moreover, the parents expressed a deep resentment of child protective service agencies, and they had a particularly poor relationship with a particular caseworker who had recently been involved with them. (It is noteworthy that several other providers in the area shared with the CAMP staff the impressions that this caseworker was especially difficult and that other families had expressed frustration in working with him.) The CAMP study was designed to evaluate the effectiveness of a cognitive-behavioral parent training intervention for abused and neglected children with disabilities and their families. The S.s were randomly assigned to one of the intervention groups.

As part of the CAMP program, a comprehensive assessment of the mother, stepfather, and child was administered. Results from selected assessment measures are presented in Table 1. Both parents were also given the Child Abuse and Neglect Interview Schedule (Ammerman, Van Hasselt, & Hersen, 1987), a semistructured interview examining the child's behavior, history, parental disciplinary practices, neglect, sexual abuse, and parental history of maltreatment and violence. It should be noted that the parents completed the Child Abuse Potential Inventory (Milner, 1986), although both profiles were deemed invalid due to a "faking-good" response style. This is consistent with the denials by both parents that they were involved with Alicia's injuries, despite converging evidence to the contrary.

Mrs. S. reported a variety of concerns about Alicia's behavior. In particular, she described Alicia as oppositional, clumsy, impulsive, intrusive, motorically overactive, inattentive, difficult to motivate, and anxious. She also reported temper tantrums, noncompliance, intermittent aggression, and irritability. An examination of her scores on the Parenting Stress Index (Abidin, 1986) revealed that Mrs. S. was experiencing a significant amount of stress related to Alicia and her behavior. Her scores on all of the scales in the Child

Table 1. Selected Results from the Assessment of Alicia's Mother and Stepfather (Case 2)

Measure	Mother	Stepfather
Beck Depression Inventory	10	5
Knowledge of behavioral principles as applied to children	13	16
Estimated IQ	77	104
Aberrant Behavior Checklist		
Irritability	18	30
Stereotype	2	0
Lethargy	13	13
Hyperactivity	29	31
Excessive speech	8	4
Parenting Stress Index (percentile)		
Total	85	80
Child domain	99+	95
Adaptability	99+	85
Acceptability	95	85
Demandingness	85	99+
Mood	95	95
Distractibility/hyperactivity	85	85
Reinforces parents	99+	90
Parent domain	40	45
Depression	15	30
Attachment	75	50
Restriction of role	5	25
Sense of competence	70	40
Social isolation	75	85
Relationship with spouse	40	55
Parent health	75	75
Life stress	40	25

Domain exceeded the 85th percentile. She also had elevated scores on several scales in the Parent Domain, including diminished attachment to Alicia, low confidence about parental abilities, social isolation, and health problems. On the Aberrant Behavioral Checklist (Aman & Singh, 1986), a measure of behavior problems specifically designed for individuals with mental retardation and other disabling conditions, she particularly endorsed items reflecting hyperactivity and irritability. Mrs. S. stated that she typically responded to Alicia's behavior problems by yelling, making threats ("I'll send you to Grandma's house to live if you don't behave"), spanking (although she denied losing control or using objects in corporal punishment), and physical restraint. She viewed these methods as only mildly effective. Mrs. S. received a low score of 13 on the Knowledge of Behavioral Principles as Applied to Children (O'Dell, Tarler-Benludo, & Flynn, 1979). This, in combination with her below average estimated IQ of 77 (as obtained from the Shipley Institute of Living Scale; Zachary, 1986), indicates that Mrs. S. had few parenting skills against a background of limited intellectual capacity. Regarding her own upbringing, Mrs. S. described that she was spanked as a child and that her mother also used threats as a way to control her behavior ("I will leave and not come back if you don't behave"). Mrs. S. was also the victim of rape at the age of 15, of which Alicia was the product.

It is noteworthy that Mr. S. participated in the assessment and the CAMP project, as it was often the case in the program (as has been reported by numerous other service providers and research projects) that fathers are typically reluctant to be active participants in such endeavors. Although both Mr. and Mrs. S. were guarded in their answers regarding physical discipline, both of them appeared to be quite sincere in their desire for help and assistance in raising Alicia. As presented in Table 1, there were some key similarities and differences between the assessment results of Mr. S. in comparison to his wife. His score of 5 on the Beck Depression Inventory (Beck, Ward, Mendelson, Mock, & Erbaugh, 1961) was low in contrast to Mrs. S. (although neither of them obtained scores indicative of clinically significant depression). His score on the Knowledge of Behavioral Principles as Applied to Children was only slightly higher than that of Mrs. S., and it was significantly lower than the means scores obtained in other studies. His estimated IQ was in the average range. Mr. S. also reported a significant amount of stress related to Alicia's behavior. He obtained a score in the 95th percentile on the Child Domain of the Parenting Stress Index. In the Parent Domain, he reported elevated scores reflecting social isolation and health problems. He expressed concerns about Alicia's noncompliance, oppositionality, frequent injuries due to "running into things," and intrusiveness. In terms of disciplinary practices, he reported yelling, using threats ("I'll tie you up in a chair"), time out (which was particularly ineffective in that she refused to stay in the time-out chair), and spanking. In general, Mr. S. felt that he and his wife were "too lenient" with Alicia. He believed that Alicia was just resistant to "authority" and was able to control herself when she wanted to. In describing his own upbringing, Mr. S. stated that he was often hit with a belt, typically by his paternal grandfather. In addition, his mother would threaten to place him in a foster home if he did not behave. Both Mr. & Mrs. S. denied alcohol and drug abuse, and they both stated that they did not engage in physical fights.

Alicia and her family lived in subsidized housing. Mr. S. had completed the 11th grade and was unemployed. Mrs. S. had dropped out of school in the 9th grade and had never been employed. Their housing was inadequate, and the home in which they lived badly needed paint and repairs. It was also dirty and unkempt. The children, however, appeared to have their hygiene and nutritional needs met. While there were no overt signs of neglect, Mrs. S. stated that she occasionally left Alicia alone up to 10 minutes at a time. On two occasions, Alicia was injured during these absences. At one point, she left the house through the back door and picked up a broken bottle, almost severing one of her fingers. Both Mr. and Mrs. S. expressed suspicion that Alicia might have been sexually abused at one point. They stated that after Alicia had visited a mentally retarded cousin at her grandfather's home she returned and was found touching her genitals. No other proof was offered that there had been sexual contact between Alicia and the cousin, although the parents were suspicious enough not to send her over there again.

Medical Issues

Peter presented with a history of multiple medical and psychiatric problems and interventions. He was born 6 weeks premature and his lungs were not fully developed, resulting in respiratory difficulty. This also required care in a special nursery involving oxygen treatment and other medical interventions. This, in turn, led to multiple caregivers' involvement in an environment with constant stimulation by individuals other than his mother. It is unclear what impact this disruption had in the early formation of infant–mother attachment. However, such separations are common in congenitally disabled and medically fragile children, and may play a role in risk for subsequent maltreatment (Ammerman, Van Hasselt, & Hersen, 1988).

As infants, both Peter and Alicia were described as being difficult to comfort. Parents are typically reinforced by an infant who cuddles, coos, and feeds well. Peter's parents, on the other hand, were frustrated by his apparent frailty and irritability and their inability to soothe and satisfy him. Chess (1970) has described infants with different personality styles and their impact on parents' coping abilities. Peter would be categorized, at best, as the "slow-to-warm-up" child who presents as negative, has intense reactions to new stimuli, and needs extensive encouragement. At other times, he could be categorized more as the "difficult" child who has unpredictable sleeping and eating habits, rejects new toys or foods, and has tantrums in response to frustration.

By the age of 1 year Peter was diagnosed as visually impaired. His parents questioned why he was not responding to toys placed in front of him. At that time, they had to cope with a child that was difficult to satisfy, had received early medical interventions (and survived), but would have an intractable visual impairment. It was about this time that Peter's father became physically abusive toward Peter and his mother, possibly in response to the frustration related to his special needs.

At age 3, Peter was diagnosed with a seizure disorder. It was first noticed when he had staring spells, cessation of activity, and drooling. This led to multiple appointments with neurologists for EEGs, another CT scan of the brain, and introduction of anticonvulsant medications. Although Peter's parents had heard of seizures, they had to learn to observe and document these episodes, give medication three times a day, watch for side effects, and return for neurology appointments. In addition, Peter was "always on the go," fidgety, and "getting into everything." Peter's father did not accept that he needed extended attention and care but contended that he would "overcome" or "outgrow" it.

By this time, Peter's parents and physicians also questioned why he was not speaking and why developmental milestones of walking and toilet training were delayed. Further evaluations revealed developmental speech and language disorders and mental retardation (which was specified as mild a year later). Having a child who could neither reason well nor clearly communicate wishes or needs when compared with other same-age children may have further impeded Mr. L.'s ability to cope.

In addition, Peter continued to contract respiratory infections resulting in bronchospasm and recurrent asthma. His medical problems not only frightened his parents but also required frequent emergency room visits, clinic appointments, and medications when ill. The fear aroused by a child displaying respiratory distress or having a seizure, and especially being unable to communicate effectively, may have reactivated the early fears of the parents about having a "vulnerable child."

By age 5, Peter was evaluated by a child psychiatrist for overactivity, impulsivity, inattention, distractibility, oppositionality, noncompliance, and temper tantrums. In spite of medication trials of pemoline and methylphenidate, his difficult-to-manage behaviors persisted. His mother reportedly was fearful of Peter's getting into dangerous situations. This fear was substantiated by his actions, including falling into a pond and taking his mother's pills on one occasion in the past.

As exemplified by Peter, children with disabilities commonly have more medical evaluations and interventions than children without disabilities. Approximately 67% of children with disabilities present with more than one condition (33% have one disability, 33% have two disabilities, and 33% have three or more disabilities) (Gottlieb, 1987). The combinations of varied forms of disabilities can result in a severely impaired child with multiple conditions. In addition, dual diagnosis is another form of multiple disability in which mental retardation and mental illness coexist. This was the case with Peter, who had multiple physical disabilities *and* severe psychiatric/behavioral problems.

The child's disability frequently leads to delayed development and requires increased intervention to optimize progress. For example, visually impaired children may have other coexisting medical conditions that interfere with normal development (i.e., hearing impairment, ambulating problems, mental retardation, seizure disorder). They also may have delays in attachment, gross motor skills, locomotion, language, and social development (Fraiberg, 1977). In the case of Alicia, it was evident that she was being raised in an environment with low levels of stimulation and active nurturance. Although there might have been congenital impairments, Alicia's development was undermined and the impact of her disabilities exacerbated (behavioral dyscontrol, social incompetence, and diminished cognitive capacity) by the deleterious family ecology.

Added medical needs can heighten vulnerability to maltreatment, since they often require so much additional time, money, commitment, and energy from parents. In children with disabilities, the potential for neglect can arise more frequently if the need for additional medical care is ignored. There are certainly more opportunities to be neglectful when more care is required. Ignoring simple child-care issues with a normal child may be far less dangerous than for a child with a disability. For example, contractures can occur in a child with severe cerebral palsy, and skin breakdown, open sores, and infection must be avoided in the child with spina bifida. Further, environmental dangers need to be identified and corrected. Examples of these include open room heaters than can lead to burns, open doors to stairways that can be a hazard for falling, and cigarettes left in ashtrays that can be used for fire setting. For those children who cannot verbally report danger or pain, considerably greater supervision and patience are needed. The injuries sustained by Alicia when she was left unattended are prime example of such risks for children who are hyperactive and impulsive. (As is often the case in maltreatment, contributory factors are not always clear. For example, Mrs. S. reported that she "never" left Alicia alone for longer than 10 minutes. This is certainly a sufficient amount of time for a child with ADHD to engage in a dangerous activity. However, Mrs. S.'s report was suspect, and it is possible that Alicia was left alone for a longer period of time.)

Recognition of physical abuse is elusive in children who already have bruises or scars due to clumsiness, ataxia, poor coordination, hyperactivity, or impulsivity, or who lack the awareness of dangers (Ammerman *et al.*, 1988). Such children may be injured as a consequence of their disabilities, or inadequate protection and supervision, rather than direct physical punishment. It may be difficult for parents to know what an adequate level of supervision is for their child with a disability, as compared to a child without a disability, in the absence of professional education and training. On several occasions, Alicia had injuries that her parents attributed to "clumsiness." Although it was the judgment of medical professionals that Alicia's injuries were not accidental, definitive proof was unavailable. The child with language impediments may be unable to communicate when physical or sexual abuse or neglect has occurred, thereby further impeding rapid identification.

Legal and Criminal Justice Systems Issues

The role of the legal and criminal justice systems in abuse and neglect of children begins with child protective service agencies. Such organizations exist in most developed countries in one form or the other. They are responsible for the investigation of suspected abuse and neglect, and for providing temporary emergency shelter for children in acute danger. In the cases of Peter and Alicia, their families had been involved with child protective services because of past abuse and neglect. For Peter, the family was monitored by a caseworker, the father was not removed from the home, and additional support services were not provided. Unfortunately, limited resources and the excessive caseloads typically carried by child protective service agencies curtail efforts to implement comprehensive interventions with many families (as occurred with Peter and his family). Although Ms. R. was found to be at high risk for engaging in physical abuse, the clinical team working with Peter and his family did not find sufficient reason to file additional reports of incidents of mistreatment. For Alicia, the family had been involved with several child protective service agencies in different counties. In fact, their recidivism and long-term contact with child welfare agencies highlights the most difficult challenge facing the child protection field: how to identify and help these families who engage in chronic, and often intergenerational, maltreatment. This group of families utilizes the largest proportion of resources, is the least responsive to standard interventions, and is the most likely to raise children at risk for emotional and behavioral problems.

Existence of a disability complicates the already-difficult process of investigating suspected cases of abuse and neglect and providing needed services. As previously mentioned, cognitive limitations of the child and injuries secondary to the disabling condition rather than abuse *per se* impede accurate identification of abuse. Also, for children with disabilities who are aggressive, physical restraint procedures may lead to bruises or hand marks that are attributed to mistreatment. (It should be noted that there is an active and contentious debate in the disability field about the use of physical restraints; currently, legislation greatly restricts and regulates their use by professionals and it is generally acknowledged that such procedures should be employed only when the children are in danger of harming themselves or others.) Of course, Mr. and Mrs. S. inappropriately used restrained as a primary management strategy, underscoring how such procedures can be abusive.

An additional problem in recognizing abuse and neglect of children with disabilities is the frequent presence of multiple caregivers for the child. These include other family members, babysitters, respite caseworkers, special education teachers, and support staff. Therefore, caseworkers must be thorough in their investigation of possible perpetrators and must also be vigilant for false allegations of mistreatment directed toward nonparental care providers.

Child protective service agencies must also contend with finding appropriate services for children with disabilities and their families. Depending on the type and extent of impairment, these might include medical and psychiatric services, parent training, and parent support groups. Accessibility to needed organizations varies considerably across localities. For low-incidence conditions, proper facilities may be unavailable in most communities. For children who are removed from the home, foster care and adoption services may be unprepared and untrained to address the special needs of children with disabilities.

The relationship between families and caseworkers is often precarious. Initially, there is a strong adversarial quality to the relationship, because caseworkers conduct investigations that may lead to criminal accusations or the removal of the child from the home. It is the primary goal, however, of child protective service agencies to protect the child and provide needed services to the child and family. Numerous forces converge to undermine obtainment of this goal. Caseworkers are typically overworked and poorly compensated, provided with limited supports and resources, often receive inadequate training (particularly involving children with disabilities), and are under intense public scrutiny. Some families are uncooperative and difficult to work with because they contend with such factors as poverty, neighborhood crime, and substance abuse. Alicia's family had substantial problems with a caseworker, and as a result they reported being skeptical of professional help. On the other hand, they did not follow up on recommendations to seek psychiatric care for Alicia. Not surprisingly, Alicia's most recent caseworker expressed considerable frustration at the family's lack of progress and improvement over the years. Balancing these competing forces is a formidable task for child protective caseworkers.

Finally, children with disabilities are usually involved in a variety of systems. These include schools (where they will have Individualized Educational Programs, or IEPs, and be involved with other professionals, such as physical therapists), base service units, and medical clinics. It is through these organizations that maltreatment is most likely to be identified. This is most clearly evident with Alicia, in that two reports of suspected abuse were filed by medical staff. Just as it is imperative that caseworkers be trained in the unique clinical issues associated with children with disabilities, it is also essential that educators and health-care providers receive training in the identification of abuse and neglect in children with disabilities.

Family and Social Issues

Peter's family history and home environment revealed vulnerabilities for potential abuse and neglect. Peter's mother grew up in a low-income home with an abusive and alcoholic father who physically mistreated her and her mother. Thus, she not only experienced this abuse but observed it frequently in the home. Peter's parents were poor and socially isolated from their own family and friends. Peter's father drank alcohol frequently and was more abusive when intoxicated. Peter's parents fought often over many issues, particularly about his special needs. They separated 1 year prior to his psychiatric hospitalization, and his father had no contact with the family after 7 months. In addition, Peter was left with multiple caretakers, whose skills were questionable, while his parents were periodically working.

Peter reportedly observed his mother being hit by his father on numerous occasions. He was also a target of severe physical punishment by his father. His mother reported "feeling like losing control" and feeling more frustrated and stressed when Peter was disruptive. This led to her use of harsh punishment on several occasions.

Alicia's family also exhibited a number of areas of concern and distress. They were poor and undereducated, leading to a variety of financial stressors. Both parents reported being socially isolated, a common characteristic of maltreating families and a significant contributor to the emergence and chronicity of abuse and neglect. Mrs. S. was intellectually limited and had never been employed. She was thus highly dependent on Mr. S. for financial support and assistance in day-to-day living. Mr. S. was authoritarian and typically had the "last word" in family decisions. This dynamic was particularly evident in issues of child care and behavior management; Mr. S.'s belief that Alicia was stubborn and "resistant to authority" and his frequent use of physical restraint were the primary management approach for both parents.

As in Peter's and Alicia's cases, the social, economic, and emotional burden on a family with a child with a disability are great. For some families, the stresses may become unmanageable. As Goldfarb, Brotherson, Summers, and Turnbull (1986) have summarized: "Obviously a disability or illness is itself a major life crisis.... But disabilities and illnesses also carry with them a number of side effects that cause stress to add up. There may be an unrelenting demand for physical or nursing care or supervision.... And in the back of everyone's mind there is an undercurrent of stress.... [There are] too many bills, [and] not enough time to get everything done" (p. 21).

The birth of a child with a disability can affect a marital relationship and the subsequent care of the child. Pueschel, Bernier, and Weidenman (1988) have found that "the birth of a handicapped child is bound to affect a husband and wife's relationship.... When the baby has special needs, an extra dimension of stress is added. Some marriages, however, have problems unrelated to the child's disability that may become more evident during this period of stress" (p. 17).

It is important to address the impact of a child with disabilities on the family system as a whole. The requirements for a family to survive stress points in which breakdown can occur have been described by Goldfarb *et al.* (1986). These family needs are in such areas as (1) economic, (2) health and security, (3) physical caretaking, (4) social, (5) recreational, (6) affectional, (7) self-definitional, and (8) educational. For example, not only are more costs incurred depending upon the type of disability, but parents may have less time to earn an income as caretaking needs increase. The family may have less recreation time, which in most families serves to reduce stress and improve cohesion and cooperation among members.

In assessing and understanding maltreatment, it is important to explore specific family stressors. Bittner and Newberger (1981) have described these stresses as child-produced, social-situational, and parent-produced. The child-produced stresses can include the following: physical disabilities, congenital disabilities, mental retardation, neurologic damage, language deficits, schizophrenia, hyperactivity, low birth weight, and prematurity (Snyder, Hampton, & Newberger, 1983). Ammerman (1991) determined that abuse is associated with the child who displays behaviors that make him difficult and also with the child whose parents perceive him as different and hard to manage. (This is not to say that these conditions directly cause abuse and neglect. On the contrary, it is evident that most children who display these features are *not* subsequently maltreated [see Ammerman *et al.*, 1988]. Rather, characteristics associated with disabling conditions [e.g., difficult-to-manage behavior problems, uncontrollable crying] may increase the likelihood of abuse in families already at risk.)

The coping styles of families who have a child with a disability vary considerably and are mediated by a number of factors. Some of the "parent-produced" vulnerabilities that affect these coping capabilities include having been abused as a child, low self-esteem, depression, substance abuse, other psychiatric illness, ignorance of child rearing, or unrealistic expectations (Bittner & Newberger, 1981).

The third set of family stressors, social-situational, include structural factors such as poverty, unemployment, mobility, isolation, and poor housing; problems in the parental relationship; and parent–child relationship difficulties (Bittner & Newberger, 1981). One such parent–child problem may be an impaired attachment resulting from the child's difficulty to be responsive and reciprocal in this relationship. It is postulated that some parents may be unable to elicit the response that they would like to elicit from their child with a disability and react with more anger, negativity, or violence than with their child without a disability (Ammerman *et al.*, 1988).

Assessment of Psychopathology

Comprehensive assessments of Ms. R. and Peter were conducted via (a) Ms. R.'s participation in the research project, and (b) the standard assessment procedures utilized by the hospital treatment team. As part of the research project, Ms. R. participated in several clinical interviews in addition to completing a variety of questionnaires evaluating psychopathology, parenting stress, social functioning, and child abuse risk. The inpatient evaluation of Peter involved clinical and psychometric assessments conducted by members of the treatment team, including an attending psychiatrist, psychiatric resident, psychodevelopmental specialist, clinical psychologist, physical therapist, and several psychiatric and pediatric nurses.

Parental psychopathology was measured using three instruments examining psychiatric disorders and personality dysfunction: the Symptom Checklist 90-Revised (SCL-90-R; Derogatis, 1983), the Minnesota Multiphasic Personality Inventory (MMPI; Hathaway & McKinley, 1940), and the Beck Depression Inventory (BDI; Beck *et al.*, 1961). The SCL-90-R contains items reflecting specific symptoms of psychiatric disturbance and yields scale scores reflecting subtypes of psychopathology (e.g., depression, paranoia). Ms. R. obtained T scores within the normal range ($T < 70$) for all of the SCL-90-R scales. Her BDI score (19), on the other hand, placed her in the moderate range of depressive symptomatology. The MMPI yielded a 4–6 two-point code, suggesting a long-standing characterological disturbance. Individuals with this profile are described as egocentric, self-centered, and narcissistic. They have difficulty in interpersonal relationships and are noted for their lack of insight into the nature of their maladjustment.

A clinical interview confirmed Ms. R.'s interpersonal difficulties. She reported having no close friends, and she was estranged from her family. Her employment history was sporadic, and she rarely remained in a job longer than 3 months. She exhibited little insight into the nature of her problems, focusing instead on the characteristics of others (including her children) that she believed were the causes of her difficulties. Although reporting several depressive symptoms, Ms. R. did not meet criteria for Axis I or Axis II psychiatric diagnoses.

Risk factors for child abuse were examined using the Novaco Provocation Inventory (NPI; Novaco, 1975) and the Child Abuse Potential Inventory (CAPI; Milner, 1986). The NPI is a measure of anger responsivity and is often used to assist in the detection of parents who exhibit poor impulse control. Ms. R.'s summative score of 182 was within the normative range on this measure. The CAPI, a measure of child abuse risk, yielded elevated scores on subscales reflecting abuse risk (288), distress (192), problems with child/self (2), and family (38). Additional measures documented further parenting difficulties. The Parenting Stress Index (PSI; Abidin, 1986) revealed high levels of stress, especially involving problems encountered with Peter. Indeed, subscale scores in the 99th percentile were noted in the following areas involving Peter: adaptability, acceptability, demandingness, mood, and hyperactivity. Furthermore, her total stress score (307) was more than 2 standard deviations above the mean for the normative sample.

Supplementary evaluations included the Child Abuse and Neglect Interview Schedule (CANIS; Ammerman, Hersen, & Van Hasselt, 1987), the Social Provisions Scale (SPS; Russell & Cutrona, 1984), and the Shipley Institute of Living Scale-Revised (SILS-R; Zachary, 1986). The CANIS is a semistructured interview designed to identify factors associated with child maltreatment. Detailed information about Peter's past maltreatment by his father (see Case 1) was adduced with the CANIS. In addition, Ms. R. reported her tendency to use physical punishment techniques (slapping, hitting with an object) to manage Peter, despite their ineffectiveness. As a child, Ms. R. was physically disciplined by her parents with hairbrushes, paddles, and belts. Ms. R.'s mother also was a victim of spouse abuse, which often resulted in facial bruising. There also was vague suspicion that Peter might have been sexually molested at the age of 4. At this time, he began to masturbate at inappropriate times and with high frequency. His father, too, masturbated frequently, often in front of the children. Peter's behavior may have been instigated by modeling of his father. On the other hand, inappropriate genital play is relatively common behavior in developmentally delayed children. Ms. R. denied any direct evidence that Peter and his father had any direct sexual contact (although Peter's observation of his father's masturbation was certainly highly inappropriate). Finally, Ms. R. described her past abuse of alcohol and other drugs, and denied current usage.

Alicia and her parents also participated in a comprehensive assessment in which there was a considerable overlap in instrumentation. As presented in Table 1, both Mr. and Mrs. S. reported significant difficulties in a number of areas of functioning and adaptation. Although their scores were relatively low in the Beck Depression Inventory, they reported significant stress related to parenting. Information from standardized measures and the semistructured interview (CANIS) revealed that both parents viewed Alicia as having a behavior problem. Their reliance on restraint as a management strategy, and the fact that they evidenced poor knowledge of basic parenting skills (as measured by the Knowledge of Behavior Principles as Applied to Children), documents a limited repertoire of problem-solving, coping, and child-management skills. Moreover, Mr. and Mrs. S. seemed to have a limited understanding of Alicia's disabilities and their effects. The viewed Alicia as having considerably more self-control than she actually manifested and attributed her misbehavior to deliberate defiance and oppositionality. Both parents used disciplinary practices (e.g., threats) that they had experienced as children. Both individual and family functioning was further undermined by poverty, a loose family structure that was at times chaotic, and a history of trauma.

The specific assessment strategies carried out in these cases reflect the general considerations that should be taken into account when working with abusive and neglectful families of children with disabilities. In particular, it is critical that the assessment be comprehensive and multidimensional. The complexity of child abuse and neglect cannot be overemphasized, and a thorough evaluation of the numerous factors that can contribute to etiology and maintenance of maltreatment is critical to effective treatment planning. A comprehensive assessment serves two purposes. First, it permits the clinician to identify deficits of functioning that can subsequently be targeted in treatment. Second, it provides a screening for severe psychopathology that may need concurrent intervention or treatment prior to addressing abuse and neglect. As such, it is necessary to use a variety of assessment strategies and multiple sources of information. These include administering questionnaires, conducting clinical interviews, and observing family interactions. Likewise, data should be gathered from professionals involved in the case, as well as significant others and extended family members. On the whole, assessment is parent-focused, given the fact that abuse and neglect is primarily defined by caregiver behavior. Other family members, however, should not be ignored. On the contrary, their involvement in assessment and treatment may make the difference between success and failure.

There are many similarities between children with and without disabilities that warrant use of similar assessment approaches. However, several special issues are associated with children with disabilities that require meticulous attention and careful consideration. The medical status of the child is very important. Many children with disabilities exhibit chronic medical conditions that require frequent monitoring. The amount of medical involvement is dependent upon the type of impairment, extent of impairment, and course of the disabling condition. All of these are critical in the family assessment of maltreatment, particularly as they pertain to neglect. Since these children require frequent medical follow-up, it is imperative that parents attend to their needs. A second consideration in assessing maltreatment in children with disabilities is to identify the types and severity of behavior problems. Many children with profound disabilities display severe behavioral disturbances that are both quantitatively and qualitatively different from those of their nondisabled peers. For example, such behaviors as head banging, eye poking, and self-scratching are especially stressful for parents and resistant to change. Physical intervention may be required to control such behaviors, thus increasing the overall likelihood of abuse occurring as a result of heightened frustration and physical proximity of the parent and child. An interview, such as the CANIS, is especially useful in gathering information about parenting practices in general and behavior-management techniques used during these kinds of situations in particular. Finally, because these behavior problems are so difficult to manage, it is important to determine whether or not the parent has the appropriate skills to deal with these behaviors.

An additional focus of assessment is the parent–child relationship and parent–child interactions. Some parents exhibit negative reactions to the birth of a child with a disability and fail to resolve these as the child matures. Hostility toward the child with a disability may contribute to the overall likelihood of abuse. In addition, children with severe disabilities are often characterized by a paucity of those behaviors that strengthen the parent–child bond. Such children sometimes do not like to be played with or touched. As a result, parents must be especially sensitive to cues and need to use a variety of techniques to engage the child. Parents who lack these skills are at especially high risk for having nonrewarding relationships with their children.

Treatment Options

When treating abusive and neglectful families, there are several variables that must be taken into account regardless of whether the child has a disability. Often, abusive parents evidence basic skill deficits that differentiate them from their nonmaltreating counterparts. For example, abusive parents are frequently inconsistent disciplinarians, who attend more often to negative child behaviors and communicate less positively with their offspring. Abusive parents' knowledge about childhood in general and their expectations about specific needs of the child also tend to be distorted. Further, there are other factors that can contribute to the etiology of maltreatment, including substance abuse, poverty, social isolation, past history of abuse, and stressful life events (e.g., marital conflict). All of these elements must be considered when designing a treatment plan.

In addition, families of children with disabilities are often faced with numerous difficult situations. Some children with disabilities display unique and recalcitrant behavior problems demanding extensive physical contact for appropriate management or intrusive management techniques. Attitudes and expectations about their children, who may develop slowly and atypically, may further complicate parenting. For instance, the wish for a "normal" child or embarrassment about their child's behaviors or appearance may arouse guilt or anger. Added to this are the extended care requirements that can increase already heightened levels of family stress. As previously mentioned, a thorough assessment is required to address the multiple issues that may be associated with the cause and maintenance of maltreatment. Data from the assessment are, in turn, used to construct an intervention approach.

Comprehensive Behavioral Treatment (CBT) was used to treat Ms. R. CBT is a skills-based intervention targeting parenting difficulties in maltreating parents of children with disabilities. It consisted of 16 sessions followed by 3 biweekly booster sessions and included five intervention components: (1) problem-solving skills and stress reduction training, (2) child management skills training, (3) parenting skills training, (4) anger control training, and (5) leisure skills training. Data from the assessments were used to determine appropriate targets for treatment. On the basis of Ms. R.'s assessment, the following areas were selected for treatment: (1) anger control training, (2) behavior management training, and (3) problem-solving skills training.

Anger control training involved having Ms. R. keep an Anger Incident Diary. She was instructed to record 10 incidents each day that were anger-provoking. Ms. R. was to describe cognitive, physical, and behavioral cues indicative of arousal. Along with this, she was to report her level of arousal using a 5-point scale. This task enhanced Ms. R.'s awareness of anger arousal and prevented such anger from building up to the point of losing control. Upon identification of self-statements associated with arousal, the next step was to teach Ms. R. to substitute positive for negative self-statements as a means of more effectively mediating anger.

As Ms. R. continued to monitor anger arousal, she became aware of Peter's behaviors that were most often provoking. In behavior management training, Ms. R. was instructed to observe and record the antecedents, behaviors, and consequences during problematic episodes. We identified that Ms. R. would spend close to 3 hours, at any one time, yelling and threatening her children in an attempt to achieve compliance. It was expected that through careful observation Ms. R. would be able to predict the onset of undesirable behaviors. In this manner, she would learn ways in which to interrupt and redirect them at the beginning, rather than allowing them to worsen beyond the point of becoming unmanageable.

A variety of coexisting problems, however, interfered with the conduct of therapy. Particularly, Mr. L. (the father of Ms. R.'s children) returned to the home. Also, Ms. R. chose to confront her father about the past occurrence of sexual abuse. These situations were crises that drew Ms. R.'s attention away from the needs of her children. Indeed, it is this pattern of "jumping" from problem to problem that necessitated inclusion of problem-solving skills training in CBT. Our treatment plan included teaching Ms. R. to reevaluate and clarify personal situations, determine priorities, and organize her lifestyle so as to prevent future problems. Unfortunately, Ms. R. missed appointments during many of these "crisis" periods. She chose to withdraw from treatment after confronting her father about being molested as a child, insisting that she "could not concentrate on anything else" at this time.

Mr. and Mrs. S. also participated in a variant of CBT in which they received 16 weekly sessions and 8 monthly booster sessions. Sessions lasted between 1 and 2 hours, and were conducted in the home. In-home treatment was provided because many families involved with maltreatment are unable to attend sessions in the clinic reliably. Transportation is often unavailable, and the lack of structure in the family interferes with making and keeping appointments in a consistent manner. Perhaps most importantly, providing treatment in the home maximizes the probability that skills will be learned and maintained in the setting that is most important for the child and family.

Mr. and Mrs. S. received training in child management skills, parent skills (i.e., nurturance), and problem-solving skills. Modeling, practice, and feedback were utilized. A re-assessment at 16 months revealed modest improvements in several areas. Alicia and her family were still followed by the child protective service agency, although no additional abusive incidents were reported.

The process of treatment for Ms. R. is most representative of these interventions with maltreating parents. Because there often are so many difficulties faced by the family, clinicians must divide their time between addressing acute crises and maintaining the focus of treatment. When the crisis is predominant, as with Ms. R., the parent may leave treatment prematurely. Thus, ensuring compliance with treatment protocols can be the primary theme in therapeutic interventions. It is also the case that the treatment of chronic child abuse and neglect (as exemplified by Mr. and Mrs. S.) often meets with only partial success. Such families are minimally responsive to intervention and require both extensive *and* long-term treatment to bring about meaningful change. It is noteworthy that the treatment provided to Alicia and her family was only modestly superior to community-treated families in the study of chronically maltreated children with disabilities (Ammerman, Hersen, & Lubetsky, 1996). Prevention of abuse and neglect through early intervention with at-risk families is the major task of the child welfare field as we enter the 21st century.

Behavior Management

Parents who engage in abusive behaviors are inconsistent disciplinarians who primarily attend to negative rather than positive child behaviors. Training these parents in the use of positive reinforcement and structured management procedures (e.g., time out, extinction) can help circumvent abusive episodes and build positive parent–child interactions (see Wolfe, 1987). This is especially true in families of children with severe disabilities. Children with disabilities can present with aversive, and at times, unique behavior problems rarely seen in children without such conditions. Managing such behaviors as self-injury (eye poking, head banging), extensive crying or tantruming, stereotypies (twirling, hand flapping), often coupled with hyperactivity and aggression, may lead to intrusive physical contact. Restraint is sometimes used if the child is in danger and is most typically employed during episodes of heightened arousal. The combination of increased emotionality and intrusive physical management may increase the possibility that more serious physical punishment will occur.

Medical and Psychiatric Interventions

Medical and psychiatric conditions must be addressed before one can attempt parent training. Prolonged and frequent medical attention is an essential part of caring for many children with disabilities and chronic illnesses. Some conditions require continuous medical visits or caretaking procedures that are both costly and stressful. Other medical procedures may be painful, generating stress for both parent and child. Teaching parents to use stress-reduction techniques can be of assistance.

Psychiatric status of the child also requires attention. Pharmacological interventions for attention-deficit/hyperactivity disorder or neurological syndromes reduce the likelihood of provocative child behavior and facilitate parent training with abusive caretakers.

Parental Attitudes and Expectations

Parental attitudes and expectations about having a child with a disability produce a further impact on parenting. The initial disappointment and discouragement upon the birth of a child with a disability can lead to insecure attachment and possibly subsequent child-abusive behavior. Sometimes parents will deny their child's disabilities and believe that he or she will outgrow any limitations. Such expectations are followed by growing frustration. Also, parents may reject their child or feel embarrassed about their child, leading to withdrawal or open hostility. Indeed, parents must first understand and accept their child's condition before they will be able to improve their behaviors.

Problem-Solving Skills

Many families that engage in maltreatment live in a continual state of crisis and chaos. Indeed, it is such a high state of emotion and stress that at times it contributes to the occurrence of abuse. Problem-solving skills training is designed to teach parents to better manage the stress associated with daily problems and to organize their lifestyle in order to minimize the impact of future problems. Stress management may include teaching parents progressive relaxation strategies and cognitive strategies, such as the previously described Anger Incident Diary. Also of import is teaching parents how to engage in enjoyable activities and effectively utilize leisure time to reduce stress.

Often parents are unaware that routine and organization can greatly lessen stress and decrease the opportunity for problems to arise. Prevention, for example, may go so far as to tie the refrigerator shut or bar the windows in order to protect a hyperactive child from injury. Other families may find that simply establishing a more structured routine prevents conflict, greatly reducing stress.

Frequently, parents create their own stress by perceiving problematic incidents as crises. Indeed, many such instances deserve immediate attention, but not at the expense of parental responsibilities. Assisting a parent in problem analysis, generating solutions, and decision-making skills will help alleviate the sense of urgency and the impatience often associated with crisis situations.

Parental Psychopathology

In some cases, abusive acts are associated with parental psychopathology. In these situations, it may be necessary to refer a parent to specialized programs (i.e., substance-abuse treatment) before involvement in parent training. In other cases, concurrent treatment modalities are an option. For example once a schizophrenic parent is stabilized on psychotropic medication, he or she may benefit from parenting skills training.

Summary

A sizable body of evidence has accrued suggesting that children with disabilities are at increased risk for abuse and neglect. Although well-controlled empirical research in this area is only now emerging, three characteristics are posited to contribute to this heightened risk: (1) disruptions in the formation of caregiver–infant attachment, (2) increased stress (often related to difficult-to-manage behavior problems and extensive care requirements), and (3) increased vulnerability. These factors, along with the other issues faced in treating families involved in the abuse and neglect of their children, must be taken into account with parents of children with disabilities.

Because of the complexity of child abuse and neglect in general, and maltreatment of children with disabilities in particular, it is critical that a multidimensional assessment be carried out. This assessment should address many areas of functioning, including the child's medical, psychiatric, and academic status. Likewise, family functioning, parental psychopathology, and parenting skills need to be closely examined. Moreover, it is essential that treatment strategies stem from such an assessment. It is impossible to utilize one treatment approach with such a heterogeneous population. Therefore, we recommend a multicomponent intervention that uses a variety of skills-based strategies designed to remediate several areas of need.

Despite the unique issues found in parents who maltreat their children with disabilities, there are many similarities between these families and maltreating families of children without disabilities. The pathways leading to maltreatment are complex and interactive. In addition, these families are very difficult to treat. Often, they have so many issues with which to deal that it is most difficult for them to focus intensely on one issue in a treatment setting. Furthermore, motivation of parents to seek and continue treatment varies considerably.

There is a pressing need for continued research in this area. For example, almost nothing is known about the treatment of neglect of children with disabilities. In addition, we know little about the maltreatment of infants with disabilities, even though, in the general population, infants are more likely than other age groups to be abused or neglected. Although most children with disabilities develop atypically, issues of developmental level and functioning are critical in designing and carrying out a treatment plan. As continued attention is accorded to this previously ignored population, the future holds promise for helping maltreated children with disabilities and their families.

Acknowledgments

Preparation of this chapter was facilitated in part by grant nos. G008720109 and H133A40007 from the National Institute of Disabilities and Rehabilitation Research, U.S. Department of Education, and a grant from the Vira I. Heinz Endowment. However, the opinions reflected herein do not necessarily reflect the position of policy of the U.S. Department of Education or the Vira I. Heinz Endowment, and no official endorsement should be inferred.

References

Abidin, R. R. (1986). *Parenting stress index* (2nd ed.). Charlottesville, VA: Pediatric Psychology Press.
Ainsworth, M. D. (1980). Attachment and child abuse. In G. Gerber, C. Ross, & E. Zigler (Eds.), *Child abuse: An agenda for action* (pp. 35–47). New York: Oxford University Press.
Aman, M. G., & Singh, N. N. (1986). *Aberrant behavior checklist: Manual*. East Aurora, NY: Slosson.
Ammerman, R. T. (1991). The role of the child in physical abuse: A reappraisal. *Violence and Victims, 6,* 87–101.
Ammerman, R. T., & Boerger, E. (1998, August). *Correlates of negative attributional styles in maltreating parents.* Paper presented at the annual convention of the American Psychological Association, San Francisco.
Ammerman, R. T., & Galvin, M. R. (1998). Child maltreatment. In R. T. Ammerman & J. V. Campo (Eds.), *Handbook of pediatric psychology and psychiatry* (Vol. 2, pp. 31–69). Boston: Allyn & Bacon.

Ammerman, R. T., & Patz, R. J. (1996). Determinants of child abuse potential: Contribution of parent and child factors. *Journal of Clinical Child Psychology, 25,* 300–307.

Ammerman, R. T., Van Hasselt, V. B., & Hersen, M. (1987). *The Child Abuse and Neglect Interview Schedule (CANIS).* Unpublished instrument, Western Pennsylvania School for Blind Children, Pittsburgh.

Ammerman, R. T., Van Hasselt, V. B., & Hersen, M. (1988). Maltreatment of handicapped children: A critical review. *Journal of Family Violence, 3,* 53–72.

Ammerman, R. T., Hersen, M., Van Hasselt, V. B., Lubetsky, M. J., & Sieck, W. R. (1994). Maltreatment in psychiatrically hospitalized children and adolescents with developmental disabilities: Prevalence and correlates. *Journal of the American Academy of Child and Adolescent Psychiatry, 33,* 567–576.

Ammerman, R. T., Hersen, M., & Lubetsky, M. J. (1996, November). Difficulties in implementing interventions in chronic child maltreatment. In J. R. Lutzker (Chairperson), *Child abuse and neglect: The cutting edge.* Symposium conducted at the annual convention of the Association for Advancement of Behavior Therapy.

Beck, A. T., Ward, C. H., Mendelson, M., Mock, J., & Erbaugh, J. (1961). An inventory for measuring depression. *Archives of General Psychiatry, 4,* 561–571.

Birrell, R., & Birrell, J. (1968). The maltreatment syndrome in children: A hospital survey. *Medical Journal of Australia, 2,* 1023–1029.

Bittner, S., & Newberger, E. H. (1981). Pediatric understanding of child abuse and neglect. *Pediatric Review, 2,* 197.

Chess, S. (1970). Temperament and children at risk. In E. J. Anthony & C. Koupernick (Eds.), *The child in his family* (pp. 121–130). New York: Wiley.

Cicchetti, O. (1987). Developmental psychopathology in infancy. Illustration from the study of maltreated youngsters. *Journal of Consulting and Clinical Psychology, 55,* 837–845.

Crosse, S. B., Kaye, E., & Ratnofsky, A. C. (1993). *A report on the maltreatment of children with disabilities.* Rockville, MD: Westat (Contract No. 105-89-1630 from the National Center on Child Abuse and Neglect), U.S. Department of Health and Human Services.

deLissovoy, V. (1979). Toward the definition of "abuse provoking child." *Child Abuse and Neglect, 3,* 341–350.

Derogatis, L. R. (1983). *SCL-90-R administration, scoring, and procedure manual.* Baltimore: Clinical Psychometric Research.

Fraiberg, S. (1977). *Insights from the blind: Comparative studies of blind and sighted infants.* New York: Basic Books.

Goldfarb, L. A., Brotherson, M. J., Summers, J. A., & Turnball, A. P. (1986). *Meeting the challenge of disability or chronic illness—A family guide.* Baltimore: Paul H. Brookes.

Gottlieb, M. E. (1987). Major variations in intelligence. In M. I. Gottlieb & J. E. Williams (Eds.), *Textbook of developmental pediatrics* (pp. 127–150). New York: Plenum.

Hathaway, S. R., & McKinley, J. C. (1940). A multiphasic personality schedule (Minnesota): Construction of the schedule. *Journal of Psychology, 10,* 249–254.

Helfer, R. (1973). The etiology of child abuse. *Pediatrics, 51,* 777–779.

Lightcap, J. L., Kurland, J. A., & Burgess, R. L. (1982). Child abuse: A test of some predictions from evolutionary theory. *Ethology and Sociobiology, 3,* 61–67.

Milner, J. S. (1986). *The child abuse potential inventory* (2nd ed.). Webster, NC: Psytec.

Novaco, R. W. (1975). *Anger control: The development and evaluation of an experimental treatment.* Lexington, MA: Heath.

O'Dell, S. L., Tarler-Benlulo, L., & Flynn, J. M. (1979). An instrument to measure knowledge of behavioral principles as applied to children. *Journal of Behavioral Therapy and Experimental Psychiatry, 10,* 29–34.

Pueschel, S. M., Bernier, J. D., & Weidenman, L. E. (1988). *The special child: A source book for parents of children with developmental disabilities*. Baltimore: Paul H. Brookes.

Russell, D., & Cutrona, C. E. (1984). *The social provisions scale*. Unpublished manuscript, University of Iowa, College of Medicine, Iowa City.

Snyder, J. C., Hampton, R., & Newberger, E. H. (1983). Family dysfunction: Violence, neglect, and sexual abuse. In M. D. Levine, W. B. Carey, A. C. Crocker, & R. T. Gross (Eds.), *Developmental-behavioral pediatrics* (pp. 256–275). Philadelphia: W.B. Saunders.

Solomons, G. (1979). Child abuse and developmental disabilities. *Developmental Medicine and Child Neurology, 21,* 101–108.

Starr, R. H., Dietrich, K. N., Fischhoff, J., Ceresnie, S., & Zweier, D. (1984). The contribution of handicapping conditions to child abuse. *Topics in Early Childhood Special Education, 4,* 55–69.

Sullivan, P. M., & Knutson, J. F. (1998). The association between childhood maltreatment and disabilities in a hospital-based pediatric sample and a residential treatment sample. *Child Abuse and Neglect, 22,* 271–288.

Wolfe, D. A. (1987). *Child abuse: Implications for child development and psychopathology*. Newbury Park, CA: Sage.

Zachary, R. A. (1986). *Shipley Institute of Living Scale: Revised manual*. Los Angeles: Western Psychological Services.

13

The Child Witness of Family Violence

Mindy S. Rosenberg, Ronita S. Giberson, B. B. Robbie Rossman, and Michelle Acker

Description of the Problem

The last two decades have been marked by a growing public awareness of family violence. Research by social scientists has suggested that family violence is widespread (Gelles & Straus, 1988). It is estimated that every year, 1.8 to 4 million women are physically abused by their partners (Novello, 1992). In fact, more women are abused by their husbands or boyfriends than are injured in car accidents, muggings, or rapes (Jaffe, Wolfe, & Wilson, 1990). A recent prevalence study by Fantuzzo, Boruch, Beriama, Atkins, and Marcus (1997) found that children were disproportionately present in households where there was a substantial incidence of female assault. Experts estimate that 3.3 to 10 million children are exposed to marital violence each year (Carlson, 1984; Straus, 1991).

Researchers have become increasingly aware that children exposed to marital violence are at risk for the development of psychological problems (Fantuzzo, DePaola, Lambert, Martino, Anderson, & Sutton, 1991; Sternberg, Lamb, Greenbaum, Cicchetti, Dawud, Cortes, Krispin, & Lorey, 1993). Jouriles, Murphy, and O'Leary (1989) found that children of battered

Mindy S. Rosenberg • Sausalito, California 94965.   **Ronita S. Giberson** • Graham B. Dimmick Child Guidance Services, Lexington, Kentucky 40507.   **B. B. Robbie Rossman** • Department of Psychology, University of Denver, Denver, Colorado 80208.   **Michelle Acker** • Professional School of Psychology, University of Denver, Denver, Colorado 80208.

Case Studies in Family Violence, Second Edition, edited by Ammerman and Hersen. Kluwer Academic / Plenum Publishers, New York, 2000.

women were four times more likely to evidence psychopathology as were children living in nonviolent homes. The types of psychological problems include internalizing (e.g., anxiety) and externalizing (e.g., acting out) behaviors (Fantuzzo et al., 1991; Hughes & Fantuzzo, 1994; Jaffe et al., 1990; McCloskey, Figueredo, & Koss, 1995); difficulties with social problem-solving skills and lower levels of social competence (Moore, Pepler, Weinberg, Hammond, Waddell, & Weiser, 1990; Rosenberg, 1987); low self-esteem (Hughes, 1988); poor school performance (Moore et al., 1990) and problems with aggression (Holden & Ritchie, 1991; Jaffe, Wolfe, Wilson, & Zak, 1986). Furthermore, recent research has found that some children are traumatized by the experience of witnessing, evidencing elevated symptoms of posttraumatic stress disorder (PTSD) (Devoe & Graham-Bermann, 1997; Kilpatrick, Litt, & Williams, 1997; Rossman, Bingham, & Emde, 1996). These findings corroborate clinical reports that describe many exposed children as experiencing trauma reactions, including difficulty concentrating, irritability, depression, hypervigilance, intrusive memories of past violence, and withdrawal from others. It appears that the negative effects of witnessing marital violence are numerous and varied, ranging from mild emotional and behavioral disturbances in the child to clinical level symptoms of PTSD and other psychiatric disorders.

In this chapter, we use the cases of Maria, Billy, and their families to highlight the significant psychological issues that emerge when children become witness to their parents' violence. We begin by describing each case and the circumstances that brought the families to our attention. Next, we expand on the medical, legal, social, and family issues, and the assessment of psychopathology, that were revealed during evaluation. We conclude with a discussion of treatment options and summary comments.

Case Study 1: Maria

The P. family came to the attention of a child and family clinic at the suggestion of an elementary schoolteacher, who was concerned about Maria P., the 7-year-old daughter. The P. family includes the mother, Mrs. P. (46 years old), father Mr. P. (48 years old), and three daughters, Maria (7 years old), Anna (5 years old), and Rosa (3 years old). Mr. and Mrs. P. had been separated for 6 months, and Mr. P. currently lived in a neighboring state. Maria's schoolteacher contacted Mrs. P. with concerns about Maria's aggressive behavior toward other children (e.g., hitting, pushing), her lack of school friends, and her difficulty concentrating on academic material. When, at the teacher's suggestion, Mrs. P. contacted the clinic, she had numerous concerns about Maria and her other children, all of whom had witnessed repeated incidents of physical violence by their father against her. Mrs. P. was especially worried about Maria, the oldest, who had witnessed the majority of marital violence. Maria cried frequently at home, had aggressive outbursts toward her sisters, and seemed confused about her feelings toward her father. Though the younger daughters were currently not displaying any behavioral or emotional signs of distress, Mrs. P. reported that in the past, both had had difficulty sleeping (e.g., waking up screaming and crying from nightmares) after which they were unable to be comforted.

In addition, Mrs. P. had concerns about her parenting skills. She reported that at times she lost her temper with her children, screaming at them for relatively minor infractions and sometimes spanking them. Mrs. P. was both physically and sexually abused as a child, and although her relationship with her children was not in a crisis state, she was afraid of perpetuating her history of physical abuse with her own children. She also felt that being sexually abused as a child contributed to her own discomfort over bathing, masturbation, normal sexual exploration, and other sexual issues with her daughters. She requested guidance in the areas of discipline, ways to encourage her children's development of appropriate social skills, and how to help them cope with her separation and planned divorce from Mr. P.

Mrs. P. met and married her husband in Arizona; she is Hispanic and he is Anglo. Whereas the marriage was her first, Mr. P. had been married once before and had five children, with whom he had intermittent contact. His first wife divorced him after years of extreme battering. Although Mrs. P. was aware of his history, she had believed his promise that he had changed. She found him to be a warm, charismatic man who shared interests similar to hers.

Once married, conflict between Mr. and Mrs. P. increased dramatically as a result of Mr. P.'s infidelities and verbal abuse, and worsened with the birth of their first child, Maria. The first violent incident occurred 3 months after Maria was born and involved Mr. P. pushing, slapping, and hitting his wife. The second incident occurred 4 months later in which Mr. P. repeatedly punched his wife's face with his fists. Following this, Mrs. P. was battered severely every few months with considerable family tension between incidents. Each battering incident left Mrs. P. with bruises on her face or torso and necessitated calling in sick to the hospital where she worked as a nurse. Their second and third children were born at intervals of two years, and although each child was planned and ostensibly desired by both parents Mr. P.'s beatings were especially severe shortly after each birth.

Maria witnessed the most extensive violence between her mother and father, but there were times when Mr. P. would force all his daughters to watch while he beat their mother. After 10 years of marriage, Mrs. P. insisted that both she and her husband attend marital counseling, which Mr. P. agreed to in order to prevent his wife from leaving. One condition of the counseling was that Mrs. P. would leave if her husband physically assaulted her. Mr. P. violated this agreement within weeks. The counselor discontinued treatment and encouraged Mrs. P. to leave, which she chose not to do at that time. The battering continued until one evening, Mr. P. beat his wife to the point of almost losing consciousness. For the first time, he threatened to hurt their children if Mrs. P. did not comply with his every demand. She left with her daughters the next day and went to live with her brother and his family in a neighboring city. The marital separation created tremendous fear and anxiety for Mrs. P. and her children: they were afraid that Mr. P. would follow them and harm them further. Mrs. P. decided fairly quickly to make the separation permanent and sought counseling for herself. She obtained a job as a nurse in a local hospital, arranged for day care for Rosa, and enrolled Anna and Maria in school. Shortly after Maria entered the new school, her aggressive behavior began to escalate, which prompted the teacher's referral to the clinic.

Case Study 2: Billy

Mrs. S brought her two sons for an evaluation at a child and family clinic at the suggestion of her mother-in-law, who was concerned that the boys might be experiencing problems stemming from the abusive family situation. Although both sons entered into therapy, we will focus on the younger boy, Billy, age 7, for the purpose of case discussion. Over the 12 years of their marriage, Mr. S. had been regularly emotionally abusive toward Mrs. S. and the children, in addition to intermittent physical abuse. For example, Mr. S. pushed and shoved his wife and once pushed her forcefully enough into a bathtub to break her hip. Mr. S. harshly disciplined and abused his older son Tom, age 11, and forced him to do many of the household chores. Mr. S. rarely touched his younger son Billy, who was not expected to help around the house and was described as his father's "favorite."

Mr. S. was described as domineering, harsh, punitive, and highly controlling. He had many rules, such as what his wife and children could and could not wear (e.g., the boys could not wear shorts) and how they were to behave. He kept the family isolated from normal contact with neighbors, other family members, and news of the outside world. He did not allow television or newspapers. Before moving to the current state, the family had lived in another state distant from Mrs. S.'s relatives, and Mr. S. had forbidden her contact with her parents. When they moved to this state, they first rented a farm outside of town. When the farm was sold, they bought land and ended up living in a trailer in the country, several miles from a neighbor and about an hour from town.

Several months before Mrs. S. came to the clinic, Mr. S.'s harshness and cruelty had escalated. There were blizzards and cold weather, with mounds of snow on the ground. Mr. S. threatened to hurt the family cat who had run out of the trailer despite having recently given birth to kittens. Mr. S. refused to look for the cat or have the kittens in the trailer, and "drop-kicked" them into the snow. The boys searched for them and found all but one frozen to death. They brought the one kitten back, nursed it, and the mother cat returned to be with it. Mr. S. wouldn't allow the cat and kitten to stay in the trailer, and at that point, also kicked out the dog. The dog survived, the remaining kitten froze to death, and they never found the mother cat.

The incident that precipitated Mrs. S. and the boys leaving began with

Mr. S. allowing Mrs. S. to go to town for much-needed groceries, and then refusing to let her go. He beat her severely twice, with the second beating witnessed by the boys, who were "terrified." Mrs. S. called 911 for assistance, and the sheriff came and took the family to a neighboring farm, where Mrs. S. called her parents, who lived at a distance of several hours. The family then relocated to Mrs. S.'s parents' home, where Mrs. S. obtained a restraining order to prevent her husband from coming to the house. Mrs. S., Billy, and Tom were seen in the clinic for over 2 years.

Medical Issues

Although medical issues were not a primary focus of concern with the P. family, there are instances where the medical profession will come in contact with this population of children and families. For example, it is relatively common for battered women to use the emergency room or other clinic facilities for treatment of injuries sustained during a battering incident (Bergman, 1976). However, battered women do not necessarily report the true cause of their injuries to health-care providers (Hilberman, 1979), and until recently, providers were not trained to ask specific questions about marital violence (Stark, Flitcraft, & Frazier, 1979). Battered women often present with vague physical complaints, minimize the extent of their injuries, and hope that health-care providers will ask the right questions or confront the causal logic of the injury. This is exactly what occurred with Mrs. S. when she was seen by a physician after being pushed into the bathtub, which broke her hip. The doctor did not question Mrs. S.'s explanation for her injury (i.e., that she broke her hip by "slipping and falling" in the tub), and Mrs. S. did not offer any additional information. Klingbeil and Boyd (1984) report that battered women typically express relief when health-care providers acknowledge directly the presence of marital violence and ask questions straightforwardly to obtain the necessary information.

Children may come to the attention of health-care providers in at least two instances. The first instance concerns the overlap between children who witness their parents' violence and experience some form of child maltreatment, including physical abuse or neglect, or sexual abuse. A substantial percentage of maritally violent families are at risk for child abuse, particularly during times when children attempt to protect the victimized parent (Barnett, Pittman, Ragan, & Salus, 1980; see Rossman & Rosenberg, 1998). In these circumstances, children may try to shield their mother from the blows of the batterer or may get in the path of flying objects and inadvertently be injured themselves. Children may also become the direct targets of either parent's anger and frustration. One of the most frequent reasons given by women for leaving a battering partner is that he threatened to abuse the children or has already injured them physically (Giles-Sims, 1983). Thus, one of the first medical issues necessitating attention is to determine whether these children have sustained physical injuries, and to treat accordingly. In situations where child maltreatment is suspected or evident, health-care providers are mandated to report to the proper authorities in keeping with the established hospital or clinic procedures for child abuse reporting.

However, it is not unusual for men who batter to restrict their wives' and children's access to health-care providers. This was the primary medical issue with the S. family; Mr. S. did not allow Mrs. S. or the children to see physicians regularly. Ostensibly, Mr. S. felt it was too expensive to have regular checkups and contact with doctors, yet the family was eligible to use medical clinic services, where the expense would have been minimal. However, the underlying concern about contact with the medical establishment was his fear that his abusive behavior would be exposed, both toward his wife and his older son. For example, as a result of the father's brutal behavior, Tom frequently sustained bruises and welts and had severe headaches. Obviously, if seen by a physician for these complaints, the doctor would have had an opportunity to intervene and report child maltreatment.

In the second instance, children may evidence the psychological sequelae of witnessing their parents' violence, although they themselves have not been physically abused. In this situation, health-care providers, particularly pediatricians and nurses, may have a unique opportunity to identify the distressed child witness, given their ongoing contact with the child and his or her family. Parents may first discuss noticeable changes in their child's behavior with pediatricians (e.g., increased aggression or withdrawal, nightmares, psychosomatic complaints) or academic problems (e.g., deceased ability to concentrate, refusal to complete homework assignments, school refusal), and it is imperative that pediatricians and nurses be aware of the possibility of marital violence as a potential causative factor.

Legal Issues

Several legal issues may emerge when working with families in which children witness marital violence. First, as noted, child maltreatment may occur when there is ongoing marital violence. In those situations, the therapist is mandated to report to child protective services and may then help the family cope with any additional legal intervention to follow. In the case of the P. family, Mrs. P.'s decision to leave her husband was precipitated by an especially severe beating coupled with his threat to harm their daughters if she did not comply with his future demands. There was no evidence of child maltreatment prior to or after the P.s' separation, so that involvement of child protective services in that capacity was unwarranted. With the S. family, the clinic providing services made two attempts to report child physical and psychological abuse to protective services. The first report was made in the family's home county protective service agency, but no case was opened and the social worker decided not to investigate. The clinic made the second report in the grandparents' county, but the caseworker could not investigate because the alleged abuse occurred when the family was out of the jurisdiction. The family wanted the report on record in the event that something happened to the children while they stayed at the grandparents' home. In this situation, the S. family "fell through the cracks" of the child protective system, and despite the therapist's concerns and urgings, social services in the first county failed to respond appropriately. Although the presence of psychological maltreatment may not be enough to initiate an investigation without evidence of significant behavioral and emotional child problems, the fact that physical abuse accompanied the psychological maltreatment should have mandated an investigation by the social worker.

If the couple decides to separate temporarily or to divorce, as in the case with both couples, the second, relatively common legal issue that arises concerns child custody rights and visitation arrangements. Making a fair custody determination in divorce cases presents enough of a challenge when marital violence is not a factor (see Weithorn, 1987), but in the context of battering relationships, contested custody determinations are fraught with myriad problems (e.g., evaluating how violence in the marital relationship affects each partner's ability to parent). As Walker and Edwall (1987) argue, the legal system can become yet another combat arena for battering men who wish to continue a relationship with their wives. In the case of the P. family, it was clear that Mr. P. did not want sole custody of his daughters and Mrs. P. did, so that contested custody was not a central focus of the divorce.

However, problems with divorce and custody were a central concern with the S. family, particularly as they related to the family's religious convictions. The family belonged to the Church of Christ, and Mr. S. was described as "fanatic" and "idiosyncratic" in his interpretation of their religion. Mrs. S. felt she was not living in a Christian home and that her husband's connection to the church and its teachings was a farce. They had not celebrated Christmas for the last 4 years of their marriage because, according to Mr. S., "there were no gifts in the Bible," yet he also ignored the original spirit of Christmas and its symbolism. The church elders strongly discouraged Mrs. S. from taking legal action to divorce her husband. According to church teachings, she had no basis for leaving the marriage. Finally, in an attempt to motivate Mr. S. to change his behavior, the church elders encouraged Mrs. S. to file for legal separation and pursue pastoral marital counseling. From Mrs. S.'s report, the pastoral counselor was aware of the physical abuse perpetrated by her husband, but since Mr. S. denied hurting his wife the counselor treated it as a difference of opinion. The pastoral counselor was not fully aware of the dynamics of marital violence or the specific forms of psychological abuse. It became readily apparent to Mrs. S. that the counseling sessions became merely an arena for Mr. S. to further abuse her emotionally and blame her for the family troubles, without the counselor's mandatory intervention. Mrs. S. withdrew from the counseling and separated herself from that church. In reaction to her filing for legal separation, Mr. S. responded in a legal, vindictive manner, stating that the boys needed a father despite the fact that he was not providing any financial support for them and even though Mrs. S. was willing to allow him visitation.

A custody battle ensued. Mr. S. chose to represent himself and wrote a fanatical letter to the judge, which included religious references and evidence of disturbed thinking. Mrs. S. informed the judge about the spousal abuse and offered the report made of child physical abuse; all of which helped to gain her custody of the boys. Mr. S. was "dazed" when the judge decided in his wife's favor because he thought he would be guaranteed custody by "acting in accordance with the Bible." Supervised visitation was allowed at first, then changed to weekly visitation.

Problems with visitation arrangements is a third legal issue that might arise when battered women seek separation or divorce. It is not uncommon for the batterer to continue to harass his ex-wife by making abusive phone calls, pumping the children for information, refusing to pick up or return the children at the designated time and place, and demanding frequent court appearances to alter visitation arrangements (Walker & Edwall, 1987). Child visitation became the primary battleground for the P. family once Mr. P. realized that Mrs. P. planned to obtain a divorce, and treatment eventually focused on the psychological issues that arose from that battle.

During the first month of the marital separation, Mr. P. focused his attention on trying to get Mrs. P. to give their marriage another chance. When it became apparent that she was not going to change her mind, Mr. P. began to "work on the girls" to influence their mother's decision. During his weekly visits and telephone calls over the next 2 months with his daughters, he began a campaign to win back his family, first by treating them as well as he could, and then through guilt. He chose Maria as the oldest and most psychologically vulnerable to tell her how he couldn't eat or sleep or work because he missed his family so much, and that he feared he would die unless they lived together again. Maria felt that her father really would die if the family was not reunited and that it was up to her to save her father's life by trying to change her mother's mind. Once Mrs. P. became fully aware of her husband's manipulative behavior, she said there would be no further contact with her or the girls unless he "straightened up," and she told him once again that she was planning to file for divorce. Mr. P. then moved to a neighboring state and was not in contact with his family again until shortly after they entered treatment.

Social and Family Issues

It is not uncommon for battered women to become increasingly isolated from their social support systems when they are involved in a violent relationship and the violence escalates over time (Browne, 1987). As ties to friends, family members, and community resources become more tenuous, there is less opportunity for them to receive the kind of feedback that could help them reevaluate their intimate relationship and take steps to stop the violence. Without the intervention of outside information and support, battered women often come to have a distorted sense of what is normal, acceptable behavior between spouses. As the violence escalates over time, battered women may become desensitized to all but extreme battering incidents.

This isolation had certainly occurred during Mrs. P.'s marriage. For example, Mrs. P. had few friends of her own while married to Mr. P. Most social contacts were through her husband's family, who either supported his negative evaluation of his wife or seemed oblivious to the escalating tension and violence in their marriage. In addition, Mrs. P. maintained limited contact with her family or origin to decrease the opportunity for arguments with Mr. P. when they visited family members and to minimize the potential for family members to confront her about her unhappy, volatile marriage. Mrs. P. had always felt socially awkward, and under the best of circumstances had difficulty making friends and reaching out to co-workers. As the violence in her marriage escalated, she became increasingly isolated from others who could provide emotional support and feedback about the dysfunctional nature of the relationship. When Mrs. P. attempted to talk with her husband about their problems, he treated her as though she were crazy and fabricating information to provoke an argument. Two years into the marriage, Mrs. P. sought help from a clergyman, who counseled her to try to be a better, more obedient wife. She came to doubt her own anguished feelings about the marriage and began to believe her husband's interpretation of their relationship problems (i.e., that any difficulties were caused by Mrs. P.'s inadequacies). It was not until Mrs. P. read a magazine article on battered wives that she realized her situation was not unique and that she must seek help.

Similar issues arose for the S. family. Mrs. S. was not allowed to work or have contact with her parents or friends. However, Mr. S. tolerated his wife's relationship with his own mother, who surprisingly, became fed up with her son's abusive behavior over time and confronted him unsuccessfully. Mr. S. attempted to behave differently around his mother but also limited his family's time with her, thereby restricting the only supportive influence from outside the nuclear family. After years of emotional degradation, isolation, and terrifying incidents of physical abuse, Mrs. S. came to question her capabilities sufficiently that she had little confidence in her ability to get a job and make a home for her sons apart from her husband. She felt trapped financially and emotionally, until the situation became so intolerable that she had to make a move.

Family Issues

Based on findings from the P. and S. family evaluations and individual interviews with the mothers and children, several family-level issues emerged for consideration in treatment. These included (1) crisis atmosphere in the home; (2) troubled parent–child relationships; and (3) strained sibling relationships.

Crisis Atmosphere in the Home

When the P. family began the evaluation phase, Mrs. P. spoke of needing to be "on guard" in the family to protect herself and her children from the possibility of her husband's violence. She described the atmosphere in the home as perpetually in a crisis state, in which she and her children needed to be prepared to leave at a moment's notice. There were times when the tension between her husband and her became so unbearable that she would not turn her back on him for fear of an unpredictable attack. Maria, in particular, tended to cling to her mother and was fearful of what her father would do if she wasn't around to monitor both parents' behavior. Occasionally at bedtime, Mrs. P. would find Maria asleep in her clothes. Maria explained that she might need to alert a neighbor to help her mother in the middle of the night, and she didn't want to be seen in her pajamas. What was most noteworthy about Mrs. P. and her daughter's vigilant behaviors is how ingrained they were, and even 6 months to a year after Mr. and Mrs. P. separated, there were many instances when both mother and daughter acted as if they were still living in the crisis atmosphere of the past.

The S. family too experienced an atmosphere of crisis after Mrs. S. and her children moved to her parents' home. They were extremely fearful that Mr. S. would do something unpredictable to punish them for their independence and "defiance" or would show up unexpectedly in their lives. Mrs. S. and her parents were worried the children might be kidnapped, and all of the family members felt apprehensive and jittery, often looking over their shoulders to see if Mr. S. was somewhere watching. The maternal grandfather in particular became quite vigilant, and at first the boys and their mother had even less freedom than they did when living with Mr. S. However, over time, and with the therapist's guidance, the S. family learned to loosen the reins intrapsychically and externally as they developed a fundamentally different way of relating that made sense for their new nuclear family.

Troubled Parent–Child Relationships

In an attempt to explain the negative effects of violence exposure, some researchers have proposed that impaired parent–child relations are the critical mechanism by which marital violence affects children. While links have been demonstrated between marital relations and the parenting relationship in nonviolent families, relatively little is known about the specific parenting of mothers and fathers in violent homes. Margolin (1995) points out that the many roles played by parents (e.g., providers of emotional support, models of emotion regulation, instructors, disciplinarians) could be undermined by marital violence and that any of these roles could be disrupted in battered women who experience depression, are distracted by basic safety concerns, or who live with fear in their own homes.

Holden and Ritchie (1991) found that battered women have high levels of parenting stress that are associated with aggressive behavior toward their children and attend to their children less than nonabused community women. However, in a more recent study, Holden, Stein, Ritchie, Harris, and Jouriles (1998) found that battered women reveal few differences in parenting behavior (e.g., providing structure, showing warmth, being emotionally available, using positive reinforcement) compared to nonabused women. However, the data source was maternal report. It is crucial that systematic observational data be the next step in looking at parenting abilities. Battering men have been found to be physically aggressive with their children (O'Keefe, 1994), mostly toward their sons (Jouriles & LeCompte, 1991). Holden and Ritchie (1991) used maternal report (which is subject to the same methodological constraints discussed earlier) to ascertain that fathers were significantly more irritable, less involved with their children, less affectionate, and less likely to reason with their children than comparison fathers. Clearly, more empirical evidence is needed to understand further the links between marital violence, parenting behavior, and children's adjustment in violent families.

The following problems were evident in the relationships between Mrs. P. and Maria and between Mrs. S. and Billy: (a) Mrs. P.'s emotional unavailability and reliance on Maria for emotional support; (b) disciplinary problems for both mothers; and (c) distorted perceptions of Maria. These are discussed in the following paragraphs.

(a) Emotional Unavailability and Reliance on Child for Support. Mrs. P.'s relationship with Maria was characterized by alternating periods of emotional unavailability and intense overinvolvement. Not surprisingly, Maria was confused by her mother's mixed messages. At times, Mrs. P. was preoccupied and did not respond to Maria's distress and need for interaction, while at other times, Mrs. P. would seek out Maria as a confidante and source of emotional support.

Before Mrs. P. entered into treatment, she found it difficult to be sensitive to Maria's emotional needs because her own desire for attention and support predominated their interactions. For example, on one occasion, Mrs. P. said, "I need a hug" to Maria and when Maria did not respond immediately because she was in the midst of doing something, Mrs. P. became upset and ordered Maria to give her a hug. At other times, Maria clearly desired affection and nurturing from her mother but was rebuffed because Mrs. P. was feeling drained or did not like the manner in which Maria sought the affection.

During her parents' violent marriage, Maria often played the role of nurturer and protector for her mother. Mrs. P. complemented this role by seeking emotional support and strength from Maria, even though she was a young child. For example, after Mr. P. had beaten her, Mrs. P. would often go to her daughters' room to comfort them because they were typically frightened and crying. However, this would often be the time that Maria would soothe her mother. Mrs. P. relates that after the final beating when she almost lost consciousness, Maria came to her, attended to her bruises and cuts, and asked, "What did Daddy do to you this time?" It was at this point that Mrs. P. realized that Maria had taken on a parental role in their relationship and vowed to stop relying on her daughter for support.

After leaving her husband, Mrs. P. actively tried to alter her own and Maria's roles in the family. She stopped turning to Maria for reassurance and discouraged Maria from continuing in the role of protector/nurturer toward her. Maria found it particularly difficult to relinquish her old role because it was the only way she knew how to be emotionally close to her mother. In an attempt to make sure that Maria understood that "things were going to be different now," Mrs. P. worked to distance herself emotionally from Maria. In response, Maria could do nothing but cling to her mother, fearing that she would lose her mother's love completely. Altering this cyclical interaction pattern of clinging/distancing/clinging became a critical treatment goal.

(b) Disciplinary Behavior. Mrs. P.'s difficulty with child discipline extended to all three daughters. She did not have a repertoire of strategies from which to draw when her children misbehaved, and she often felt "at a loss" as to how to respond. She would alternate between overreaction to her child's slightest infraction (e.g., not clearing the table immediately after dinner) and failing to respond to more severe misbehavior (e.g., Maria hitting her sister on the head with a doll). Because Mrs. P. was unable to set firm, consistent limits with her children, they did not have a clear understanding of what was expected from them. Moreover, as Mrs. P. allowed Maria to continue her aggressive behavior toward her sisters and peers without any form of intervention, her behavior escalated and Mrs. P. became even more frightened, angry, and uncertain of what to do next.

Mrs. P. recognized that she felt "out of control" with her daughters on multiple occasions, although these feelings did not lead to any abusive incidents. She described how difficult it was for her to control her anger once she allowed herself to feel any anger at all and stated that "any anger led to big anger." Mrs. P.'s ability to discipline her children effectively was further complicated by her guilt over exposing her children to a violent marriage. She reported feeling a sense of explosive rage that sometimes came over her in response to fairly minor misbehavior on the part of her daughters. She would yell and scream at her daughters or leave the room rather than physically harm them. The children would cry in response to her anger, which increased her guilty feelings and further compromised her ability to manage their behavior appropriately. She thought of herself as a "terrible" parent and often wondered, "How can anyone as mixed up as me be a good role model?"

Disciplinary issues were evident with the S. family as well. Mr. S. had favored Billy so blatantly over Tom, whom he scapegoated and physically abused, and when he was no longer the central disciplinarian in the family, Mrs. S. and her parents needed to figure out new ways of guiding the boys' behavior. Since physical abuse and harsh discipline were the strategies the boys were used to (Tom in particular), taking away privileges, setting limits without physical punishment, and talking things through were not as effective and powerful tools for a period of time.

However, both Mrs. S. and her parents were committed to nonphysical strategies of responding to the boys and maintained a united front to disallow aggression in the home. Tom had great difficulty controlling his aggressive behavior and Billy knew exactly how to get Tom's "goat." Mrs. S. worked hard to maintain a positive view of both her sons, but Tom's aggression reminded her a great deal of her husband. She saw her older son as overly sensitive to rejection and easily frustrated; he would quickly get into verbal arguments at home and school, but then cry afterward. Billy, on the other hand, continued to behave as though he should have special privileges, which he had been granted by his father. It took Mrs. S. some time to get through to Billy and have him understand that he was going to be treated as fairly as his brother and be held to the same standard of behavior. For Billy, the loss of special treatment was both a relief and a loss, as he struggled with his feeling that losing his "special-ness" meant that he wasn't as loved as he used to be. Tom struggled with his belief that he was "bad" because of his father's harsh treatment. Both children began to understand over time that their father's extreme behavior toward them and their mother didn't reflect accurately their true natures.

(c) Distorted Perceptions of Children. Mrs. P. held noticeably different perceptions of Maria from those of Anna and Rosa. In general, Mrs. P. tended to perceive Maria in an unrealistically negative light while her perceptions of Anna and Rosa tended to be overly positive. The effects of these divergent perceptions contributed to several problems in Mrs. P.'s relationship with Maria. Mrs. P. tended to hold inappropriate expectations for Maria's behavior; she misinterpreted positive information about her daughter and identified her as the problem child who needed harsher punishment than the other girls. Not surprisingly, there was intense sibling rivalry between Maria and her sisters as a result of their mother's differential treatment.

Because Mrs. P. had very different perceptions of her three children, her interactional style with each child also was quite different. These varied styles, in turn, affected the children's behavior, which further reinforced Mrs. P.'s perceptions of them. For example, Mrs. P. had extremely high expectations of Maria, but at the same time perceived her to be minimally competent in daily activities (e.g., household tasks, self-help skills). Maria was acutely aware of these expectations, felt pressured to succeed at everything she did, and dreaded the possibility of performing below standard. Consequently, Maria often appeared dependent on others to show her what to do and needed enormous guidance and reassurance before approaching new situations. These behaviors only served to reinforce Mrs. P.'s perceptions of Maria as a child who was barely able to get along in the world without a great deal of prodding and attention. Indeed, Maria was rarely praised for her efforts. A second example of this phenomenon could be found in the way Mrs. P. played with her daughters. She was far more playful and spontaneous with her two younger daughters than she was with Maria, and in turn, Anna and Rosa were playful with her while Maria was solemn and self-conscious with her mother. Again, these differences in interactions only served to reinforce Mrs. P.'s perceptions that her younger daughters were "alive and well" while Maria was a problem child.

Mrs. P. not only perceived Maria as helpless but also as "weird." She had very little psychological understanding of her daughter and tended to project many of her negative feelings about herself onto her child. In fact, Mrs. P. had difficulty perceiving any of Maria's positive qualities and would misinterpret positive feedback about Maria from teachers or other adults who knew her. For instance, when a teacher wrote that Maria did a "good job" on an assignment, Mrs. P. interpreted the feedback to mean that Maria could have done an excellent job if she tried harder and that "good" was meant to let Maria know that she wasn't working up to her capabilities. In contrast, Mrs. P. saw Anna and Rosa as resilient "healthy" children and tended to portray them in an overly positive light. Mrs. P. did not recognize that Anna's behavior could become too aggressive at times or that she liked to get Maria in trouble with their mother. Rosa was depicted to be an "angel," a child who could do no wrong. In terms of discipline, Mrs. P. also tended to treat Maria differently from her other daughters, with Maria typically receiving the harsher punishment.

Strained Sibling Relationships

Mrs. P.'s differential treatment of her daughters led to intense sibling rivalry between Maria and Anna in particular. The rivalry took the form of resentment, aggression, and competition for their mother's approval and attention. Although Maria and Anna each provoked the other, Anna's behavior tended to be more subtle while Maria's behavior usually involved physical aggression. Maria was blamed more often for "starting" the fight and was told that she "should know better" since she was older than her sister. Mrs. P.'s response served to intensify the conflict between the sisters, and it appeared that the three of them were locked in an escalating battle without end.

Strained sibling relationships between Billy and Tom were a significant part of the S. family's life. Mr. S.'s differential treatment of his sons contributed to combative interactions between the two boys and Tom's painful feelings of his father's rejection in the face of Billy's exalted position. The boys needed to share a bedroom when they moved to their grandparents' house, which further escalated their angry and complicated relationship. The residual pattern of paternal favoritism remained in regard to visitation arrangements. Tom didn't want to have contact with his father, whereas Billy did want to see his father and felt extremely guilty about it, since no one in the household had positive feelings about Mr. S. The escalation of the boy's fighting was a central issue at the beginning of therapy, and it was necessary for Mrs. S. and her parents to maintain a united, patient but firm front with Billy and Tom.

Child Issues

Although there are multiple issues that could serve as the treatment focus for child witnesses to marital violence (*cf.* Rosenberg & Rossman, 1990; Rossman & Rosenberg, 1998), the following areas of concern emerged for Maria and Billy during the evaluation sessions: (1) coping with the traumatic memories of the father's violence and its emotional consequences; (2) alternating between feeling a profound sense of powerlessness and feeling overly powerful to control people and events; and (3) having problems with emotion regulation and expression.

Coping with Traumatic Memories

Maria was more strongly affected by her father's violence toward her mother than the other children in the family. She witnessed more abusive incidents than her sisters, and because she was the oldest, she was better able to understand the seriousness of the violence and its implications for her mother's safety. When Maria came to the attention of the clinic, she evidenced many symptoms associated with posttraumatic stress disorder. For example, she experienced intrusive, repetitive memories of the violence that interfered with her daily functioning. Maria would often talk about the abuse to others—for example, her schoolteacher. Although she was a good student, the intrusive memories interfered with her concentration and overall school performance. Maria would frequently daydream in class and the teacher felt that she was in "another world" for a significant proportion of the school day. In therapy sessions, Maria described nightmares in which women and little girls were beaten and carried away by monsters; she awoke from these nightmares screaming and shaking with fear. She repeatedly narrated several of the more severe incidents of abuse, but her affect was noticeably flat and she appeared numb. On other occasions, Maria had difficulty recalling violent incidents or refused to talk further about her experiences.

During the evaluation sessions, Maria's play revealed that she saw the world as a dangerous place, full of unpredictable events. She introduced over and over again in her play sudden tragedies and accidents, as for example, when a family drove their car off an unexpected cliff. There were recurrent themes of needing to be careful in order to avoid these tragedies, although even those play characters who were extremely careful experienced a variety of destructive outcomes. Through play therapy, Maria could begin to work through her experience of unpredictable violence. However, in contrast to real life, she would now be able to create and control the dangers around her.

Power and Powerlessness

In the evaluation sessions, Maria often expressed her own sense of powerlessness to control other people or events through play. At the same time, Maria felt a strong responsibility to "make things better" for family members and friends. It was important for Maria to have a great deal of control over what happened to others. Many times she was able to "save" people in miraculous ways, which made her feel strong and happy. However, another frequent theme in these sessions involved several traumatic events occurring one after the other. On one occasion Maria exclaimed, "I can't rescue all these people all by myself, I'm only a little kid!" She began to get angry at the people, stating that it was they who made her feel so bad about herself (i.e., incompetent). After throwing the doll figures around the playroom, she began to cry and talk about how sad and lonely she felt. The juxtaposition of her feelings of responsibility and power to influence people and circumstances with her overwhelming sense of powerlessness contributed to a decreased sense of self-efficacy and self-worth, aggressive behavior, and depressive symptoms.

Another way in which Maria grappled with her feelings of powerlessness was by clinging to external structure. Her way of finding safety in an unpredictable world was to follow carefully all rules, and she often became upset over seemingly minor deviations from any rules. Maria's schoolteacher described this behavior as "perfectionistic," but Mrs. P., who was frequently frustrated by Maria's rigidity, perceived this behavior as additional evidence of Maria's "strangeness." An example of Maria's need to follow rules precisely was an occasion when she cried inconsolably because she was unable to complete a homework assignment on the "proper" paper. A goal in therapy was to help Maria gain some flexibility and feel more comfortable with herself without this excessive dependence on structure.

Issues of power and powerlessness arose for Billy in different ways than for Maria. Billy derived his (false) sense of power from having his father involved in the family. Mr. S. protected Billy and allowed him an exalted status in the family that was not challenged successfully by his mother or brother. When the nuclear family constellation changed, Billy felt a sense of powerlessness, as his status was redefined to that of a loved and cared-for child, but one not favored over his brother or given immunity for behavioral transgressions. On some level, Billy believed his father's explanations that his mother and brother deserved the treatment they received, and that Billy as the "good" one of the bunch. In therapy, Billy struggled between his feelings of being overly powerful and unrealistically powerless until he was able to come to some understanding of his own sense of efficacy in his world.

Emotion Regulation and Expression

Maria and her sisters were acutely aware of their mother's emotions, and in fact, Mrs. P.'s brother compared them to puppets. He reported that both children seemed not to have their own emotions when they were around their mother; instead, they simply watched and then mimicked her mood when she came to pick them up. For Maria, this fine-tuned sensitivity to her mother's and others' emotions interfered with her ability to identify, understand, and communicate what she was feeling, even in the most innocuous situations.

Initially, Maria's tendency was to "gloss over" and deny her feelings of anger, sadness, and fear. She would report that "everything was fine," despite clear evidence to the contrary (e.g., tears in her eyes, a negative behavioral report from her teacher). This style was so pronounced that at times Maria contradicted herself in one breath in an effort to avoid expression of her distress. For example, she would state, "School's pretty bad, but I like it," or "It makes me sad, but I feel better." This tendency was compounded by Mrs. P.'s discomfort with her own feelings of sadness, anger, and fear, or those feelings expressed by her children. She rarely allowed Maria to articulate her negative feelings fully and focused almost exclusively on the positive side of every issue that Maria raised (e.g., "But how can you feel that way, things are getting better") or moving quickly to problem solving (e.g., "You should try again").

Maria had difficulty expressing her emotional needs directly and modulating her own distress. She often reacted to distress by becoming angry and aggressive or intensely sad. Maria often sought nurturance from her mother in indirect or inappropriate ways. For example, she would squeeze between her mother and one of her sisters on the couch, clinging to her mother. She had difficulty trying to soothe herself and relied primarily on emoting strategies, such as crying, biting her nails, screaming, or aggressive behavior. In general, Maria had few effective coping strategies when she felt emotionally needy and overwhelmed.

Not unexpectedly, Maria had particular difficulty expressing anger in appropriate ways and she tended to alternate between aggressive and passive behavior when she felt angry. The aggression in her daily experiences was mirrored in her early fantasy play. When Maria came to the attention of the clinic, she hit and pushed both sisters on a regular basis. Prior to the teacher's recommendation for therapy, Mrs. P. walked into Maria's bedroom one evening and found her trying to strangle Anna. While Maria's aggression toward her younger sisters was often an expression of anger (whether it was justified anger toward them or displaced anger toward her mother), Maria sometimes hit her peers at school without provocation, and apparently, without anger. She explained that she "hit them so they won't think I'm afraid of them." A focus of therapy was to help Maria express her anger more appropriately and directly and to respond to peers assertively.

Adult emotions and moods were experienced as unpredictable and confusing to Maria, and she struggled to understand why adults (and she herself) often displayed sudden changes of mood. She initially explained her play characters' behavior in magical terms, such as "he was put under a spell by an evil wizard" or "he drank a magic potion and became a different person" or "a poltergeist entered his body." The confusion in her play mirrored her feelings about her father and his rapid swings between warmth and aggression. Clearly, an important therapeutic goal would be to help Maria explore these different aspects of her father and begin to integrate her discrepant memories of him.

Emotions and emotional material were a central focus of concern for Billy. He avoided anything to do with emotions, would change the subject, distract, get up, and move around the playroom, or become tired. Whatever little emotion he did express was predominantly negative (e.g., anger). A central therapeutic goal was to help Billy be able to identify a range of different emotions (i.e., learn emotion words) and how the words might relate to feelings in his body; help him tolerate different affects in the face of his anxiety and express his emotional experience to others so that they could understand. This was an extremely difficult yet rewarding aspect of therapy, because it was so clear that Billy's family experience contributed to a developmental impairment in his emotional functioning.

Assessment of Psychopathology

Both the P. and S. families were evaluated over a series of sessions, which included several interview sessions with the mothers to gather information about developmental history, family history, and current family functioning. Child Behavior Checklists (CBCL, Achenbach & Edelbrock,

1985) were completed for each of the children. For the P. family, phone interviews were conducted with Maria and Anna's schoolteachers, Rosa's baby-sitter, Mrs. P.'s individual therapist, and her brother. School visits were made to observe Maria and Anna in their classrooms and to meet their teachers. All three children were seen individually and jointly in play sessions to observe their interactions. Family sessions were also conducted to observe the quality of interaction between Mrs. P. and her daughters and among the girls themselves in the presence of their mother. Similar procedures were conducted with the S. family.

After the initial evaluation procedures were completed, it became clear that Anna and Rosa were functioning well psychologically but Maria was in emotional turmoil. The therapist recommended psychological testing to further assess Maria's cognitive and socioemotional functioning. She was administered the following assessment instruments: the Wechsler Intelligence Scale for Children—Revised (WISC-R) (Wechsler, 1974); the Pictorial Scale of Perceived Competence and Social Acceptance for Young Children (Harter, 1985), Conger Children's Sentence Completion Test (Rohde, 1975), and the Rorschach (1951).

Initial psychological evaluations were completed on both the S. boys. We will discuss the younger son, Billy, because he was the child who witnessed violence primarily and did not experience the physical abuse that his brother suffered. Billy was administered the following assessment instruments: (1) the Wechsler Intelligence Scale for Children–Revised (WISC-R); (2) Rorschach; (3) Thematic Apperception Test (TAT) (Murray, 1943); (4) family drawings; (5) Conger Sentence Completion; (6) Spielberger State-Trait Anxiety Questionnaire for Children (Spielberger, Edwards, Montouri, & Lushene, 1970); and (7) the Bene–Anthony Family Relations Test (Bene & Anthony, 1957).

Maria's Evaluation Findings

Maria's developmental history was unremarkable. She met all developmental milestones at the appropriate ages, and was generally a healthy infant and toddler. She was toilet-trained at approximately 2 years, 2 months and maintained bladder and bowel control without regression. As far back as she could remember, Mrs. P. felt that Maria was particularly sensitive to her marital arguments. She would cry as soon as anyone raised their voice, and it was often difficult to console her once she became upset. Mrs. P. also described Maria as a "slow-to-warm-up" child, who tended to approach novel situations with trepidation until she spent enough time to feel comfortable and know what to expect. On the Child Behavior Checklist, Mrs. P. reported elevations in Maria's behavior on the Depression,

Somatic Complaints, and Aggression subscales. Maria's teacher generally supported Mrs. P.'s perceptions, although the teacher had a more balanced perspective of Maria's strengths and limitations.

On the WISC-R, Maria obtained a full scale IQ of 117, which placed her in the high average range of intelligence. A significant difference of 20 points emerged between her verbal IQ of 106 and her performance IQ of 126. Whereas there were many possible explanations for this difference, two appeared especially plausible. First, Maria's "slow-to-warm-up" style was painfully evident during the initial play and testing sessions and appeared to compromise her ability to demonstrate the extent of her knowledge. She was noticeably shy, and hesitated to guess or elaborate on her answers to verbal subtests. She found the nonverbal performance subtests much easier, perhaps in part because she did not have to interact verbally with the examiner. Because of Maria's hesitant style, the examiner felt that her verbal IQ underestimated her true ability. A second, related explanation is the fact that Maria is bilingual, having learned both English and Spanish simultaneously as a young child. It is not uncommon for bilingual children to score significantly higher on nonverbal than verbal measures of intelligence (see Kaufman, 1979). A third, and least likely explanation for Maria's significant verbal–performance discrepancy was that she had a learning disability. However, Maria consistently achieved good grades in school and there was no indication that she was having particular difficulty in any of her subjects. According to her teacher, Maria's academic problems at school stemmed from her frequent day-dreaming in class. Once the teacher redirected her attention to work, Maria was easily able to complete her assignments. Follow-up educational testing by the school to assess for learning disability confirmed its absence.

Maria's performance was quite even within the verbal and performance domains. All verbal subscores clustered around the average to slightly above average range while her performance subscores were significantly higher. Maria's profile did not evidence any relative strengths or weaknesses.

Maria's scores on the Pictorial Scale of Perceived Competence and Social Acceptance were compared to norms for children her age. Her mean score for perceptions of physical competence was highest, followed by her mean cognitive competence score; both were similar to scores obtained by same-age peers in the normative sample. Maria's perceptions of maternal and peer acceptance were much lower than those reported by same-age peers, and appeared to be an accurate reflection of the relationship with her mother and friends when she entered therapy. Interestingly, Maria's answers on the sentence completion test that related to friendships contradicted the responses she gave on perceptions of peer acceptance. For

example, in completing the sentence stem, "The thing I do best is ...,"
Maria answered "make friends," which was clearly in contrast to her
experience at school and in the neighborhood. Additional sentence completion items suggested that Maria's potential for self-awareness was quite
good for her age (e.g., "The worst thing about me is ... I get angry at my
sister"). She was clearly struggling to make sense of the often discrepant
perceptions she had of her father and her parents' relationship (e.g.,
"When I see my mother and father together ... I feel good"; "I like my
father but ... he was kind of mean"; "What I want to happen the most is ...
love in my family").

Maria's responses on the Rorschach lent additional support to the
idea that she was depressed, placed too low a value on herself, and was
consumed with extreme anger that at times masked her sad and lonely
feelings. Her protocol reflected her cautious manner and suggested that
she invested a great deal of effort into processing information and was
likely to approach stimuli with caution and thoroughness. She tended to
rely on her inner world of thoughts and feelings for gratification, but she
clearly did not have the psychological resources to cope with her overwhelming pain and turmoil. Her repertoire of coping strategies was limited and somewhat rigid. Her affect was not well modulated, and under
stress she had little or no sense of being able to control her explosive
feelings.

Maria's record contained several special scorings of morbid and aggressive where she attributed depressed or angry affect to her percepts.
For example, she perceived "a sad cat" and "a lonely bat" on Card IV; "a
hungry cat," "a mean wolf," and "someone who's mad" on Card IX; and
"a mad dragon" on Card X. She tended to perceive her social environment
as marked by aggressiveness and was likely to express aggression directly.
The form quality for each of these percepts was compromised. There were
relatively few human responses (one-tenth of the record) in contrast to
animal responses, suggesting that even for her age, there was some detachment from people in her environment. In general, the form quality of
Maria's responses suggested that she was not perceiving reality in the
same way as other children her age, and form quality deteriorated in the
presence of uncontained affect. Her responses indicated the presence of
complicated internal conflicts and possibly excessive rumination.

In summary, Maria was functioning in the high average range of
intelligence, although the combination of her hesitant response style and
bilingual background may have underestimated her true verbal abilities.
She was clearly experiencing emotional turmoil in the form of depression,
anxiety, and anger that exceeded her available psychological resources
and interfered in multiple domains of her life (e.g., academic, social, and

familial spheres). The family evaluation revealed several areas of concern, including the family's isolation from potent support systems, a pervasive crisis atmosphere in the home, Maria's troubled relationship with her mother and father, Mrs. P.'s problems with discipline, and the family's difficulty with emotional expression.

Treatment Recommendations for Maria and Her Family

Based on the evaluation findings and psychological testing, the therapist recommended two levels of intervention with the P. family. First, child play therapy sessions with Maria were indicated to address the emotional turmoil that resulted in her anxiety, sadness, and aggressive behavior. These sessions would focus on an exploration of Maria's inner experience with the ultimate goal of helping her understand and integrate her traumatic memories and affects of living with her father's abusiveness toward her mother and the emotional chaos it caused her and her family. Additional goals were to help Maria express her emotional needs more directly and appropriately, find effective ways to communicate anger, build social skills to encourage more positive peer relationships, and in general, help to boost her self-esteem.

Second, parenting sessions were recommended to extend and strengthen Mrs. P.'s parenting skills, and to develop more appropriate perceptions and expectations of her children. Intermittent family and mother–daughter sessions were also indicated to focus on communicating, decreasing sibling rivalry, and improving Mrs. P.'s relationship with Maria.

Billy's Evaluation Findings

Billy's early development was reported as normal. He was healthy and reached developmental milestones as expected. He was described as the more outgoing of the two boys, even at a young age. Even though Billy was clearly favored by the father, both boys "walked on eggshells" around him. Billy could never be certain when his father would "explode" and "pop off" at his mother or older brother, which left him anxious and jumpy in general. Although Billy appeared to be quite depressed at times, his mother and grandmother's responses on the CBCL did not identify this as a significant problem. Billy's grandmother reported borderline clinical significant results on the CBCL's aggression and somatization subscales. In discussion with Billy's new teacher, the evaluator found that the teacher was not as concerned about his aggression in the classroom and reported that he was always courteous with her. She acknowledged that he did get into vigorous verbal arguments with classmates at times.

During the initial evaluation session, Billy was reserved and reluctant to explore the playroom and warmed up slowly over time. He continued to appear very anxious, however, and was extremely concerned about his performance and unwilling to take risks. On the WISC-R, Billy obtained a full scale IQ of 116, placing him in the high average range of intelligence. His verbal and performance IQs were 112 and 117, respectively. While his subtest scores were not particularly scattered, he performed best on the vocabulary subtest, which is a good predictor of school performance. He did significantly less well on the arithmetic subtest. It was likely that his high test anxiety level impaired his functioning on this task. Billy generally received Cs or below in school until his family moved in with his grandparents. At that time, he began receiving As and Bs, which was commensurate with his abilities.

Although Billy was generally anxious on structured cognitive tasks, he was extremely anxious with less structured tasks containing emotional material or ambiguous stimuli. He exhibited a striking aversion to discussion emotional issues of any type. For example, it seemed he had difficulty getting out the words in response to emotional content, or he would simply avoid emotional topics, attempt to change the subject, or distract in other ways. On those occasions when Billy did respond with affect, it was primarily negative (e.g., anger toward his brother or mother). On the Rorschach and TAT, Billy tended to rob situations and stimuli of their affect, responding with concrete stories and images or highly intellectualized answers. He had great difficulty being creative or using his imagination. His discomfort with and minimization of affective cues was not surprising given the high levels of parental conflict i his family. His general coping style was to isolate feelings from his thoughts.

At the time of evaluation, most of the anger that Billy expressed was directed toward his brother and mother, although infrequently he also expressed some anger and disappointment with his father. Billy's minimization strategies, which tended to isolate affect from thought content, probably helped him cope with his family's problems in the short term. However, these defenses left him without ways to manage strong negative affect other than to distance from it or explode. These defensive strategies may also have been very energy-consuming. Mrs. S. described Billy as frequently tired during the day, sleeping most of the way home following evaluation sessions and tending to sleep for more hours than other children his age. This is atypical for 7-year-olds and was flagged for further observation. As reported earlier, neither mother nor grandmother reported Billy depressed, as measured by the CBCL.

Billy's self-perceptions were mixed: he felt helpless and powerless to exert control in his daily life, but at the same time he was able to feel pride in some of his accomplishments. Thus, he was not a child with classic low self-esteem, where typically helplessness and powerlessness are present with self-regard eroded. Feeling mastery in some developmental domains might have helped him socially. Billy evidenced relatively strong social skills—contrary to his brother—and by all accounts, had little difficulty making and maintaining friends. The Bene–Anthony Family Relations Test suggested that he was able to mobilize social support from many members of his family, who fortunately, were emotionally available for him as well. Billy felt a particularly strong attachment to a 3-year-old male cousin, with whom he was able to act playfully and protectively. However, he seemed to be confused about how to integrate his original nuclear family with his new family circumstances, which now included his grandparents but not his father (except for ongoing visitation).

One final area of concern was noted for Billy. He had great difficulty handling rules of any kind. He seemed to have the understanding that whoever was in control and more powerful physically made the rules, and that this person could change instantly. In addition, his father's rules hadn't necessarily pertained to him, since his father demanded compliance from his mother and brother and often let him slack off. Therefore, Billy often ignored or opposed others' rules, expecting that the rulemakers would either lose interest or let him get away with his behavior.

In summary, Billy was an attractive 7-year-old of above-average intelligence. He evidenced no cognitive deficits but had great difficulty with emotional material. He tended to isolate intellectual content from emotional cues. Emotional or ambiguous stimuli were associated with high anxiety levels for Billy. Billy's splitting of affect from content left him unable to modulate strong negative affect, particularly anger. He expressed few positive emotions but did interact socially with some positive affect. While Billy appeared to feel powerless over events in his life, he was not overly self-critical and could feel proud of some accomplishments. He was uncertain about his new family composition and how to integrate his past family circumstances with his new family members and dynamics.

Treatment Recommendations for Billy and His Family

While Billy did not appear to be severely disturbed, he was clearly experiencing emotional distress and confusion about his family situation. Individual treatment was recommended to work on his sense of powerlessness, high anxiety level, lack of appropriate risk taking, modulation of emotional expression, strained relationships with his mother, brother, and father, and understanding of the marital violence and divorce. Tom was also seen in individual treatment, and both boys were seen with their mother in family sessions. Contact was also maintained with the maternal grandparents, since Mrs. S. continued to live with her parents for some time.

Treatment Options

Maria and the P. Family in Treatment

Over a 1-year period, Maria made excellent progress toward the treatment goals identified by her therapist. By the end of therapy, Maria's play had grown significantly less aggressive and she had had no aggressive outbursts at home or at school for quite some time. Her fantasy play, which was concerned with injury in various settings, also became more realistic: she was able to cope with problems facing her fantasy characters without resorting to magic or unrealistic rescue solutions. Maria was no longer preoccupied with death and violence, either in her play or in her outside world. She seemed to have gained some distance from her traumatic memories of violence and was able to talk about her experiences in a more integrated way.

For example, at the beginning of therapy, Maria never let the dangers in her play world harm her characters. The endings to her fantasy stories usually involved some magical form of intervention that reversed the potentially violent outcome and provided a more acceptable conclusion. Pynoos and Eth (1986) refer to this type of coping as "denial in fantasy," which is a strategy used by some children to modulate their anxiety after experiencing a traumatic event. In Maria's play, children were run over by cars but were miraculously spared; characters were captured by villains but saved at the last moment; meals appeared magically just before characters starved. Maria was remarkably resistant to attempts to consider what would happen if her play situations played out naturally (i.e., if the play had a negative ending). Only much later in therapy was she able to tolerate and talk about the distress created by these traumas and the violent events that she witnessed. Once this occurred, her play became less magical and more realistic. Over time, Maria also introduced fewer dangers and tragedies into her play.

Maria also felt increasingly comfortable and secure with her place in the family and reported that her relationship with her mother was much improved. She was able to express her feelings and experiences more appropriately to her mother, who was in turn better able to meet Maria's emotional needs. For example, during family sessions, Maria was able to tell her mother how she felt hurt and angry when she was made to be the bad one in the family and her sisters were the "good guys." Mrs. P. was able to listen to Maria and validate her feelings without becoming defensive. Maria's sense of competence and self-esteem grew immensely over the course of therapy, and she was able to understand and feel proud about the gains that she had made.

Maria was observed in her classroom several weeks before terminating therapy. Her teacher reported that Maria was an excellent student, and although she continued to have "perfectionistic tendencies," they did not interfere significantly with her work. On the day that she was observed, Maria earned an early recess as a reward for completing all her assigned work correctly. As Maria cleared her desk and prepared to go outside, two female classmates yelled, "Come on, Maria, let's go play jumprope," and Maria hurried out with them. Although the teacher found her shy at times, Maria was able to make friends in her class and was reported to be happier and far less preoccupied with family matters than she had been a year earlier. Thus, the teacher's perspective clearly supported the therapist's (and Maria's) view of the hard work that was accomplished during individual therapy.

Throughout treatment, the girls' contact with their father continued to be stressful, particularly for Maria. Mrs. P. struggled to distance herself emotionally from her husband but continued to express sadness over his inability to "pull himself together" and confusion over the role he should play in their daughters' lives. Mr. P.'s phone calls to Maria were often tense, as he tried to extract information from her about Mrs. P.'s current life. After talking with her father, Maria frequently fought with her mother and sisters. Occasional visitation was arranged, but after the first visit, Mr. P. did not comply with the agreements (e.g., he took the girls away from the site that he been prearranged for visitation and was several hours late in returning the children), and there was some concern about the possibility of kidnapping. Mrs. P. found it extremely difficult to set firm limits with her husband and struggled to decide how to proceed with his blatant disregard for the visitation arrangements. She contacted the court and visitation was suspended temporarily until arrangements for supervised visitation were made. Mr. P. decided to enter individual therapy at that time and agreed to supervised visitation until he demonstrated his willingness to establish a more constructive relationship with his children rather than using them as revenge against Mrs. P. Maria's anxiety and symptomatic behaviors slowly decreased after Mr. P. entered therapy and made a commitment to understanding and changing his violent interpersonal relationships. However, supervised visitation continued until after the P. family terminated treatment and the P.'s divorce was finalized.

Mrs. P. also made significant progress during the parenting sessions, the dyadic work with Maria, and the family meetings. A major focus of Mrs. P.'s work was to help her see the connection between her past experiences and her present interactions. Mrs. P. wanted intensely to have what she called "clean and clear" interactions with others. For her, this meant responding to others with feelings that were not entangled with previous experiences in her history. "Clean and clear" responses were those that occurred immediately and were honest rather than distorted by guilt, self-doubt, or fear of rejection.

A second focus of the therapeutic work with Mrs. P. was to help her with the process of integrating opposite characteristics, such as good and bad. This splitting seemed to serve a defensive function for her in that Mrs. P. would often begin feeling overwhelmed if she tried to integrate the two extremes. If Mrs. P. was feeling good, then she did not want to contemplate anything unhappy or "bad." Doing so meant running the risk of losing her good feeling. Over the course of therapy, Mrs. P. grew in her ability to integrate opposites. For example, she began to have increasingly realistic perceptions of the positive and negative attributes of all her daughters, rather than seeing Maria as "sick," and Anna and the baby as "healthy." Mrs. P. also became able to view herself and her experiences more accurately, beginning first with her professional self-image and developing a realistic assessment of her strengths and weaknesses. Further along in therapy, she was less likely to perceive herself and her life either with a "Pollyanna-like" quality or with unrelenting pessimism, as she had when therapy began. Rather than dissolving into misery and helplessness, Mrs. P. was able to say as she faced a new problem, "Maybe I'll be able to make a balance with this as I have with other things." Whereas in the past previously small concerns ballooned easily into larger concerns, Mrs. P. grew increasingly able to modulate her emotional responses and maintain a balanced perspective.

At the end of therapy, Mrs. P. was able to change her way of relating in many aspects of her life. In the area of discipline, she experienced a great sense of relief when she was able to give logical consequences for the girls' misbehavior, without being filtered through her own psychological problems. She worked hard to control her anger and be firm rather than harsh in her disciplinary interactions with her daughters. She also began to model more appropriate ways of communicating emotions to the girls and over time felt less threatened and angry by Maria's emotional needs. As discipline became less problematic, Mrs. P.'s relationship with Maria slowly began to improve. Most importantly, Mrs. P. no longer relied on Maria for emotional support and was able to accommodate to Maria's need for connection and affection. Gaining distance from Maria enabled Mrs. P. to begin perceiving her more accurately and positively. Mrs. P.'s empathy for and understanding of her daughter grew, and she was less likely to see Maria as "weird." She began to participate in community events, made several new friends, and toward the end of therapy, she began to date men. As Mrs. P. progressed in each of these areas, her sense of competence as a woman and mother also grew, and she began to take real pride in herself and in *all* of her children.

Billy and the S. Family in Treatment

Billy, his mother, and his brother were seen in weekly therapy sessions for slightly over 2 years. His mother and grandmother made a significant commitment to treatment. Billy's initial work began with a focus on building his sense of control over his environment while providing him an opportunity to express his feelings about his father's abusive behaviors toward his mother and brother and their pets.

As Billy became more comfortable and open in the therapeutic relationship, and as the issues were highlighted by his father's inconsistent and sometimes unannounced visitations, Billy began to bring in themes that reflected his ambivalence toward his father. With great difficulty, Billy began to express extreme negative feelings toward his father and his confusion over his father's motivations. Billy had become accustomed to being "special" to his father, and he felt both relieved and guilty about occupying this position in the family while his brother and mother so obviously suffered from his father's treatment. Billy would comment that his father didn't know how to be loving and that he neglected Billy emotionally. He expressed his ambivalence by saying "After all, he's still my dad even if I don't like what he does." He was able to retain positive feelings about his father's ability to teach him skills and willingness to take him and his brother camping.

As the possibility of divorce became more imminent, Billy spent more time in therapy dealing with his family situation and sorting out his feelings about his father. He began to explore the differences in his life since moving away from his father, and the differences for his mother and brother. This endeavor led to new empathy and perspective-taking skills, as he began to understand his mother's and brother's experience of living with Mr. S. He concluded that their life was better away from their father: "I'm not always on tippy-toes and I have more freedom." Billy was now able to listen to the radio and participate in Boy Scouts and other extracurricular activities that he thoroughly enjoyed. These had been forbidden previously by his father.

Billy was able to make great strides in several psychological domains during treatment. He continued to develop a positive sense of self, including an understanding of things he could and could not control. He continued doing well in school and was becoming involved in school activities, including sports. As he gained a better sense of his family situation and his role in it, he expressed his desire to live with his mother, saying, "She's so much better, you can talk to Mom," and "If Mom and Dad got back together, it would be a disaster." He began to perceive himself, his mother, and his brother as a family unit, and he began making efforts to get along better with his brother. He was particularly pleased when his brother would practice sports with him at home. Over time, Billy's anxiety level decreased noticeably, and he was able to work within a set of rules, whether playing a game in session or doing chores at home. He felt less threatened in expressing a range of emotion and began integrating more feeling with his thoughts. He was willing to express his opinions, even unpopular ones. Mrs. S. worked hard to increase the positive home atmosphere and reward the boys both for achievement and for being good citizens in the family. Through family meetings and continued open communication, Mrs. S. and the boys distributed chores and identified desired ways of relating that felt fair and satisfactory to all. At the time of termination, the family and therapist agreed that much change had been accomplished and that it was time for the family to try its new wings.

During treatment, Mrs. S. also made great strides. She had obtained additional professional training that resulted in a good position as she reentered the job market and the ability to move her family into an independent living situation. She developed and clarified her role as a parent to the boys and felt a great sense of accomplishment. She also gained a clear sense of the positive power she could exert in the family and her rights regarding divorce and custody issues. She expressed wonder and dismay at the time she had spent in the abusive relationship with her husband, and she endeavored to understand what had happened psychologically during the course of their marriage. She approached termination of therapy with a newfound sense of optimism about her son's and her own future; she acknowledged that they still had struggles ahead but would face them together.

Summary

In many ways, both Maria's and Billy's stories clearly illustrate the finding that witnessing marital violence can be a profoundly disorganizing experience for children, with significant effects on their cognitive, emotional, and behavioral functioning. Child witnesses experience these effects directly (i.e., actually witnessing violence perpetrated against a loved one) and indirectly (i.e., parent–child relationships that become distorted and compromised as a result of marital violence). Consequently, it is important for therapists to maintain a systems framework during evaluation and treatment of child witnesses and their families.

Child witnesses to marital violence live in a world of extremes and they come to understand and respond to their environment in terms of dichotomies. Children may experience their parents as emotionally unavailable or overavailable, controlled or explosive, ignoring or overreacting. They may alternately try to deny or ruminate on memories of violence, feel powerful or profoundly powerless, minimize negative emotions or explode with anger and sadness. Child witnesses develop ways of coping that may be quite adaptive in the context of living in a violent family. However, over time these coping strategies begin to interfere with the child's emotional health and become maladaptive in interactions outside the family. The content of therapy is not limited to helping children confront and integrate their traumatic memories but also to focus on their distorted cognitions, emotional reactions, and behavioral responses with the goals of increasing flexibility, modulation, and balance. Therapists must not underestimate the deleterious effects of witnessing violence on children's psychological well-being and must seize the opportunity to guide child witnesses and their families toward healthier intra- and interpersonal relationships.

References

Achenbach, T. M., & Edelbrock, C. S. (1985). *Manual for the Child Behavior Checklist and Revised Child Behavior Profile*. Burlington: University of Vermont.

Barnett, E. R., Pitman, C. B., Ragan, C. K., & Salus, M. K. (1980). *Family violence: Intervention strategies*. Washington, DC: U.S. Department of Health and Human Services (Publication No. [OHDS] 80-30258).

Bene, E., & Anthony, J. (1957). *Manual for the Bene–Anthony Family Relations Test*. London: National Foundation for Educational Research in England and Wales.

Bergman, A. (1976). Emergency room: A role for social workers. *Health and Social Work, 1*, 1.

Browne, A. (1987). *When battered women kill*. New York: Free Press.

Carlson, B. E. (1984). Children's observations of interparental violence. In A. R. Roberts (Ed.), *Battered women and their families: Intervention strategies and treatment programs* (pp. 147–167). New York: Springer.

Devoe, E., & Graham-Bermann, S. (1997, June). *Predictors of posttraumatic stress symptoms in battered women and their children*. Paper presented at the Second International Conference on Children Exposed to Family Violence. London, Ontario, Canada.

Fantuzzo, J. W., DePaola, L. M., Lambert, L., Martino, T., Anderson, G., & Sutton, S. (1991). Effects of interparental violence on the psychological adjustment and competencies of young children. *Journal of Consulting and Clinical Psychology, 59*, 258–265.

Fantuzzo, J. W., Boruch, R., Beriama, A., Atkins, M., & Marcus, S. (1997). Domestic violence and children: Prevalence and risk in five major U.S. cities. *Journal of the American Academy of Child and Adolescent Psychiatry, 36*, 116–122.

Gelles, R. J., & Straus, M. A. (1988). *Intimate violence.* New York: Simon & Schuster.

Giles-Sims, J. (1983). *Wife battering: A systems theory approach.* New York: Guilford Press.

Harter, S. (1985). *The self-perception profile for children.* Unpublished manuscript, University of Denver.

Hilberman, E. (1979). The battered woman. *Emergency Medicine, 2,* 24.

Holden, G. W., & Ritchie, K. L. (1991). Linking extreme marital discord, child rearing, and child behavior problems: Evidence from battered women. *Child Development, 62,* 311–327.

Holden, G. W., Stein, J. D., Ritchie, K. L., Harris, S. D., & Jouriles, E. N. (1998). The parenting behaviors and beliefs of battered women. In G. W. Holden, R. Geffner, & E. N. Jouriles (Eds.), *Children exposed to marital violence: Theory, research, and intervention.* Washington, DC: American Psychological Association.

Hughes, H. M. (1988). Psychological and behavioral correlates of family violence in child witnesses and victims. *American Journal of Orthopsychiatry, 58,* 77–90.

Hughes, H. M., & Fantuzzo, J. W. (1994). Family violence: Child. In R. T. Ammerman, M. Hersen, & L. Sisson (Eds.), *Handbook of aggressive and destructive behavior in psychiatric patients* (pp. 491–508). New York: Plenum.

Jaffe, P. G., Wolfe, D. A., Wilson, S. K., & Zak, L. (1986). Family violence and child adjustment: A comparative analysis of girls' and boys' behavioral symptoms. *American Journal of Psychiatry, 143,* 74–77.

Jaffe, P. G., Wolfe, D. A., & Wilson, S. K. (1990). *Children of battered women.* Newbury Park, CA: Sage.

Jouriles, E. N., & LeCompte, S. H. (1991). Husband's aggression toward wives, and mother's and father's aggression toward children: Moderating effects of child gender. *Journal of Consulting and Clinical Psychology, 59,* 190–192.

Jouriles, E. N., Murphy, C. M., & O'Leary, K. D. (1989). Interspousal aggression, marital discord, and child problems. *Journal of Consulting and Clinical Psychology, 57,* 453–455.

Kaufman, A. S. (1979). *Intelligent testing with the WISC-R.* New York: Wiley.

Kilpatrick, K. D., Litt, M., & Williams, L. M. (1997). Posttraumatic stress disorder in child witnesses to domestic violence. *American Journal of Orthopsychiatry, 67,* 639–644.

Klingbeil, K. S., & Boyd, V. D. (1984). Emergency room intervention: Detection, assessment, and treatment. In A. R. Roberts (Ed.), *Battered women and their families: Intervention strategies and treatment programs* (pp. 7–32). New York: Springer.

Margolin, G. (1995, January). *The effects of domestic violence on children.* Paper presented at the Conference on Violence against Children in the Family and the Community, Los Angeles.

McCloskey, L. A., Figueredo, A. J., & Koss, M. P. (1995). The effects of systemic family violence on children's mental health. *Child Development, 66,* 1239–1261.

Moore, T., Pepler, D., Weinberg, B., Hammond, L., Waddell, J., & Weiser, L. (1990). Research on children from violent families. *Canada's Mental Health Journal, 38,* 19–23.

Murray, A. H. (1943). *Thematic Apperception Test Manual.* Cambridge: Harvard College.

Novello, A. C. (1992). From the surgeon general. U.S. Public Health Service. *Journal of the American Medical Association, 267*(23), 3132.

O'Keefe, M. (1994). Linking marital violence, mother– child, father–child aggression, and child behavior problems. *Journal of Family Violence, 9,* 63–78.

Pynoos, R. S., & Eth, S. (1986). Witness to violence: The child interview. *Journal of the American Academy of Child Psychiatry, 25,* 306–319.

Rohde, A. R. (1975). *Sentence completion method: Its diagnostic and clinical applications to mental disorders.* New York: Ronald.

Rorschach, H. (1951). *Psychodiagnostics.* New York: Grune & Stratton. (Original work published 1921)

Rosenberg, M. S. (1987). Children of battered women: The effects of witnessing violence on their social problem solving abilities. *Behavior Therapist, 4,* 85–89.

Rosenberg, M. S., & Rossman, B. B. R. (1990). The child witness to marital violence. In R. T. Ammerman & M. Hersen (Eds.), *Treatment of family violence: A sourcebook* (pp. 183–210). New York: Wiley.

Rossman, B. B. R., & Rosenberg, M. S. (198). *Multiple victimization of children: Conceptual, research, and treatment issues.* Binghamton, NY: Haworth Press.

Rossman, B. B. R., Bingham, R. D., & Emde, R. N. (1996). Symptomatology and adaptive functioning for children exposed to normative stressors, dog attacks, and parental violence. *Journal of the American Academy of Child and Adolescent Psychiatry, 36,* 1–9.

Spielberger, C. D., Edwards, C. D., Montouri, J., & Lushene, R. (1970). *The State-Trait Anxiety Inventory for Children.* Palo Alto, CA: Consulting Psychologists Press.

Stark, E., Flitcraft, A., & Frazier, W. (1979). Medicine and patriarchal violence: The social construction of a "private" event. *International Journal of Health Services, 9,* 461–489.

Sternberg, K. J., Lamb, M. E., Greenbaum, C., Cicchetti, D., Dawud, S., Cortes, R. M., Krispin, O., & Lorey, F. (1993). Effects of domestic violence on children's behavior problems and depression. *Developmental Psychology, 29,* 44–52.

Straus, M. A. (1991). *Children as witnesses to marital violence: A risk factor for life long problems among a nationally representative sample of American men and women.* Paper presented at the Ross Roundtable on Children and Violence, Washington, DC.

Walker, L. E. A., & Edwall, G. E. (1987). Domestic violence and determination of visitation and custody in divorce. In D. J. Sonkin (Ed.), *Domestic violence on trial: Psychological and legal dimensions of family violence* (pp. 127–152). New York: Springer.

Wechsler, D. (1974). *Manual for the Wechsler Intelligence Scale for Children—Revised.* New York: Psychological Corporation.

Weithorn, L. A. (Ed.). (1987). *Psychology and child custody determinations: Knowledge, roles, and expertise.* Lincoln: University of Nebraska Press.

14

Psychological and Emotional Abuse of Children

Marla R. Brassard, Stuart N. Hart, and David B. Hardy

Description of the Problem

Psychological maltreatment is increasingly recognized as a core issue in all forms of child maltreatment and as the unifying concept that connects the cognitive, affective, and interpersonal problems that are related to physical abuse, sexual abuse, and all forms of neglect (Brassard, Germain, & Hart, 1987; Brassard, Hart, & Hardy, 1993; Hart & Brassard, 1987). It is the repeated pattern of behavior or extreme incident that expresses to children that they are worthless, unwanted, unloved, or only of value in meeting another's needs that causes the lasting damage to their selves and their psyches.

The psychological concomitants, more than the severity of the acts themselves, constitute the real traumas and are responsible for the damaging consequences of sexual abuse (Abramson & Lucido, 1991; Friedrich, Burke, & Urguiza, 1987; Nash, Hulsey, Sexton, Harralson, & Lambert, 1993)

Marla R. Brassard • Faculty of Health and Behavioral Studies, Teachers College, Columbia University, New York, New York 10027.   **Stuart N. Hart** • Department of Counseling and Educational Psychology, School of Education, Indiana University-Purdue University, Indianapolis, Indiana 46202.   **David B. Hardy** • Tri-Country Youth Program, Greenfield, Massachusetts 01301.

Case Studies in Family Violence, Second Edition, edited by Ammerman and Hersen. Kluwer Academic / Plenum Publishers, New York, 2000.

and physical abuse (Claussen & Crittenden, 1991; Hart & Brassard, 1989; Vissing, Straus, Gelles, & Harrup, 1991). In cases of neglect it is not simply the parents' failure to provide adequate care but the pervasive psychological unavailability, with the complete rejection this communicates, and the lost opportunities for healthy interpersonal involvement that place a child at risk for severe developmental disorders (Crittenden, 1988; Egeland, Sroufe, & Erickson, 1983; Farber & Egeland, 1987).

Psychological maltreatment is gaining increasing research and legal attention after decades of being ignored. Historically, the lack of an adequately operationalized definition made it problematic to identify psychological maltreatment and to provide appropriate protective services to those families in need. A number of facts confounded the issue: psychological maltreatment is manifested in both acts of commission and acts of omission; there is an absence of physical evidence; it both occurs with other forms of maltreatment and exists alone; it can be defined only within an interpersonal context; and salience is dependent on the developmental stage of the victim. In addition, the high rates of co-occurrence with other forms of abuse and neglect made many child abuse professionals question the benefits of identifying psychologically maltreating families as a separate group. Considerable progress has now been made. There are accepted definitions of psychological maltreatment (American Professional Society on the Abuse of Children, 1995; U.S. Department of Health and Human Services, 1988, 1998), measures with known reliability and validity (see Brassard & Hardy, 1998 for a review), clear evidence of harm to victims when occurring alone or with other forms of maltreatment (Hart, Binggeli, & Brassard, 1998) even at low levels of intensity (Barnett, Manly, & Cicchetti, 1993), and growing evidence that this is by far the most frequent form of maltreatment. What is still lacking is application of this knowledge by child protective services and the courts, and a societal commitment to provide the services needed to support all families in child rearing, particularly those who are clearly in danger of failing at this most important task.

Accurate estimates of the incidence of all forms of child maltreatment are extremely difficult to obtain and this is particularly true of psychological maltreatment. The absence of agreed-upon definitions, the use of different populations, and different methodologies all contribute variance to these estimates. For example, the American Humane Association (1988) reported an incidence of only .54 cases per 1,000 children in one study, while another published study reports 900 cases per 1,000 children (Bouchard, Tessier, Fraser, & Laganiere, 1997). For a more extensive review of this issue see Brassard and Hardy (1997).

Although there is little agreement in the literature on the incidence of psychological maltreatment, one area of common agreement is the high level of co-occurrence of psychological maltreatment and other forms of abuse and neglect. There now exists a sizable body of research that suggests that most maltreated children experience more than one type of maltreatment (Barnett *et al.*, 1993; Briere & Runtz, 1988, 1990; Egeland & Sroufe, 1981) and that psychological maltreatment is particularly likely to co-occur with other forms of abuse and neglect.

Claussen and Crittenden (1991) investigated the co-occurrence of physical and psychological maltreatment in 175 families referred to child protective services (CPS), 175 control families, and 39 families receiving mental health services. Results indicated, that in the CPS sample, 91% of the physical abuse and 89% of the physical neglect cases also reported co-occurring psychological maltreatment. In the control sample, 93% of those reporting physical abuse and 91% of those reporting physical neglect also reported psychological maltreatment. The rate of co-occurrence was so high that the investigators recommended that assessments of psychological maltreatment be performed on all cases of physical abuse and neglect that are investigated.

Claussen and Crittenden (1991) reported that psychological maltreatment occurred at a rate of five times that of physical abuse in their community control sample. A number of retrospective studies on adult women (Briere & Runtz, 1988, 1990; Moeller, Bachman, & Moeller, 1993) have also documented the high rate of co-occurrence of various forms of maltreatment, with psychological maltreatment reported more frequently than other types of abuse and neglect. Briere and Runtz affirm that 90% of the women in their study reported experiences of psychological maltreatment.

While it is hard to compare results across studies because of differing definitions, populations, and methodologies, there does seem to be developing a consensus among researchers in the field that psychological maltreatment is the most frequent form of child maltreatment, that it occurs in most families that exhibit other forms of maltreatment, and that it can occur in families that exhibit no other forms of maltreatment.

In an attempt to establish an adequately operationalized definition of psychological maltreatment, we used a combination of categories of psychological abuse and neglect conceptualized by ourselves and other researchers (Baily & Baily, 1986; Brassard *et al.*, 1987; Garbarino, Guttman, & Seeley, 1986; U.S. Department of Health and Human Services, 1988). We have subsequently empirically identified and articulated five distinct subtypes of psychological maltreatment and related them to adverse child outcomes (Brassard *et al.*, 1993; Hart & Brassard, 1989). These subtypes are also embodied in the *Guidelines for the Psychosocial Evaluation of Suspected Psychological Maltreatment in Children and Adolescents* (American Professional Society on the Abuse of Children, 1995).

Spurning is a type of verbal battering that is a combination of rejection and hostile degradation. The parent may actively refuse to help a child or even to acknowledge the child's request for help. Spurning also includes calling a child debasing names, labeling the child as inferior, and publicly humiliating the child.

Terrorizing is threatening to physically hurt, kill, or abandon the child if he or she does not behave. It also includes exposing a child to violence or threats directed toward loved ones and leaving a young child unattended.

Isolating entails the active isolation of a child by an adult. The child may be locked in a closet or room for an extended length of time, or the adult may limit or refuse to allow any interaction with peers or adults outside the family.

Exploiting/corrupting involves modeling antisocial acts and unrealistic roles or encouraging and condoning deviant standards or beliefs. This includes teaching the child criminal behavior, keeping a child at home in the role of a servant or surrogate parent in lieu of school attendance, or encouraging a child to participate in the production of pornography.

Denying emotional responsiveness includes ignoring a child's attempts to interact and reacting to a child in a mechanistic way that is devoid of affectionate touch, kiss, and talk. Parents who behave in this way communicate through acts of omission that they are not interested in the child and are emotionally unavailable.

Consequences of Psychological Maltreatment

There now exists over a decade of empirical research that attests to the destructive consequences of psychological maltreatment and establishes its centrality in all forms of child abuse and neglect. In an extensive review of the research literature on psychological maltreatment, Hart *et al.* (1998) identified 29 separate negative developmental outcomes that are related in the literature to psychological maltreatment. Low self-esteem, depression, high levels of negative affect, and poor, often hostile interpersonal relationships are characteristic of victims of psychological maltreatment. Psychological maltreatment appears to be a particularly harmful form of abuse and neglect. For example, Erickson and Egeland (1987) suggest that other than physical injury leading to death, psychological unavailability may be the most damaging form of maltreatment. In another study, Vissing *et al.* (1991) demonstrated that verbal aggression from parents was more closely related to adverse developmental outcomes, such as elevated rates of physical aggression, delinquency, and interpersonal problems, than was physical abuse, and that in combination they created an even greater risk factor.

Case Descriptions

Introduction to Case 1

The case described here is based on an actual family that participated in our research project on psychological maltreatment (Hart & Brassard, 1989); however, all names and identifying characteristics have been changed to ensure confidentiality. The D'Niale family is a multiproblem family that has clearly experienced for several generations the problems related to poverty, unemployment, substance abuse, criminal activity, domestic violence, and the physical abuse and neglect of children.

The D'Niale family was chosen as a case study because the family as a whole functioned as a powerful but destructive force that undermined the healthy development of identity, self-esteem, and autonomy in all of its members. With its constant crises and pathogenic functioning, the family failed to provide even the bare minimum of psychological support, cognitive stimulation, and encouragement that is necessary for normal child development.

The second criterion that led to selection of this family as a case study is that during our assessment we witnessed incidents of all five subtypes of psychological maltreatment. We will describe the examples we identified and attempt to articulate the connections between the specific parental behaviors and the developmental outcomes exhibited in the children's behavior.

In July 1987 the state department of social services (DSS) received a report from a preschool teacher concerning the possible abuse of a 4-year-old named Joey D'Niale, who had arrived at school with multiple bruises. During the investigation, Joey's mother, Blanche D'Niale, blamed her mother, Beatrice Gelid, who in turn blamed Blanche, and both finally resorted to blaming Joey's 20-month-old brother, Sonny Jr. Charges of physical abuse were substantiated, although a perpetrator was not identified.

Blanche D'Niale and her family were not new to DSS; they had been in and out of the system since shortly after the birth of Blanche's first child in 1980. Joey had personally received services from eight social service agencies in addition to the protective services received from the department. The D'Niale family file at DSS was also cross-indexed with the files of several members of Blanche's extended family, indicating that interfamily as well as intrafamily patterns of maltreatment existed.

Assessment

Our family research assessment, described more extensively later in this chapter, lasts about 4 hours. It involves the collection of information on physical condition of the home, mother's psychological functioning, her satisfaction with her relationships, current life stressors, and information on her family of origin. The mother is also videotaped interacting in a structured task with one of her children.

Although Blanche was more than cooperative throughout the assessment—which not only taxes one's endurance but demands significant self-disclosure—there were constant interruptions created by her 20-month-old son, Sonny Jr.

Oscillating between ignoring him entirely, threatening to break his fingers, promising to buy him presents, and demanding that he not act like a baby, her responses only seemed to escalate his oppositional and aversive behavior. Sonny Jr. became extremely active, continually climbing on and poking the two members of our assessment team, crumpling up completed questionnaires, and then spilling milk all over the table.

Blanche's mother arrived and immediately monopolized the assessment. She insisted on answering questions on marital satisfaction and parenting practices that were clearly directed toward Blanche, often contradicting or discounting Blanche's responses. Her insensitive and intrusive behavior toward Blanche was markedly similar to Blanche's behavior toward her own children.

In our assessments, we always start with an attempt to identify who the significant players in the family and home are and how they are related. This proved to be no easy task in the D'Niale family. The family has moved seven times in the last 2 years, with the composition of the household changing constantly, as extended family members move in and out. The structure of Blanche's family matched what her caseworker described as an "extremely enmeshed matriarchy." The stable relationships in the family seem to exist between Blanche, her sister Barbie Gelid, her mother Beatrice Gelid, and her recently deceased maternal grandmother. Blanche is currently married to Sonny Jr.'s father, but all three of her children have different fathers and all of her relationships with men seem unstable and full of conflict—a configuration that closely resembles her description of both her sister's and mother's relationships with men.

Characteristics of Family Members

Blanche D'Niale: Blanche is a white woman of 29 years of age. She evidenced mild to severe deficits on all assessment measures. Her intellectual ability fell in the borderline to mentally retarded range. On the Beck Depression Inventory, Blanche's score of 27 placed her in the moderate to severe range for depression. She has no job skills and has been living on welfare since the birth of her first child.

Blanche was easily engaged in the assessment process, and she talked freely about the problems in her family and marriage. In our Family of Origin Interview Blanche reported that she was born and has lived all of her life within several blocks of her current apartment. Shortly after Blanche's birth her mother abandoned her to the care of her maternal grandmother, where she lived for 5 years until her grandmother overdosed on drugs. She remembers those 5 years as the happiest of her life. In the subsequent years of her childhood she was shuffled from one home to another as family members proved unable to provide adequate care for her. The descriptions of her early experiences seem split between reports of horrendous abuse and neglect and reminiscences of idealized family relationships.

At the time of the assessment, Blanche had minimum social support and much consequent stress. Her current relationship was physically violent and occasionally life-threatening to both parties. She reported major conflicts over child rearing and was awaiting the beginning of her husband's jail sentence. On the Locke-Wallace Marital Satisfaction Scale, Blanche's score of 56 is over 2 standard deviations below average. She indicated that she wished she hadn't married and that she was "very unhappy" in her marriage.

There were noticeable skill deficits in Blanche's parenting. She consistently placed age-inappropriate expectations on her children's behavior, at times infantilizing them and at times expecting them to act like adults. She told her 2-year-old son to go into the kitchen and get some juice and a plate of cookies for her guests, and then later reprimanded her 5-year-old for drinking out of a glass and not a spill-proof plastic cup. She stated that Sonny Jr. helped with the housework because even at the age of 2 he realized it was too much work for her to do alone. Blanche seemed to possess little understanding of the developmental needs of children, especially those needs that are related to healthy social and psychological development. Despite constant interruptions, Blanche answered all of our questions without hesitation. However, her responses indicated a severe lack of integration and an almost total absence of reflective thought. She repeatedly contradicted herself, denying the obvious and producing answers that were inconsistent. The most striking example of this was her response when asked how she would raise her children differently from the way she was raised. She answered that she would not abuse her children as she had been abused while simultaneously making threatening gestures with a lit cigarette to Sonny Jr., who was attempting to climb into her lap. Although she was not able to identify any sources of satisfaction in her parenting role or any strengths in her relationships with her children, Blanche claimed that she enjoyed being a parent and "loves children." She is currently trying to conceive another child.

Sonny D'Niale: Sonny is a chronic alcoholic who suffers from alcohol-related seizures and episodes of violent acting out. One month prior to our visit, upon discovering there was no cold beer in the apartment, he dragged the refrigerator onto the back porch and sent it plunging into the alley four floors below. At the time of the assessment he was unemployed, had just been convicted on charges of breaking and entering, and was awaiting sentencing. We were able to obtain little information on his family of origin other than that his father was an alcoholic and his brother had recently overdosed on narcotics. Although Blanche had little positive to say about her husband, she did emphasize that he is an involved father and has good relationships with both of her sons.

Sonny Jr.: Sonny Jr., just over 2 years of age, has a small but solid stature similar to his father's. He was in constant movement for the 4 hours that we were present, engaging in continual limit-testing and oppositional behavior. The toys in the house bore testimony to his destructiveness, for all of the toy cars were without windows or wheels and there was an extensive collection of dolls and stuffed animals with missing ears or limbs. He constantly bullied his older brother and continually punched, kicked, and poked both members of the assessment team. For some reason, Sonny Jr. seemed to be favored by his mother, and despite overwhelming evidence to the contrary, she proudly exclaimed that he is the brightest and best behaved of her children.

Joey: Joey is Blanche's 5-year-old son. He is a severely withdrawn child who shies away from interaction with both family and strangers. His development is markedly delayed, and since infancy he has been involved in various developmental intervention programs. However, his attendance has been poor and his progress has been limited. His protective service records contain numerous complaints by service providers that Blanche neglects to follow through on recommendations and fails to take Joey to scheduled appointments. While Blanche seems to appreciate the involvement of agency staff in her life during periods of crisis, she seems committed to keeping the attention focused upon herself, and actively sabotages attempts to address Joey's needs.

Joey has experienced much early trauma in his home. He was not only physically abused by his mother, grandmother, and younger brother but in addition witnessed the battering of his mother by his stepfather, the rape of his mother by a neighbor, and the death of a child-care provider, and he was burned out of his home by arsonists. After we were there for several hours, Joey did cautiously approach us and happily played with the drawing materials we provided. His quiet gentleness provided a stark contrast to the constant acting out of his little brother.

When assessed at school, Joey obtained an IQ of 91 on the Wechsler Preschool and Primary Scale Intelligence Test, which placed him at the bottom end of the average range of functioning. His readiness skills were assessed with the Woodcock-Johnson Tests of Academic Achievement, in which he scored in the low average range. On the Perceived Self-Competence Teacher Form, Joey's teacher rated him very low on peer acceptance and low on the cognitive competence scale. On the Child Behavior Checklist (CBCL) his ratings placed him in the clinical range on the internalizing scale. His scores were above the 98th percentile on the anxious, socially withdrawn, and obsessive-compulsive subscales. On the CBC the teacher also reported that Joey was less hardworking, behaved less appropriately, seemed less happy, and learned less than his special education peers. The teacher's comments about Joey reflect her ratings on the various scales. She wrote: "Joey is a very passive little boy who shows very little emotion. He communicates through whispers and physical gestures. He plays alone or next to peers. He has a tendency to observe other children at play and he tunes out others at group time."

Francine: At age 8, Francine is Blanche's oldest child. When Francine was 5 months old, an anonymous report that Blanche was leaving her child unsupervised for long periods at home was filed through the child abuse hotline. During the investigation the social worker reported that she witnessed Blanche yelling at the infant in an abusive fashion and that the child was not receiving adequate physical care. Blanche agreed to relinquish custody of Francine to her mother, Beatrice. The neglect and abuse continued under the custody of Beatrice. Early in 1983, charges of neglect were substantiated when a local hospital reported that Francine had received emergency services for the ingestion of toxic substances three times in as many months. Then, in 1985, charges of physical abuse were substantiated against Beatrice when Francine appeared at school with a bruised face.

Affirming her continued involvement in her daughter's life, Blanche explained that she is often recruited to help with the disciplining of Francine, who acts like a "juvenile delinquent." Describing a recent incident in which Francine ran away from her grandmother's home, Blanche stated, "That was no way to treat my mother. I hunted her down and beat her. I only hope she has learned something." Although we were unable to obtain any information from Francine's school, it is documented that she received special education services and that the school has filed complaints of educational neglect.

Psychological Maltreatment in the D'Niale Family

Spurning was clearly evidenced in the D'Niale family. Blanche continually belittled her children, calling Joey a sissy, a baby, "stupid," and an assortment of other degrading names. She referred to Sonny Jr., who spent the 4 hours of our visit in a soiled diaper, as "stinker" and "my little shit." Blanche's lack of knowledge of child development and unrealistic expectations of her children continually created opportunities for disappointment and frustration, which she would then angrily vent upon her children. Joey's anxiety and low self-esteem and Sonny Jr.'s angry acting out are clearly related to Blanche's repeated verbal attacks.

Terrorizing seemed to be one of the D'Niale family's most frequently used means of asserting control and power. The use of corporal punishment is an unquestioned aspect of parenting for Blanche. She claimed, "Even my social worker says it's all right to hit your kids as long as you use your bare hand. I never use my fist, and when I kick them I always use the side of my foot, never the front."

During the assessment Blanche used threats of physical punishment that bordered on brutality. When Sonny Jr. spilled a glass of milk, a not-uncommon occurrence for a 2-year-old child, Blanche responded with the threat, "Clean that up or I'll break your fingers." She repeatedly threatened to break bones and noses, to burn with her cigarette, and to put Joey out with the garbage.

There appears to be a clear causal relationship between Joey's social withdrawal, Sonny Jr.'s hypervigilance, Francine's habitual running away, and the climate of terror that is created by the verbal and physical assaults that family members inflict upon one another. Since this situation is supplemented with experiences of rape, death, fire, and homelessness, it is easy to understand how the D'Niale children exhibit various patterns of maladaptation and psychological distress.

The D'Niale family exhibited several isolating behaviors. Blanche listed her mother, her sister, and her sister-in-law as her three best friends and commented that the family tends not to socialize with outsiders. Frequent conflicts with their neighbors are the norm. Blanche never lets her children play with other children in the neighborhood and has been cited repeatedly for keeping her children home from school. Several times during the assessment she advised us to ignore the children and made unsuccessful attempts to confine the children to their bedroom. The deficits in social competence that all of the children display are related to this extensive restriction of opportunities to interact with peers and adults outside the family.

Exploiting and corrupting behavior was seen in Sonny Sr.'s models of criminal behavior, alcohol abuse, and violent acting out. Blanche used threats and extortion to control her children's behavior, reported keeping the children home from school when she wanted company, and used the children for protection when Sonny was drunk and abusive. In the D'Niale family, the multigenerational pattern of chronic unmet needs and crisis addiction, coupled with extremely limited emotional, financial, and intellectual resources, has led to both overt and unintentional exploitation of others.

The chronic omission of appropriate emotional responses in the D'Niale family constituted extreme denied emotional responsiveness. Reflecting her depression, Blanche generally exhibited a flat affect, with an occasional outburst of hostility that seemed more related to her internal processes than an appropriate response to ongoing interactions. A startling example of her denied emotional response, with an element of corruptive behavior, occurred during our visit. Joey had been attempting to draw at the coffee table, but Sonny Jr. kept tearing up the paper Joey was working on. Without protest, Joey moved his paper to the sill of the open window, where he could draw while shielding the paper from his little brother. Sonny Jr. responded by going over and slamming the window sash down upon Joey's hands. Joey turned toward Blanche, crying. She shot him an annoyed glance and admonished him, "You are three years older, you have to learn to hit back."

With so much loss, pain, and anger in Blanche's relationships, it is understandable that she does not possess the necessary emotional resources to respond adequately to the needs of her children. However, the extent of her emotional neglect of her children almost certainly places them at risk for serious psychological maladaptation. While there are undeniably strong bonds in the D'Niale family, it is a family that is devoid of healthy attachments, and the qualities of care and protection that are so essential to human development are noticeably absent. Without extensive therapeutic interventions these maladaptive patterns of attachment will most likely persist, creating problems and disruptions in relationships throughout the D'Niale children's lives. In addition, their disorganized and problematic patterns of attachment jeopardize the establishment of future relationships that can provide corrective experiences.

Case 2: Harm Sway

Harm Sway sits in a cell in a maximum-security prison. He is 17 years old and in the third year of a 30-year sentence for killing his grandparents when he was 14 years old.

This case is based on a true story of the influences and effects of child maltreatment, particularly intragenerational psychological maltreatment. We first provide highlights from records of social agencies that came to know Harm and had the opportunity to intervene to influence his development. The information comes from reports of his early and later school experiences, for which available records were sparse, and from his two admissions to a psychiatric center, arrest by police, legal defense, and sentencing by court, for which records were more complete. At the end of the chapter, interventions that could have been applied will be suggested. Permission to present this case was given by the lawyer who handled Harm's original trial and is handling his appeal process.

Early School Period: Kindergarten and First Grade

Harm lived with his mother and father for the first 6 years of his life and with his mother and stepfather during his 11th year. He lived with his maternal grandparents from age 6 through 10 and again from ages 12 through 14.

At age 5 Harm was referred for psychological evaluation by his kindergarten teacher because of maladaptive behaviors including hyperactivity, attention deficits, aggression toward peers, low academic achievement, and playing with feces in the bathroom. The school psychologist referred him to a psychiatric facility.

When Harm was first admitted, his mother indicated she didn't know what to do with him because he had too much energy. Psychiatric center personnel diagnosed him as suffering from major depression (single episode) and having an attention deficit disorder with hyperactivity. He was found to have anger toward his father and mother, a pervasive sense of hopelessness and despair, and self-esteem at almost nonexistent levels. In the early period of his treatment he seemed quite angry and struck out frequently at peers and staff. He was unable to identify things of importance to him, and while indicating favorite adult-family members, he stated he was treated unfairly by adults and said (they) "be bad to little kids."

Family history and dynamics were given little attention. His early development was reported to be normal but marked by repeated moves and the birth of two younger sisters. Although Harm had no history of serious illnesses, he had hit his head hard enough to raise a knot, had broken his nose three times, and had stitches on his face during these years (these were not attributed to, but could have been caused by, physical abuse and neglect).

Medication (Mellaril), family therapy, and talk therapy were applied. Placement in a self-contained class for the emotionally disturbed in school was recommended. After approximately 2 months, he was discharged to his parents. The discharge noted that his family was supportive. Harm was seen by the psychiatric center as an outpatient upon returning home, but this was found to be ineffective.

Harm returned to the first grade and was placed in a special class for emotionally handicapped students. He became increasingly oppositional and aggressive (for example, he choked a peer) in school, his academic work deteriorated, his mood was sometimes quite labile, and he tended to withdraw and isolate himself. This school behavior and his home behavior resulted in readmission to the psychiatric center in February of that school year, when he was 6½ years old. His mother indicated, "My son has gotten so aggressive that he is unmanageable." At home he displayed increased aggression and was openly defiant of parental authority. A number of times he removed the newborn baby from the crib and once intentionally dropped her on the floor. He hit and choked his siblings, cut his sister's hair off while she was sleeping, poured hot water on one of his sisters, and asked his mother how many pills he would have to take to die.

Individual and group psychotherapy and "family involvement" to focus on the psychotherapy were applied upon rehospitalization. The diagnosis was major depression, recurrent, representing a serious emotional disturbance. Treatment goals included alleviation of depression and elimination of self-injurious and aggressive behavior. Mellaril and Pamelor were prescribed. He was discharged after 6 weeks. It was recommended that Harm return to a regular first-grade class and continue individual therapy and medication.

Later Parochial and Public School Placements

Harm was in a parochial school during the periods when he lived with his maternal grandparents, which covered most of the remainder of his school years, with the exception of portions of the fifth, sixth, and eighth grades when he was in public school. Parochial school records provided only very limited information on academic achievement, which was satisfactory. His public school records also generally indicated satisfactory progress. Some achievement problems were noted in fifth and sixth grades. In the eighth grade, there were minor incidents of use of foul language, a teacher's impression that he was going to damage a piece of laboratory equipment, his failure to start his homework in class at the teacher's request on one occasion, and numerous tardies. While these factors were mentioned in his school records along with notification of two in-school suspensions for his tardies, other disciplinary, special needs, and intervention histories were not in evidence.

Arrest and Investigation by Police, Lawyers, and Experts after Grandparents Are Killed

At 14 years of age, Harm shot and killed his grandparents at their home with one of his grandfather's guns, and within hours he returned to the crime scene and gave himself up to the police. Following this event, for the first time in his life, Harm's developmental history was carefully studied. For the most part, this study was carried out by his legal defense team because of its strong interest in determining his motivation and its implications.

Harm's life was pervaded by psychological maltreatment and physical abuse from infancy through his arrest as reported by Harm, his mother, aunts, sister, and the principal of his parochial school. The highlights of the maltreatment are presented here separately first for the periods with his mother, father, stepfather, and siblings, and then with his grandparents, followed by some clarification of the intergenerational connectedness of these experiences. Descriptions of Harm's treatment in and across settings, and in the parochial school setting, indicate that he was spurned, terrorized, isolated, corrupted, and exploited, denied emotional responsiveness, and denied needed mental health services, and that this maltreatment was at levels that would be considered severe according the APSAC practice guidelines (American Professional Society on the Abuse of Children, 1995).

Harm was slapped or spanked hundreds to thousands of times a year by his mother or father during his first 5 years of life. He reportedly was beaten by his stepfather when living with his mother. The physical abuse described also constitutes psychological maltreatment terrorizing, and partly because the punishment was nearly always for minor behavioral concerns, it constitutes spurning and corrupting. Extensive additional psychological maltreatment occurred. His mother criticized his behavior throughout his life, constantly telling him he was doing something wrong, and gave him little or no loving touch, hugs, kisses, or warmth, which was much different from and poorer than the treatment she gave his sisters. When hospitalized a second time for psychological problems, Harm's father virtually abandoned him by refusing to visit him there or contact him for years. He observed his mother being beaten by his stepfather. Harm's mother sent him to live with her parents who had abused her, and she rejected him when he asked to come back to live with her (shortly before the killings) even though she knew he was being abused by her parents in the same ways they had abused her.

Harm's life with his grandparents continued and in fact increased and expanded this pattern of abuse. He was beaten by his grandfather with a belt approximately weekly during the early 5-year period and with a razor strap approximately every 1 to 2 weeks during the later 2 to 3 year period. He was also punched and kicked by his grandfather. This physical abuse was for actions such as playing with the wrong children, snacking, "smarting off," not doing a job correctly, and for doing anything wrong at school (for which he had usually already been punished). His grandfather made him get the belt or razor strap with which he would be beaten; told him if he cried while being beaten he would be beaten for crying; and told him if he ever fought back he would kill him—come at him when he was asleep and kill him. Harm's beatings by his grandfather were almost always precipitated by his grandmother encouraging the beatings, and observed by her without intervention. Harm's grandfather constantly put him down, calling him "stupid" and "an asshole" and saying he had no future, would amount to nothing, and would never get a job—all in response to minor infractions. His grand-mother constantly nagged, yelled at him, and criticized him for minor infrac-tions. His grandparents fought and argued constantly, and they displayed no affection or physical contact with each other. They allowed him no relations or friendships outside of the church–school community; they allowed him no visits from friends in their home or by telephone, and no use of the telephone unless they were listening; and they denied him opportunities for contact initiated by his father and mother. Generally, they showed no interest in any of his perspectives, ideas, or desires. His grandparents denied him the medication and counseling that had been prescribed by the psychiatric institute, and he was denied any special programming for his learning dis-ability in the church school. Harm's grandfather taught him to use guns and told him handguns were for killing people.

Harm's mother had been maltreated by her parents in many of the very same ways Harm was, including the following: beatings by her father that her mother encouraged, even through lies about her, and that she observed without intervention; extreme sexual taboos by her mother and sexually demeaning language by her father; verbal put-downs; isolation; tutoring in use and specific purposes of guns; control through fear and intimidation; incessant nagging by mother; no choices; having to get the belt when she was to be beaten and told that she would be killed in her sleep if she ever fought back. The abuse by her father was reported to a social service agency at one point with very little impact on the family. She was suicidal when she was 15 years old, and she ran away from home at 15 and again at 16 years of age. When her own adult life was in turmoil, she sent Harm to live with her parents, and shortly before he killed his grandparents she told him she was aware he was being abused.

Harm shot and killed his grandparents after an argument with them about an internal school suspension notice for tardies, received by mail. During the argument, his grandfather hit him and threatened him. Harm tried to escape his grandfather's physical attack. He considered suicide, something he had thought about several times before. He expected another beating or to be killed (he had been told what would happen if he resisted). In his memory, no one had ever taken seriously his needs, his distress, or fears, and no one was willing to protect him from people who mistreated him—in fact, they seemed always to take the side of those hurting him. It appears he acted impulsively, in a state of fear and confusion.

Medical Issues

Although there is no published research that deals directly with the medical aspects of psychological maltreatment, there is a growing litera-ture that suggests a relationship (Hart et al., 1998). For example, rejection (spurning) and denied emotional responsiveness have been found to be associated with asthma, allergies, and other respiratory ailments (Jacobs, Spilken, & Noeman, 1972) and hypertension (McGinn, 1963). Due to the high rate of co-occurrence with other forms of maltreatment, any medical problems associated with psychological maltreatment are usually attributed to the more visible injuries resulting from the other abuse.

We did not have medical histories on the D'Niale family and are not able to comment on the medical issues related to the case, with the exception of noting that Blanche D'Niale had been reported to CPS on charges of medical neglect for not attending to Joey's ear infections. In Harm's case, he was hospitalized at age 5 and 6 for severe psychiatric difficulties that included life-threatening aggressive acts toward his siblings and suicidal behavior. Instead of recognizing that early suicidal/homicidal behavior is almost always accompanied by severe child maltreatment in the cases that have been studied (see Rosenthal & Rosenthal, 1984), family circumstances were considered to play a small role in his difficulties and he was given a diagnosis without a serious inquiry into how such a young child could be displaying such significant symptomatology.

Legal Issues

Psychological maltreatment is a relatively new legal concept in family law (see Corson & Davidson, 1987; Melton & Corson, 1987) and when unconnected to physical abuse/neglect or sexual abuse rarely leads to government intervention (Hart, Brassard, & Karlson, 1997). The federal Child Abuse Prevention and Treatment Act of 1974 included a "mental injury" category in its definition but left further definition to the states (see Corson & Davidson, 1987, for a review). State statutes vary dramatically in the degree to which the term *mental injury* is specified, with most delegating the drafting of regulations to child protective services. When CPS does not assume this role, social workers are left to their own devices in deciding whether psychological maltreatment is serious enough to warrant state intervention.

Increasingly, courts recognize how important it is to protect children from psychological harm (Hart, Brassard, & Karlson, 1997). Courts are only permitted to interfere with the fundamental right of parents to rear their children if they can demonstrate that the parents' methods have impaired or are likely to impair their child's physical or mental well-being. In cases of sexual abuse, courts feel comfortable acting on the basis of presumed harm because of clear guidelines for maltreating behavior and community acceptance of those standards. While such a societal consensus has not developed in criminal law around psychological maltreatment, divorce and child custody litigation and child protective service actions brought by the state under the category of children in need of services, or CHINS, are creating case law where psychological maltreatment is held to be a compelling factor in court decisions. These precedents, coupled with judicial and bar experience with such cases, may be a force to develop societal consensus on the right of children to be protected from psychological maltreatment (Hart, Brassard, & Karlson, 1997).

We have found CPS reluctant to pursue psychological maltreatment cases unless it co-occurs with another form of abuse and neglect. Agency action in the D'Niale case is typical. The department was concerned about medical neglect, educational neglect, physical abuse, and lack of adequate supervision. When each of these issues had been successfully dealt with, the CPS case was closed, despite awareness of continuing psychological abuse and neglect. In Harm Sway's case, the family never came to the attention of CPS because his severe behavioral difficulties were viewed as constitutional impairments and not manifestations of the severe psychological and physical abuse he was experiencing.

Social and Family Issues

Much research has been done on the social influences and family characteristics associated with child maltreatment in its various forms (Brassard et al., 1987; Garbarino, 1998; Gil, 1970; Wolfe, 1987). Unfortunately, we know very little about families where maltreatment occurs but that do not come to the attention of child protective services. Our own research and the clinical observations of others indicate that many of the factors related to other forms of maltreatment are also associated with psychological maltreatment. However, patterns of these factors unique to psychological maltreatment have yet to be identified. The combination of poverty, substance abuse, maternal depression, marital violence, and instability, and the absence of adequate problem-solving and parenting skills in the D'Niale family constitute a cluster of problems that is quite typical in families where child maltreatment occurs and is likely to be identified.

Assessment of Psychopathology

In most states and provinces the identification of psychological maltreatment requires evidence of both psychologically maltreating caregiver behavior and mental injury to the child attributable to the caregiver maltreatment. Some jurisdictions allow evidence of probable harm to the child. The *Guidelines for the Psychosocial Evaluation of Suspected Psychological Maltreatment of Children and Adolescents* (American Professional Society on the Abuse of Children, 1995) is recommended as guide for clinicians, in concert with local laws and regulations, in their assessments.

As part of a 3-year federal grant from the National Center on Child Abuse and Neglect, we found that psychological maltreatment can be differentiated into the five distinct subtypes described earlier (the subtypes described in the APSAC guidelines as well). We also found that it is possible to distinguish between maltreatment and appropriate parenting through the use of a multidimensional scaling of parenting practices. Maltreating mothers of preschool and school-aged children can be discriminated from carefully matched control mothers using ratings of psychological maltreatment displayed during videotaped parent–child interactions on age-appropriate tasks (Brassard *et al.*, 1993). These video scale observation measures were significantly related to child interpersonal competence after CPS maltreatment status and maternal and child variables described in the following paragraphs had been accounted for (Hart & Brassard, 1989).

Blanche D'Niale, a participating mother in the research project, obtained moderate scores on all five of the psychological maltreatment subscales, combining to give her a high total scale score. She did not obtain a single point on our good parent scales, which measure prosocial and prodevelopment behavior of the mother exhibited during the videotaped session.

Using Belsky's (1984) model of the determinants of parenting, we assumed that Blanche's ability to parent would be determined by (a) her personal resources (history of care and development in childhood, personality, competencies, and presence and degree of psychopathology); (b) the social support available to her and stress she has to contend with (marital satisfaction, life stress and hassles, and family and community support for her child-rearing efforts); and (c) the ease or difficulty involved in rearing her particular children (a function of constitutional factors and behavioral shaping of interactional patterns over time inferred from current developmental status and case records). Therefore, these were the variables we examined in order to assess prognosis for treatment and to attempt to understand the extent of family dysfunction we observed.

In Harm Sway's case we also looked for the five subtypes of psychological maltreatment and found Harm, over the course of his life, to have chronically received severe levels of all five subtypes of maltreatment from his successive caregivers. To document mental injury we used the APSAC guidelines, finding evidence that major developmental milestones were not achieved at age 5 and 6 when he was hospitalized (e.g., impaired capacity to regulate his emotional state; a likely attachment disorder seen in his fear of his caregivers; highly antagonistic sibling and peer relationships) or that he had a serious emotional disturbance as evidenced by meeting criteria for an Axis 1 disorder using the American Psychiatric Association's *Diagnostic and Statistical Manual of Mental Disorders* (1994). At the very early age of 5 Harm met criteria for a major depressive episode as well as attention-deficit/hyperactivity disorder (ADHD) and was hospitalized twice for the severity of these psychiatric problems. He was not reevaluated until after his arrest for murder, so we do not know his mental state from ages 6 to 14.

Treatment Options

Much of the treatment research and clinical experience with maltreating families suggests that they are very difficult to work with and that often our efforts are unsuccessful, with families continuing to abuse and neglect their children both during and after treatment (Cohn & Daro, 1987). Primary prevention does not appear to be very effective at reducing rate of child maltreatment (Daro, 1988; MacMillan, MacMillan, Offord, & Griffith, 1994). While none of the evaluated treatment or prevention studies targeted psychological maltreatment specifically, some evidence suggests that families identified by CPS primarily for psychological abuse and neglect may be among those families most resistent to treatment (Cohn & Daro, 1987). This finding may be due in part to the small number of substantiated cases that involve stand-alone psychological maltreatment (U.S. Department of Health and Human Services, 1998), making it likely that these cases are quite severe. Thus, we know very little about effective prevention or treatment for child maltreatment and even less about psychological maltreatment in particular.

The most promising research findings have to do with maltreated children's response to intervention. They suggest that some of the emotional distress and socioemotional delays associated with maltreatment can be mitigated through group or individual psychotherapy or a close, compensatory relationship with an adult (see Cohn & Daro, 1987; Egeland, Jacobvitz, & Sroufe, 1988; Kolko, 1998), which may also prevent maltreatment of future offspring (Egeland *et al.*, 1988; Main & Goldwyn, 1984).

We have been developing a comprehensive treatment model derived from a combination of ecological/systemic theory, psychoanalytically influenced organizational theory, and social learning theory. The pattern of isolation and limited openness to new information from the environment that exists in the D'Niale family is common in maltreating families. Absence of exposure to other models of parenting maintains the belief that abusive behavior is appropriate and that acts of abuse are ultimately the fault of the child (Azar, 1989; Kaufman, 1988; Spinetta & Rigler, 1972). It not only allows maltreatment to occur undetected but also weakens the social supports necessary to mediate family stresses and increases the likelihood that abusive and maladaptive problem-solving strategies will be employed (Garbarino, 1977; Polansky, Chalmers, Buttenweiser, & Williams, 1981; Wahler, 1980).

Owing to this pattern of isolation from social supports and inadequate problem-solving skills, the D'Niales, like other multiproblem families, are caught in cycles of "perpetual crisis" (Kagan & Schlosberg, 1989). Continual experiences of abandonment, trauma, and anxious arousal divert the family from productive problem solving and reinforce chaotic behavioral patterns of violent acting out, denial, projection, and hopelessness.

Because multiproblem families are often less resistant to outside intervention during crisis period, within our treatment model each crisis is used as an opportunity to build a supportive, consistent relationship with the family. As we work with the family to deal with the crisis on the concrete level, we not only demonstrate and teach appropriate problem-solving skills but also present more rewarding models of interpersonal relationships and provide opportunities for family members to come to terms with past traumas.

Critical to engaging the D'Niale family in treatment is establishing a relationship with Blanche. As with other parents, Blanche's unresolved issues from her childhood have enormous impact of her own parenting. In maltreating families, the unmet psychological needs of the adults prohibit their empathizing with and protecting their children (Erickson, 1988; Fraiberg, 1983). Parents abused as children need assistance in learning new models of relating to and communicating with others. They must have an opportunity to work through, cognitively and affectively, the painful experiences of childhood trauma that prevent them from forming nurturing relationships with their children. Whether conceptualized as transference issues (Fraiberg, 1983), dysfunctional representational working models of relationships (Bretherton, 1985; Sroufe & Fleeson, 1986), unresolved issues in parents' families of origin (Bowen, 1978), or a cognitive developmental immaturity (Newberger, 1980), many maltreating parents are not psychologically able to assume the role of adult and parent because of unmet needs and concomitant delays in their own cognitive and emotional development.

In many maltreating families, including the D'Niale family, parents often need extensive individual attention and nurturance before interventions with other family members can occur. As the therapeutic relationship with Blanche is developed and stabilized, this individual attention will be balanced by attempts to reach out and engage Sonny in the treatment process. Marital issues are an important part of the treatment of maltreating families, and the existence of drug or alcohol problems in families greatly impedes all interventions to improve their functioning and eliminate abuse (Daro, 1988; Murphy, Jellinek, Quinn, Smith, Poitrast, & Goshko, 1991; Wolfner & Gelles, 1993). A lack of skills for solving both interpersonal and concrete problems exacerbates the psychological neediness and social isolation that these families experience. The treatment provider needs to offer parents assistance in acquiring specific skills, such as (a) parenting (child management, knowledge of child development and how to facilitate it); (b) relationship forming and maintaining (communication, social skills, problem solving, perspective taking); (c) anger management; and (d) basic life skills and empowerment (money management, assertiveness with institutions such as welfare, hospitals, schools). Behavior therapists have demonstrated the effectiveness of their interventions with some maltreating parents in these areas (Goldstein, Keller, & Erne, 1985; Lutzker, 1983, 1990; Lutzker & Campbell, 1994; Lutzker & Rice, 1987; Wolfe, 1987).

Because child maltreatment is usually seen as a symptom of parental dysfunction, most interventions have focused on stopping the abuse rather than assisting children with the associated emotional distress and developmental impairments (Baglow, 1992). Failure to address children's emotional response to the maltreatment leaves them vulnerable to repeating problematic patterns of relating in all of their relationships, most notably in relationships with their own children (Mann & McDermott, 1983). Therapeutic work with children in general is still in its childhood (Kazdin, 1988), but there are promising models and research findings with victims of child maltreatment that suggest this is a fruitful area for exploration (see Kolko, 1998).

Both Sonny Jr. and Joey have been referred to therapists who specialize in work with abused and neglected children. As with their parents, interventions will focus on the working through of traumas, the development of corrective relationships, and skill development in the areas of interpersonal relations, affect modulation, and behavior control. We also encouraged Mrs. D'Niale to have each boy placed with particular teachers that we felt could provide the structured, supportive environment we thought they needed and potentially a compensatory, close relationship as well.

The problems and crises of the D'Niale family are so numerous and severe that it is quite easy for professionals dealing with this type of family to become as overwhelmed and hopeless as the family members themselves. It is a vital aspect of the treatment process to realize the family resources that are available and personal strengths of its members (Karpel, 1986). These strengths are not always readily apparent, yet they must be identified, actively validated, and used as building blocks.

Interventions Possible but Not Applied in the Case of Harm Sway

As noted earlier, few attempts were made to intervene in Harm's life in a way helpful to him. Admission and treatment at the psychiatric center and placement in a special class during part of the first grade are the only formal efforts recorded or described. Harm's mother indicated that she made an attempt to follow through on the medication and therapy prescribed by the center. However, she ended up sending Harm to live with her parents, who, in turn, and at the recommendation of the principal of Harm's parochial school, denied him medication, therapy, and special education services.

Numerous opportunities to intervene constructively in Harm's life presented themselves. Some of those will be mentioned here. There is a strong tendency in our society to use labels or descriptions for conditions, as though they provide explanations, rather than to look for causes. The psychiatric center that worked with Harm did this in labeling him as depressed and ADHD, and did not sufficiently investigate the child-care and developmental experiences of his early life, which were so abusive and would have made it likely for him to develop the personal and interpersonal problems he displayed. The psychiatric forensic evaluation conducted at the request of the prosecution followed the same pattern in the results it provided: labeling Harm as a person with a "conduct disorder," as though it were a problem within him rather than learned behavior; failing to mention that child abuse is a recognized precipitating factor for this problem; and failing to recognize any legitimacy in Harm's fear of his grandfather at the time of the killings. In Harm's case, and the case of others like him, it is imperative that child development histories be thoroughly investigated. We must distinguish distortions in thinking, feeling, and behavior due to learning and attempts to meet basic needs under threat and stress from pathological mental conditions, endogenous disabilities, or inherent evil.

Taking a historical view, many interventions, preventive and corrective, could have been of significant help.

First, social services could have worked with the family when Harm's grandfather was reported for abusing his mother and when his mother ran away from home and stayed with friends. They could have helped her protect herself and prepare for better parenting.

A risk assessment in hospital of Harm's mother's readiness and characteristics for parenting would have revealed the need for her family to receive "home visitor" services. Had she lived in Hawaii or one of the other states where this program exists, the combination of trust building, advocacy, and mentoring fundamental to this service could have significantly altered Harm's upbringing.

Extended family members aware of the physical and verbal abuse of Harm in his early years and his mother's lack of emotional connection to him could have pressed harder for him to be sent to live with them—something they contemplated—or could have involved social services.

Both Harm's first school and the psychiatric center should have seriously investigated the causes of his emotional and interpersonal problems. Such serious problems do not develop by magic. In the vast majority of cases, the individuals were not born with a flaw making their development inevitable. Factors in their environment—experience—have primarily or at least significantly influenced these developments. An intervention model for schools and mental health services to work backwards from possible consequences of psychological maltreatment to determine its relevance to extant emotional and behavioral problems and possible interventions has been suggested previously (Hart, 1987).

A baby-sitter who noted significant bruising on Harm's body due to the beatings from his grandfather shortly after placement in his care should have reported this to social services. Young people in general, and baby-sitters in particular, should be prepared to act when they suspect child abuse. Many states and local areas have formal programs to certify adolescent baby-sitters. Child abuse information and reporting procedures should be included in these programs.

Faculty, Harm's parochial school could have intervened to help him and his grandparents. Harm's teacher, principal, and peers, collectively, considered that he was having more trouble in school than most students, acted impulsively, had quick mood swings and became easily upset, and was an angry child who hated authority. Instead of aligning with his grandparents to double up on the physical punishment and condemnation Harm was given for minor infractions, the school personnel and students could have offered compassion, understanding, respite, a peer support system, and realistic opportunities for development of coping strategies and self-respect. If one teacher really cared and had become a trusted advocate and mentor for him, it might have made a significant difference in his life. These combined factors, which represent the core of the home visitor model, have been established empirically to work with troubled adolescents (Shore & Massimo, 1979). The principal of the school could have called in social services when he knew there was the danger of something terrible happening because of Harm's problems and his grandfather's treatment. Indeed, he had warned the grandfather of this the night before the killings but took no other action. School personnel across the nation continue to be ill-prepared to recognize or intervene in cases of child maltreatment. This should be remedied through preservice and in-service education.

The prosecution and judiciary in Harm's case had the opportunity to recognize that this 14-year-old was trying to survive, was immature and distorted in his perspectives, and represented little danger to anyone other than his abusers (even his parochial school principal recognized that Harm had shown a remarkable ability to control himself in confrontational situations). Instead, they cooperated to have Harm tried as an adult, give him a long sentence, and eventually send him from a youth correctional and services institution to an adult prison. Across the nation, in cases such as this, courts appear to prefer punishment over rehabilitation, and stronger punishment can be applied to adults than to children and youth (Mones, 1991). Sentences and placement should take the long-term best interests of society into consideration. Offenders at this age will be released some day as young or middle-aged adults. An extended period in adult prison is likely to create a dangerous criminal rather than rehabilitate the individual after maladjustment and abuse.

Understandable acts of violence against an enemy need to be taken seriously by society. Just models of adjudicating "effects of battering" cases or primitive self-preservation cases such as Harm's need to be developed. They need to promote rehabilitation and prevention. For example, Hart, Brassard, & Karlson (1997) has suggested that when tried as an adult and given long sentences, such youth should be placed in a therapeutic juvenile correctional setting and their cases automatically reviewed by the court when they reach age 21, before transfer to adult prison. At that point, the court should have the opportunity to suspend, reduce, or otherwise modify the sentence according to the nature and degree of rehabilitation achieved.

Harm remains in prison, still a victim of abuse. His statement as a young child continues to ring true: Adults "be bad to little kids."

Summary

Psychological maltreatment is gaining increasing research and legal attention after decades of being ignored. Considerable progress has now been made. There are accepted definitions of psychological maltreatment, valid and reliable measures, compelling evidence of harm to victims, and indications that this is by far the most frequent form of maltreatment. What is lacking is application of this knowledge by CPS and the courts to protective cases, the development of empirically validated interventions for families and for child victims that address psychological maltreatment, and a societal commitment to address the serious problem of child maltreatment and its implications for mental health and public safety.

Acknowledgments

The authors would like to thank Carey Dimmitt for her comments on an earlier draft of this manuscript, the Massachusetts Department of Social Services for their ongoing assistance in our work, the D'Niale family for their willingness to share their experiences with us, and Harm and his attorney for giving us permission to share his troubling case with the public.

References

Abramson, E., & Lucido, G. (1991). Childhood sexual experience and bulimia. *Addictive Behaviors, 15*, 529–532.

American Humane Association. (1988). *Highlights of official child neglect and abuse reporting 1986*. Denver: Author.

American Professional Society on the Abuse of Children. (1995). *Guidelines for the psychosocial evaluation of suspected psychological maltreatment in children and adolescents*. Chicago, IL: Author.

American Psychiatric Association. (1994). *Diagnostic and statistical manual of mental disorders* (4th ed., DSM-IV). Washington, DC: Author.

Azar, S. T. (1989). Training parents of abused children. In C. E. Schaefer & J. M. Briesmeister (Eds.), *Handbook of parent training* (pp. 414–441). New York: Wiley.

Baglow, L. J. (1992). A multidimensional model for treatment of child abuse: A framework for cooperation. *Child Abuse & Neglect, 14*, 387–395.

Baily, F. T., & Baily, W. H. (1986). *Operational definitions of child emotional maltreatment*. Augusta: Maine Department of Social Services.

Barnett, D., Manly, J. T., & Cicchetti, D. (1993). Defining child maltreatment: The interface between policy and research. In D. Cicchetti & S. Toth (Eds.), *Child abuse, child development, and social policy* (pp. 7–74). Norwood, NJ: Ablex.

Belsky, J. (1984). The determinants of parenting: A process model. *Child Development, 55*, 83–96.

Bouchard, C., Tessier, R., Fraser, A., & Laganiere, J. (1997). La violence familiale envers les enfants: Prevalence dans la basse-ville et etude de validite de la mesure. In R. Tessier, C. Bouchard, & G. M. Tarabulsy (Eds.), *Enfance et famille: Contextes de development*. Quebec, Canada: Presses de l'Universite Laval.

Bowen, M. (1978). *Family therapy in clinical practices*. New York: Jason Aronson.

Brassard, M. R., & Hardy, D. B. (1998). Psychological maltreatment. In M. E. Helfer, R. F. Kempe, & R. D. Krugman (Eds.), *The battered child* (5th ed., pp. 392–412). Chicago: University of Chicago Press.

Brassard, M. R., Germain, R., & Hart, S. N. (1987). *Psychological maltreatment of children and youth.* New York: Pergamon.

Brassard, M. R., Hart, S. N., & Hardy, D. B. (1993). The psychological maltreatment rating scales. *Child Abuse & Neglect, 17,* 715–729.

Bretherton, I. (1985). Attachment theory: Retrospect and prospect. In I. Bretherton & E. Waters (Eds.), *Growing points in attachment theory and research: Monographs of the Society for Research in Child Development, 50* (1–2, Serial No. 209). Chicago: University of Chicago Press.

Briere, J., & Runtz, M. (1988). Multivariate correlates of childhood psychological and physical maltreatment among university women. *Child Abuse & Neglect, 12,* 331–341.

Briere, J., & Runtz, M. (1990). Differential adult symptomology associated with three types of child abuse histories. *Child Abuse & Neglect, 14,* 357–364.

Claussen, A., & Crittenden, P. (1991). Physical and psychological maltreatment: Relations among types of maltreatment. *Child Abuse & Neglect, 15,* 5–18.

Cohn, A. H., & Daro, D. (1987). Is treatment too late: What ten years of evaluative research tell us. *Child Abuse & Neglect, 11,* 433–442.

Corson, J., & Davidson, H. (1987). Emotional abuse and the law. In M. R. Brassard, R. Germain, & S. N. Hart (Eds.), *Psychological maltreatment of children and youth* (pp. 185–202). New York: Pergamon Press.

Crittenden, P. (1988). Family and dyadic patterns of functioning in maltreating families. In K. Brown, C. Davies, & P. Stratton (Eds.), *Early prediction and prevention of child abuse* (pp. 161–189). New York: Wiley.

Daro, D. (1988). *Confronting child abuse: Research for effective program design.* New York: Free Press.

Egeland, B., & Sroufe, L. A. (1981). Attachment and early maltreatment. *Child Development, 52,* 44–52.

Egeland, B., Sroufe, L. A., & Erickson, M. (1983). The developmental consequences of different patterns of maltreatment. *Child Abuse & Neglect, 7,* 459–469.

Egeland, B., Jacobvitz, D., & Sroufe, L. A. (1988). Breaking the cycle of abuse. *Child Development, 59,* 1080–1088.

Erickson, M. F. (1988). *School psychology in preschool settings.* Paper presented at the annual meeting of the National Association of School Psychologists, Chicago.

Erickson, M. F., & Egeland, B. (1987). A developmental view of the psychological consequences of maltreatment. *School Psychology Review, 16,* 156–168.

Farber, E. A., & Egeland, B. (1987). Invulnerability among abused and neglected children. In E. J. Anthony & B. C. Cohler (Eds.), *The invulnerable child* (pp. 253–288). New York: Guilford Press.

Fraiberg, S. (Ed.). (1983). *Clinical studies in infant mental health: The first year of life.* New York: Basic Books.

Friedrich, W., Burke, R., & Urguiza, A. (1987). Children from sexually abusing families: A behavioral comparison. *Journal of Interpersonal Violence, 2,* 391–402.

Garbarino, J. (1977). The human ecology of child maltreatment: A conceptual model for research. *Journal of Marriage and the Family, 39,* 721–735.

Garbarino, J. (1998). The role of economic deprivation in the social context of child maltreatment. In M. E. Helfer, R. F. Kempe, & R. D. Krugman (Eds.), *The battered child* (5th ed., pp. 49–60). Chicago, IL: University of Chicago Press.

Garbarino, J., Guttman, E., & Seeley, J. (1986). *The psychologically battered child: Strategies for identification, assessment, and intervention.* San Francisco: Jossey-Bass.

Gil, D. B. (1970). *Violence against children: Physical child abuse in the United States.* Cambridge, MA: Harvard University Press.

Goldstein, A. P., Keller, H., & Erne, D. (1985). *Changing the abusive parent.* Champaign, IL: Research Press.

Hart, S. N. (1987). Mental health neglect: Proposed definition. In M. R. Brassard, R. Germain, & S. N. Hart (Eds.), *Psychological maltreatment of children and youth* (pp. 3–24). New York: Pergamon.

Hart, S. N., & Brassard, M. R. (1987). A major threat to children's mental health: Psychological maltreatment. *American Psychologist, 42,* 160–165.

Hart, S. N., & Brassard, M. R. (1989). *Developing and validating operationally defined measures of emotional maltreatment* (NCCAN Research Grant Final Report). Unpublished.

Hart, S. N., Brassard, M. R., & Karlson, H. (1997). Psychological maltreatment. In J. Briere, L. Berliner, J. A. Bulkley, C. Jenny, T. Reid (Eds.), *APSAC handbook on child abuse and neglect* (pp. 72–89). Thousand Oaks, CA: Sage.

Hart, S. N., Binggeli, N., & Brassard, M. R. (1998). Evidence for the effects of psychological maltreatment. *Journal of Emotional Abuse, 1,* 27–58.

Jacobs, N., Spilken, A, & Noeman, M. (1972). Perception of faulty parent–child relationships and illness behavior. *Journal of Consulting and Clinical Psychology, 39,* 49–55.

Kagan, R., & Scholsberg, S. (1989). *Families in perpetual crisis.* New York: Norton.

Karpel, M. (Ed.). (1986). *Family resources: The hidden partner in family therapy.* New York: Guilford Press.

Kaufman, K. (1988). *Child abuse assessment from a systems perspective.* Unpublished paper. Available from the author at Children's Hospital, Department of Pediatrics, Ohio State University, Columbus, OH 43210.

Kazdin, A. (1988). *Child psychotherapy,* New York: Pergamon Press.

Kolko, D. (1998). Integration of research and treatment. In J. Lutzker (Ed.), *Handbook of child abuse treatment and research* (pp. 159–181). New York: Plenum.

Lutzker, J. R. (1983). Project 12-Ways: Treating child abuse and neglect from an ecobehavioral perspective. In R. F. Dangel & R. A. Polster (Eds.), *Parent training* (pp. 260–297). New York: Guilford Press.

Lutzker, J. R. (1990). Project 12-Ways: Treating child abuse and neglect from an ecobehavioral perspective. In R. F. Dangel & R. F. Polster (Eds.), *Parent training: Foundations of research and practice* (pp. 260–297). New York: Guilford Press.

Lutzker, J. R., & Campbell, R. (1994). *Ecobehavioral family interventions in developmental disabilities.* Pacific Grove, CA: Brooks/Cole.

Lutzker, J. R., & Rice, J. M. (1987). Using recidivism data to evaluate Project 12-Ways: An ecobehavioral approach to the treatment of child abuse and neglect. *Journal of Family Violence, 2,* 283–289.

MacMillan, H., MacMillan, J., Offord, D., & Griffith, L. (1994). Primary prevention of child physical abuse and neglect: A critical review. *Journal of Child Psychology and Psychiatry and Allied Disabilities, 35,* 835–856.

Main, M., & Goldwyn, R. (1984). Predicting rejection of her infant from mother's representation of her own experience: Implications for the abuse-abusing intergenerational cycle. *Child Abuse & Neglect, 8,* 203–217.

Mann, E., & McDermott, J. F., Jr. (1983). Play therapy for victims of child abuse and neglect. In C. Schaefer & K. O'Connor (Eds.), *Handbook of play therapy* (pp. 283–307). New York: Wiley.

McGinn, N. F. (1963). Perception of parents and blood pressure. *Dissertation Abstracts International, 24,* 872.

Melton, G. B., & Corson, J. (1987). Psychological maltreatment and the schools: Problems of law and professional responsibility. *School Psychology Review, 16,* 188–194.

Moeller, T., Bachman, G., & Moeller, J. (1993). The combined effect of physical, sexual, and emotional abuse during childhood: Long-term health consequences for women. *Child Abuse & Neglect, 17,* 623–640.

Mones, P. A. (1991). *When a child kills: Abused children who kill their parents.* New York: Pocket Books.

Murphy, J. M., Jellinek, M., Quinn, D., Smith, G., Poitrast, F. G., & Goshko, M. (1991). Substance abuse and serious child maltreatment: Prevalence, risk, and outcome in a court sample. *Child Abuse & Neglect, 15,* 197–211.

Nash, M., Hulsey, M., Sexton, M., Harralson, T., & Lambert, W. (1993). Long-term sequelae of childhood sexual abuse: Perceived family environment, psychopathology, and dissociation. *Journal of Consulting and Clinical Psychology, 61,* 276–283.

Newberger, C. M. (1980). The cognitive structure of parenthood: The development of a descriptive measure. In R. Selman & R. Yando (Eds.), *New directions of child development: Clinical developmental research* (Vol. 7, pp. 45–67). San Francisco: Jossey-Bass.

Polansky, N. A., Chalmers, M., Buttenweiser, E., & Williams, D. (1981). *Damaged parents: An anatomy of child neglect.* Chicago: University of Chicago Press.

Rosenthal, P. A., & Rosenthal, S. (1984). Suicidal behavior in preschool children. *American Journal of Psychiatry, 141,* 520–525.

Shore, M. F., & Massimo, J. (1979). Fifteen years after treatment: A follow-up study of comprehensive vocationally oriented psychotherapy. *American Journal of Orthopsychiatry, 49,* 240–245.

Spinetta, J. J., & Rigler, D. (1972). The child abusing parent: A psychological review. *Psychological Bulletin, 77,* 296–304.

Sroufe, L. A, & Fleeson, J. (1986). Attachment and the construction of relationships. In W. W. Hartup & Z. Rubin (Eds.), *Relationships and development* (pp. 51–72). Hillsdale, NJ: Erlbaum.

U.S. Department of Health and Human Services. (1988). *Study findings: Study of national incidence and prevalence of child abuse and neglect, 1988.* Washington, DC: National Clearinghouse on Child Abuse & Neglect.

U.S. Department of Health and Human Services, Children's Bureau. (1998). *Child maltreatment 1996: Reports from states to the national child abuse and neglect data system.* Washington, DC: U.S. Government Printing Office.

Vissing, Y. M., Straus, M., Gelles, R. J., & Harrop, J. (1991). Verbal aggression by parents and psychological problems of children. *Child Abuse & Neglect, 15,* 223–238.

Wahler, R. G. (1980). The insular mother: Her problems in parent–child treatment. *Journal of Applied Behavioral Analysis, 13,* 207–219.

Wolfe, D. A. (1987). *Child abuse: Implications for child development and psychopathology.* Beverly Hills: Sage.

Wolfner, G. D., & Gelles, R. (1993). A profile of violence toward children: A national study. *Child Abuse & Neglect, 17,* 197–212.

III

Violence toward Adults

15

Wife Battering

Mary Ann Dutton and Edward W. Gondolf

Description of the Problem

Wife battering has been described as the social problem of the 1990s. National surveys conducted in 1975 and 1985 suggest that domestic violence exists at "epidemic" proportions (Straus & Gelles, 1990): nearly 2 million women battered a year. At least one act of violence occurs per year in 16% of all married couples. Nearly one-third of all married couples experience physical abuse at some point. Sixteen percent of murder victims were killed by family members, and spouse murders make up the largest category of family murders (41%) (Dawson & Langan, 1994). They are typically related to a long history of wife battering (Fagan & Browne, 1994).

According to a national survey, the incidence of battering may have decreased as much as 20% since the mid-1970s (Straus & Gelles, 1986). This alleged reduction is most likely related to increased public awareness of battering (Klein, Campbell, Soler, & Ghez, 1997), the advent of women's shelter programs, and more decisive intervention from the criminal justice system. At the same time, local social services, particularly battered women shelters, and the national domestic violence hotline have been overwhelmed by requests for assistance. The women requesting services

Mary Ann Dutton • Bethesda, Maryland 20814.   **Edward W. Gondolf** • Mid-Atlantic Addiction Training Institute, Indiana University of Pennsylvania, Indiana, Pennsylvania 15705.

Case Studies in Family Violence, Second Edition, edited by Ammerman and Hersen. Kluwer Academic / Plenum Publishers, New York, 2000.

have needs far more acute and complex than in the past. Consequently, a wider range of social service staff is encountering wife battering firsthand or is being called upon to assist in wife battering cases.

Despite these alarming trends, wife battering has a long history as a deep-seated social phenomenon. Several social historians have documented the informal and formal sanctions that have encouraged wife battering (Davidson, 1978; Martin, 1976; Pleck, 1987). In early 19th-century America, a husband was permitted to discipline his wife physically without prosecution for assault and battery. The legendary "rule of thumb" law derived from English common law eventually restricted the instrument of wife beatings to a stick no thicker than the man's thumb. Only in the last 20 years have courts finally considered wife battering to be a criminal offense.

Such "selective inattention," as it has been called (Pleck, Pleck, Grossman, & Bart, 1978), has important social implications. It was not until the women's movement of the 1970s identified and responded to wife battering that it emerged as a social problem (Tierney, 1982). Social scientists, physicians, social workers, psychologists, and clergy had virtually overlooked and even denied that wife battering existed prior to this time.

More recently, the efforts to deal with wife battering have been increasingly "professionalized." Grassroots activists have been replaced by trained clinicians and social workers at many shelters. Family service and mental health agencies have increasingly developed programs for battered women and for batterers. In the process, the explanations and treatments for wife battering have become increasingly psychological in emphasis. The popularity of family systems theory, in particular, has led to a view of wife battering as an interactive dysfunction between two individuals. The women may, in this light, be equally involved as perpetrators or provocateurs.

The feminist opposition has objected to what it refers to as "victim blaming" implied by the family systems theorists and practitioners. According to feminists, the social sanctions for wife battering and the control and subjugation imposed on battered women warrant a different picture. If women are violent, it is largely in retaliation or defense against their secondary status in and outside the home (Saunders, 1986). Recent laboratory research of couples involved in domestic violence found that partner's behavior has little influence on batterer's abusive behavior (Jacobson & Gottman, 1998). Whatever the woman's part, it does not typically have the same impact as the man's (Pagelow, 1985; Stets & Straus, 1990).

Recent federal legislation, the Violence Against Women Act of 1994, created many new funding mechanisms for domestic violence initiatives in prosecutors' offices, police, and the courts, in addition to increasing resources for shelter programs. Research evaluating the impact of these federal programs is currently under way.

In sum, professional social service workers are faced with a difficult challenge with regard to wife battering. They must first address the systemic oversight or neglect of the problem inherent in their profession. Second, they must confront their own resistance to dealing with what is an uncomfortable and unwieldy problem in itself. Third, they must assess what has been a controversial and oftentimes inconclusive field (see Gondolf & Fisher, 1988).

To assist in this important and necessary endeavor, we attempt to summarize some of the leading issues facing social service professionals. We accept the assertion of domestic violence experts that wife battering is a distinct behavioral syndrome (Walker, 1984) that may be compounded by psychological disorders or substance abuse but not explained by them. *Wife battering* here refers to the physical assault of women by their husbands or partners that is accompanied by a constellation of psychological abuse, marital rape, child abuse, and even threats of homicide to make for an abusive relationship—that is, a "reign of terror." The varied aspects of abuse are discussed more specifically in the following chapters. Our effort is to identify the prevailing and most current treatment considerations, but our recommendations tend to reflect the feminist approach, to which we subscribe. In sum, we address wife battering primarily as a power dynamic between victim and perpetrator.

Case Description 1

Joan is a low-income Caucasian woman who has faced many problems in her life, beginning in early childhood. Her mother, a prostitute and an alcoholic, gave Joan to her grandmother to raise. They lived in a poor rural community. She was sexually abused during childhood by her grandfather until the age of 8 years when he died suddenly. Beginning in adolescence, Joan began to hitchhike to the nearest town, spend the evening at a bar, spend the weekend with someone whom she picked up at the bar, and hitchhike home again at the end of the weekend. Her alcohol abuse and promiscuous sexual behavior placed her at risk for additional violence victimization. She was sexually assaulted on two separate occasions and physically assaulted numerous times, usually by the men with whom she had casual sexual encounters. Joan quit school in 10th grade and never returned to complete her GED.

Joan met her husband, Ben, when she was in her early twenties. He seemed to her to be a strong man who knew what he wanted, and he wanted to marry her within a month of their meeting. Joan was reluctant but was persuaded by his apparent intense affection for her. Evidence of Ben's violent nature was apparent from the beginning. He expressed intense anger in response to Joan's spending time with another man shortly after she and Ben met. While Ben expressed his strong interest in Joan, he continued to see other women. Joan felt that it was only fair that she do the same thing. When Ben found out about it, he dragged her from the other man's house, "claiming his woman." Joan was both confused and flattered by his attention. Shortly thereafter, Ben said he wanted to marry Joan and she agreed. He moved in with her and her grandmother.

After the marriage, Ben's chronic polydrug habit became apparent. His generally violent behavior was known by local law enforcement officers as well as by other members of the community. His violence toward Joan consisted primarily of threats and sexual abuse. He routinely held guns to her head, threatening to "blow her away." Occasionally, he would actually fire the gun outside a window or toward a pet. He even pulled the trigger once with the gun aimed at himself, but there was no bullet in the chamber. Ben's sexual abuse included forced fellatio. He typically didn't have to use much force, because Joan was afraid of what would happen if she refused to comply with his demands.

Joan did not call the police, go to a shelter, or fight back against Ben's violence. Her grandmother was aware of the violence, although she kept it hidden from most other family members when they visited the home. Joan was afraid to leave because she believed her grandmother and the pets were also in danger of being hurt by Ben. Ben attempted to keep Joan isolated from family members when they came around by demanding that she remain with him in the bedroom. Even when she was allowed to be in their presence, she did not freely socialize with them for fear of Ben's reaction to her appearing to have a good time.

The couple lived primarily on Ben's disability income and income from his sporadic employment. Joan took several low-paying jobs, but each time left within a few weeks when Ben demanded that she do so. Joan knew that Ben's family members were aware of his violence, because he had been violent toward them since his adolescence. One of his brothers had also seen him point a gun at Joan. Joan attempted to confide secretly in the wife of one of her husband's brothers, but because she too was being abused Joan felt there wasn't much she could do to help. Joan knew that the local police were aware of Ben's violent tendencies and that they usually avoided rather than confronted him. Ben usually carried a loaded gun at all times.

Joan became chronically depressed and suicidal. She also drank heavily and used marijuana. On several occasions, her husband took a gun from her that she stated was intended to kill herself. Once, Joan was taken to a psychiatric hospital and admitted for several days. She never talked about the threats or sexual abuse by Ben who visited her daily, usually complaining that she was in the hospital and not at home. Joan's severe depression was diagnosed, but there was no attempt to assess for current risk of intimate violence. She was prescribed an antidepressant medication. Joan's suicidal impulses quickly decreased over the several days of her hospitalization and she was discharged in a much improved condition. Shortly after her discharge, Ben refused to give Joan money to refill her medications and she discontinued use of them.

Case Description 2

Georgia is a middle-class African-American woman whose career as a nurse was one that she cherished and at which she excelled. She was seen by her colleagues and co-workers as a caring professional and a person who was liked by nearly everyone, although her relationships didn't usually extend beyond the work setting. Georgia's first marriage ended in divorce when her husband began having an affair. She attempted to confront him about it, but after an unsuccessful resolution she separated from her husband, taking her two small children. Her husband never fought for custody and maintained no contact after the divorce.

Georgia met Larry a couple of years later and was initially attracted by his romantic nature. He not only courted her with flowers and nice dinners but spent time with the girls and offered to take them all on outings most weekends. Georgia was lonely. She felt that being a single mother of two small children and holding a stressful full-time job without the support of an extended family had taken its toll. She was delighted to meet a man who seemed to share the same family values as she.

Larry and Georgia dated for 6 months before he moved into her home. He held a full-time job working as a mechanic. She came to realize that Larry didn't have many friends but attributed that to his being a socially shy and private man. Larry wasn't as ambitious as Georgia might have liked, but she felt that his family orientation more than made up for what was lacking in his career. Georgia felt that their combined income would easily support the family, although they still had to be careful of expenses. Georgia did not ask Larry to pay rent or contribute to the household expenses once he moved in, although he bought groceries most of the time. She felt that it wasn't fair for Larry to pay the mortgage or the utilities because his name was not on any of them. If they married, Georgia assumed they would share their finances at that point.

Shortly after Larry moved into Georgia's home, they had their first real argument. Larry called Georgia a "bitch" and yelled at her. She was initially surprised by his behavior and a little wary, but brushed it off as a time of transition for both of them. Georgia's father had been a man with a temper, and she was intimidated by such men. Larry began to assume more responsibility with the girls, picking them up from day care and watching them during the occasional evenings when Georgia had to work. She occasionally took an extra shift to make some additional money now that Larry was available to stay with the girls. They seemed to like him and he seemed more than willing to spend time with them.

Several heated arguments between Larry and Georgia occurred before he first physically struck her 9 months after they began living together. Larry slapped Georgia during an argument and then immediately apologized, saying he didn't know what had gotten into him. She was stunned, but not physically hurt, and felt confused by his behavior. He promised that he would never do anything like that again. It was 3 months before he did. This time, he hit Georgia with the back of his hand, causing a bruise to her face. Georgia took time off work for a couple of days and then tried to cover up the mark with makeup. She felt embarrassed and vowed to tell no one about what had happened. Georgia had had similar feelings as a child when hearing her father scream at her mother when she had friends in the house. This time, Larry didn't apologize until the next morning when he saw the bruises. He admitted losing control and apologized. Both times the violence occurred after the girls were in bed sleeping.

Georgia began to think there might be a problem, but she knew that Larry was under a lot of pressure from his work. She wanted to help him but wasn't sure what to do. When they talked, Larry said that he felt left out and wanted to feel more like a member of the family. He said that if they got married and owned the house together, he might feel more secure and less worried about losing her. Although initially reluctant, Georgia put his name on the mortgage after he agreed to a plan for him to pay her some money over the next year. They wrote it down and both signed it. They were married a few weeks later in a quiet ceremony with only a few friends. There were no more violent episodes for 6 months, although during arguments Georgia noticed that she became vigilant, looking for any signs that Larry was again going to "lose control." It took a little longer each time to relax and feel comfortable again, but she began to believe that Larry had changed. She trusted that getting married was indeed what Larry needed to feel secure in their relationship.

After 6 months, Georgia became pregnant, even though she was using birth control. She felt ambivalent about the pregnancy, but Larry seemed elated. Georgia was uncomfortable with the idea of abortion and felt that having a child together would cement her relationship with Larry. On a few occasions during the pregnancy, Larry slapped Georgia. She was upset but did not feel as frightened as in the past. She believed he would not hurt her because of the pregnancy. When the baby arrived, Larry was an adoring father, spent time with the baby, and shared in the child care.

It was 6 months later that a major violent episode occurred. Georgia was late coming home from work. She had stayed after her shift to spend some time with co-workers celebrating a birthday. She knew that Larry would be there to take care of the girls in the evening after picking them up from day care. Georgia rarely went out, especially without Larry, but she felt she needed to spend some time relaxing. Since the new baby had arrived, she was more tired than usual and feeling a little depressed.

When Georgia walked in the house, the girls were asleep. Larry was in the living room waiting for her. She could tell right away he was angry, but she was unprepared for what came next. Larry hit Georgia on her head and across her back, pinned her against the wall, pulled her hair, and shoved her to the floor. He did not hit her face. Georgia was stunned and terrified. She had never seen Larry like this. He accused her of being with another man. He also made a statement that would stay with Georgia long after. Larry said that if she didn't pay attention to him, at least he had his three daughters. He commented that even Susan took care of him better than did her mother. Georgia felt a shock go through her body when he said that and froze—unable to move. She felt terrified, confused, panicked. She didn't know how to explain what was happening. Larry calmed down and went into the other room, leaving Georgia alone. She went into the second bedroom, where she stayed all night. Larry left her alone until he went to work the next morning. Georgia gathered the girls and left to go to a motel. She had 2 days off work and needed some time to think.

Medical Issues

The very nature of wife battering includes assault that often injures. In a study of Texas shelter women (Gondolf & Fisher, 1988), it was found that nearly half of the battered women who had contacted a shelter reported head injuries, 13% had bones broken by their batterers, 42% had sought medical care for battering injuries sometime during their relationship, and 10% required hospitalization. More than half of 833 female patients at two emergency departments, two hospital walk-in clinics, and one private hospital reported experiencing violence from an intimate partner during their lifetime and 15.3% reported such violence during the previous year (Abbott, Johnson, Koziol-McLain, & Lowenstein, 1995).

Injury, however, is not the only health-related consequence of domestic violence. Victims of domestic violence are treated not only in emergency medical but also in primary care settings. In one study, the lifetime and 1-year prevalence rates for domestic violence were 38.8% and 23%, respectively (Hamberger, Saunders, & Hovey, 1992). Interestingly, neither demographic nor health factors accurately predict who among an adult female patient population has been a victim of domestic violence (Saunders, Hamberger, & Hovey, 1993). Women who have been victimized by violence have more health problems, use the health care system more frequently, and rate their health problems as being worse more often than those who are not abused (Koss, 1994; Koss, Woodruff, & Koss, 1990).

Domestic violence victims face pregnancy-related risks as well. A prospective study of 691 pregnant women found that 17% reported physical abuse during pregnancy (McFarlane, 1993). In some cases, abuse begins during pregnancy. Of women who reported no prior abuse, 8% indicated they had been abused beginning in their second or third trimester (McFarlane,

1993). The health consequences of abuse during pregnancy apply to both the mother and the unborn fetus. Injuries during pregnancy can result in placental separation, antepartum hemorrhage, fetal fractures, rupture of the uterus, preterm labor, and low birth weight (Parker, McFarlane, & Soeken, 1994). Miscarriage may also have been the result of violence.

HIV is another medical issue with relevance for battered women. A recent study (Wingood & DiClemente, 1997) found that among 165 sexually active African-American women, those in abusive relationships were less likely than others to use condoms and more likely to experience verbal abuse, emotional abuse, and threats of physical abuse when discussing condom use. Additionally, they felt more worried about acquiring HIV. Another study (Goodman, Rosenberg, Muesser, & Drake, 1997) found evidence that victimization is associated with increased HIV-related risk behaviors among seriously mentally ill women.

Because of the battered woman's fear of retaliation, her self-doubts and suspicion, and the batterer's surveillance of her, a battered woman is generally reluctant to disclose the abuse to a physician. She often tries her best to take care of herself, until the injury is too serious to be ignored. Neither Joan nor Georgia ever told a physician about the abuse. Batterers frequently strike where bruises will not show, and excuses are made to friends who notice a black eye or a limp: "I bumped into a door," or "I fell down the steps." Battered women who do go to a hospital emergency room often give a misleading account of the circumstances. Therefore, much about the abuse is likely not to be disclosed.

A study of several hospital emergency rooms revealed that hospital staff tend to view battered women's unwillingness to talk as "unresponsiveness" or "evasiveness." Prevention, referral, and priority are not given to these cases. In fact, battered-women cases are typically viewed by hospital personnel as "dirty work"—that is, detracting from the "real" emergencies. These cases also have complicated social dimensions that demand a kind of involvement that hospital staff often feel unequipped for (Kurz, 1987).

These sorts of oversights can be addressed in the following ways, according to the recommendations of several reports on the subject (Warshaw & Ganley, 1995). First, battered women need to be identified as such. Because the medical presentation of domestic violence is so varied, it is not adequate just to inquire of those persons who are suspected to be abused. Instead, routine screening for all persons seeking medical care is recommended (Warshaw & Ganley, 1995).

Second, once abuse has been identified assessment is necessary. It is important to include attention to immediate safety needs, chief complaint and present illness, physical examination and preservation of evidence, expanded assessment (in primary care setting), safety and lethality assessment, suicide and homicide assessment, and mental health assessment (Warshaw & Ganley, 1995).

Third, intervention involves validating the abused woman's experience with the professional, letting her know of their concern. Providing information and safety planning are essential. Contacting the police and child abuse reports may also be indicated (Warshaw & Ganley, 1995), but should always be considered within the context of safety planning for the abused woman. Identified battered women need to be referred to specialized domestic violence programs that can help address the emotional and social issues they are facing (Rich & Burgess, 1986). Some emergency rooms present a card to the battered woman indicating the hotline of a women shelter, and staff outline other social service and criminal justice options that may help in establishing safety.

Finally, careful documentation of the injuries and their suspected cause can serve as vital court evidence and aid in obtaining needed referral assistance. Some emergency rooms have begun to keep a special file of all suspected battered women, which enables prompt response to inquiries and recognition of repeat cases. Documentation involves charting information in the medical record, photographing injuries, making body maps indicating injuries and old scars, and keeping laboratory records (Warshaw & Ganley, 1995).

Legal Issues

Many battered women do not initially consider their battering to be a crime and consequently have little contact with the legal system. Some women may have a vague sense that if the injury is severe enough, they could press charges. Other battered women expect that the police will do little except complicate matters. Police, in turn, often believe that battered women or their batterers will attack intruding police and eventually drop the charges if arrests are made (Bolton & Bolton, 1987).

These notions are gradually changing as proarrest policies are established across the country. Statutes requiring mandatory arrest have been enacted in 15 states and the District of Columbia, although in some jurisdictions police officers still do not have full arrest powers in misdemeanor domestic violence cases they did not witness (Schmidt & Sherman, 1996). Although early data indicated that proarrest markedly decreased battering recidivism (Sherman & Berk, 1984), replication data indicate a more complex picture. These data suggest that arrest reduces domestic violence among employed people but increases it among unemployed people and may reduce it in the short term, but not the long term (Schmidt & Sherman, 1996).

Helping a women to secure the legislated police action and court response is a service that many women's shelters offer or coordinate. A growing number of women are beginning to call the police and press charges on their own, in response to the increased public awareness and improved police response. Over half of the women (64%) in a large Texas study had previously contacted the police on at least one occasion; one-fifth (19%) had previously taken legal action (Gondolf & Fisher, 1988).

The most common legal action sought by battered women is an *order of protection*. This court injunction, which goes under a variety of names in different states, is separate from filing criminal charges that attempt to bring about punishment. The court injunction prohibits the batterer from a designated proximity of the woman for up to 2 years. If the batterer violates this specification, he may be subject to immediate arrest and prosecution. However, it is still questionable how long the batterer will stay in jail or what his sentence will be.

These court orders may be useful in communicating a decisive message to the batterer, especially if he is likely to be intimidated by the judicial system. The police or court action is often an essential step in convincing the batterer that he has a problem, as well as a necessary means of interrupting an otherwise escalating situation (Gondolf, 1987a). The court orders also provide the battered woman with some leverage against the batterer if she does eventually return to the relationship. Two recent studies of the impact of protective orders (Harrell, Smith, & Newmark, 1993; Keilitz, Hannaford, & Efkeman, 1997) found that many battered women found them to be helpful, although even a permanent order did not significantly reduce the likelihood of contact during the following year (Harrell et al., 1993). A substantial number of battered women stated that their reason for not returning to obtain a permanent order, after having filed for a temporary order, was because the abuser had stopped bothering them (Keilitz et al., 1997).

There are, of course, some serious shortcomings to court orders. One is that they are particularly difficult to enforce. Consequently, the order may give a woman an illusion of safety when none exists. Orders also seldom resolve an abusive relationship without further intervention or separation. Most importantly, an order of protection may initially incite the batterer to take what he considers to be a retaliatory measure. Following through to get a permanent order does not appear to deter most types of abuse (Harrell et al., 1993), although "being the subject of the court's attention can influence the abuser's behavior" (Keilitz et al., 1997).

Ideally, the legal measures of arrest, persecution, and orders of protection need to be coordinated with other social services. In most communities, shelter advocates are available to help women negotiate with the legal system to try to get the most protection from it. While reform of the criminal justice system remains uneven, it does provide an essential first step in ending wife battering. Domestic violence issues are relevant for many other areas of the law, including matters related to children, other civil issues (e.g., tax, property, torts), the workplace, and immigration (Goelman, Lehrman, & Valente, 1996).

Family Issues

Wife battering, like other forms of family violence, raises a variety of family issues. But unlike child and elder abuse, it threatens the very foundation of the family structure—the marriage partnership. A fundamental family issue, therefore, is whether the family is to exist or continue as a two-parent family. Traditionally, there has been a tendency for those working with battered women to advocate for separation of the batterer from the battered woman and children. This can be achieved temporarily through an order of protection, discussed in the previous section, which orders the man from the home. Also, separation is frequently obtained through shelter residence, in which the woman and children leave home for safety and support. Georgia, for example, separated from her violent husband. Ultimately, it may mean a legal separation and divorce.

A number of separations usually occur over a period of time. Studies of battered women show that they tend to engage in a progressive process of change, including several temporary separations prior to either terminating the relationship completely or experiencing a cessation of the violence (Okum, 1988). The separation offers a time to gain support, recover from emotional and physical injuries, and weigh their options clearly. It also gives the women some leverage over the man in what might otherwise be a gross imbalance of power and control. Saying "I'll leave again" may prove to be a kind of defense (Bowker & Maurer, 1985).

The consequences of leaving, even temporarily, weigh heavy in the balance. For many battered women, separating from a violent man means a loss of income, housing, and transportation—the essentials of survival (Strube, 1988). The majority must care for children as well, with little or no assistance. No matter how threatening and violent the relationship, it may still provide the women with a sense of economic security. Children may long for the father, and women too may feel attachment as a result of their long emotional investment. In other words, they experience a kind of "psychological entrapment" (Brockner & Rubin, 1985). Some women may even experience an increased sense of batterer-induced dependency resulting from repeated assaults on self-esteem and physical integrity (Dutton & Painter, 1993).

A separation, moreover, brings with it complicated custody problems and property rights. These can often incite conflicts and impose couple contact in a way that puts the woman at further risk. Often an advocate is essential in negotiating these issues and assisting in child visits or the dividing of the property. Mediation is rarely recommended in cases involving domestic violence (Fisher, Vidmar, & Ellis, 1993).

Perhaps the most neglected family issue is the impact of family violence on the children (Roy, 1988). The children are first and foremost affected by the violence they see between their parents. The battering presents a role model, especially for the boys, but it also creates a state of terror and insecurity among both sexes. The consequences of witnessing marital violence on children include behavioral problems, difficulties with cognitive and social problem-solving ability, and interference with coping and emotional functioning (Rosenberg & Rossman, 1990). The violence affects children differently at different developmental stages. It nonetheless has a uniform emotional disruption on children not unlike that on children brought up in war-torn countries (Roy, 1988). The boys in particular tend to act out aggressively, and the girls characteristically fall into a state of suspicion and distrust.

A substantial portion of children who witness wife battering also are abused themselves (Edleson, 1996). As many as half of a Texas sample of battered women reported child abuse (Gondolf & Fisher, 1988). A national probability sample of couples found that fathers who frequently abuse their wives also frequently abuse their children and that mothers who are themselves abused abuse their children at higher rates that nonabused women (Straus, 1990).

The children are affected not only by the violence but also by the separations and the moves that accompany the effort to gain safety. Leaving their home, changing schools, and fleeing under cover deprive children of social support and stability.

One of the most frequently asserted explanations for family violence is "intergenerational transmission." That is, children from violent homes are very likely to be in violent homes as adults. While there remains some debate over whether women might be prone toward victimization in this way, men overwhelmingly have violent backgrounds. A range of studies show that from 60% to 80% of batterers come from violent homes. Further, the link between childhood victimization and violent criminal behavior has been demonstrated (Maxfield & Widom, 1996; Widom, 1989).

Helping children who have witnessed wife abuse is essential in order to improve the child's adjustment and to help prevent that child from reexperiencing battering as an adult. A variety of curricula and counseling techniques have been and are being developed to help children first to identify their emotional struggles and second to learn alternatives to the violence that has so encompassed them (Jaffe, Wolfe, & Wilson, 1990; Peled & Davis, 1995; Peled, Jaffe, & Edleson, 1995; Roy, 1988).

Assessment of Psychopathology

There are those who claim that psychopathology has been sorely neglected in a field that is so strongly influenced by sociological and criminal justice perspectives (Hamberger & Lohr, 1989). The efforts to establish some typifying characteristics or profile of battered women and battering men have been in vain. The diversity of both the battered and the batterer leads us to conclude that at best we might identify a typology of batterers and perhaps battered women in which only a small portion have major psychiatric disorders.

Specific concerns in psychological assessment include (1) alcohol abuse, (2) traumatic effects of battering, and (3) personality issues. A disproportionate percentage of wife-battering cases include alcohol abuse. Experts in the field, however, view alcohol abuse as a compounding factor and often a result of battering. It provides an excuse for the violence but is not its cause (Gelles, 1974). Alcoholic batterers have been shown to batter as much as 40% of the time without being under the influence of alcohol. The battering and injury it causes tend to be more severe after drinking (Kantor & Straus, 1987; Roberts, 1988; Van Hasselt, Morrison, & Bellack, 1985). Further, being a victim of violent crime, including battering, increases the risk for serious alcohol and drug-use problems (Kilpatrick & Resnick, 1993).

Both acute and chronic effects of traumatic experiences, including domestic violence, have been well recognized (Dutton, 1992; Herman, 1992; van der Kolk, McFarlane, & Weisaeth, 1996). Repeated exposure to violence—such as found in chronically abusive relationships or when a woman has been abused during childhood as well as in her intimate relationship—and other pretrauma risk factors (e.g., alcohol and drug problems, family history of psychiatric disorder, poverty) may result in more serious outcomes. The role of trauma symptoms typically associated with parental abuse among perpetrators of intimate abuse has been recognized recently (Dutton, 1995).

Personality disorder has been considered an important dimension for understanding differences among perpetrators of intimate violence. Although all batterers do not exhibit personality disorders, several distinct personality disorders have been recognized (Dutton, in press; Hamberger & Hastings, 1986; Holtzworth-Munroe & Stuart, 1994; Saunders, 1992). Special treatment considerations may be warranted based on different personality disorders (Dutton, in press). With few exceptions (see Saunders, 1996), research on differential treatment effectiveness remains scant.

Profile of Battered Women

The diagnosed psychopathology of battered women does not conform to any particular pattern. In a study of psychiatric patients, the self-identified battered women arriving in a psychiatric emergency room had a diversity of diagnoses (Gondolf, 1990), whereas the diagnoses of other kinds of victims were relatively similar. Interestingly, the battering was not specifically addressed in any of the psychiatric cases. No referrals were made, safety was not evaluated, nor were the women informed of their options. Those women who were not currently suicidal, delusional, or threatening counterattack were released to return to their batterers. With increased education in the health-care profession (Warshaw & Ganley, 1995), these responses to domestic violence are beginning to change.

The variation in battered women's psychopathology (ranging from none to severe) can be understood from two perspectives. First, the effects of battering vary across victims. This variation depends on a number of violence-related and other factors, including severity of violence and abuse, subjective appraisal of life threat, time since exposure to violence, chronicity of battering, the extent of social support in the recovery environment, and the presence of prior victimization, including childhood trauma (Dutton, Perrin, & Chrestman, 1995; Green, 1990). Second, women with serious psychopathology are exposed to violence and abuse at high rates (Goodman et al., 1997). Even though their psychopathology does not cause the violence against them, it may render them more vulnerable to violence in the context of their ability to protect themselves. The absence of psychopathology or symptoms associated with domestic violence may be explained by exposure to relatively less severe violence over a shorter period of time, well-developed coping skills, access to adequate resources, and strong social support.

Common symptoms of exposure to domestic violence include depression, posttraumatic stress disorder, anxiety, and dissociation (Campbell & Lewandowski, 1997; Dutton, 1992; Follingstad, Rutledge, Berg, Hause, & Polek, 1990; Kemp, Green, Horowitz, & Rawlins, 1995). These symptoms characterize the effects of trauma generally. Little is known about the longitudinal course of the effects of battering, although ending the violent relationship or cessation of violence within the intimate relationship has been associated with the reduction of symptoms (Campbell, Miller, Cardwell, & Belknap, 1994).

The popularized notion of learned helplessness has also been used to explain the reactive symptoms. The abuse and battering "condition" the battered women to feel helpless. They become pessimistic and passive, and even blame themselves for the violence. Research efforts to document this profile, however, have not been able to establish that battered women as a group are any more depressed or passive than nonbattered women (Launius & Lindquist, 1988; Walker, 1984).

In a study of Texas women, battered women were active help-seekers despite the severity and duration of their abuse. A more active profile based on the coping and help-seeking may be that of a survivor. In our case examples, both Joan and Georgia made varied attempts to stop the violence against them, employing many personal strategies, such as talking with friends about the abuse and confronting the batterer, even if they used few formal strategies such as calling the police. Many women use formal and informal help-seeking strategies such as calling the police, petitioning for a civil protection order, seeking divorce and separation, discussing the violence with a physician, getting counseling, and using a shelter or crisis hotline. No one strategy or series of strategies appears as the "most" successful (Bowker, 1983). Social services staff might, therefore, see their initial and perhaps primary function as facilitating and furthering this process: encouraging and aiding the woman's involvement with a variety of informal and formal help sources and assuring the appropriate response of the helpers.

Profile of Men Who Batter

The diagnosed psychopathology of batterers is shown to be less diversified than that of battered women. The research with psychiatric patients identified as batterers shows them to be disproportionately diagnosed as having personality disorders (Gondolf, 1990). A series of studies using the MCMI have suggested that the vast majority of batterers in counseling programs show symptoms of a variety of personality disorders, but that no single overriding profile exists. Instead, these studies have generally found distinct types of personality profiles among batterers (Gondolf, 1997; Hamberger & Hastings, 1986; Saunders, 1992; Tweed & Dutton, 1996). Based on MCMI profiles, one study grouped these types as *little pathology*, *narcissistic/antisocial*, *avoidant/dependent*, and *severe pathology* (Gondolf, 1997).

We have to differentiate among batterers to account for the sometimes contradictory or inconclusive efforts to formulate a batterer profile. One empirical study based on behavioral descriptions of batterers established a typology of batterers that suggests a continuum of violence (Gondolf, 1988b). Those identified as "sporadic" batterers were those who were less frequently abusive and were more likely to apologize and regret their battering. The "chronic" batterers battered more frequently and severely, and were more likely also to be abusive to the children.

A recent study found that batterers—like nonviolent but distressed men as well as happily married men—can be categorized based on their physiological reactivity to conflictual interactions in the laboratory setting as Type I or Type II reactors (Gottman, Jacobson, Rushe, Shortt, Babcock, La Taillade, & Waltz, 1995; Jacobson, Gottman, & Shortt, 1995). The proportion of men in all three categories in whom heart rate was reduced at the onset of conflict (Type I) ranged from 20–28% of the sample, whereas those whose heart rate accelerated (Type II) ranged from 72–80% of the sample (Jacobson et al., 1995). Type I batterers were found to be more verbally aggressive during laboratory interactions, reported more violence toward others, had more elevated scales reflecting antisocial behavior and sadistic aggression, and were lower in dependency than Type II batterers (Gottman et al., 1995).

Although batterers as a group cannot be considered to have an "abusive personality," one author (Dutton, in press) has argued that the pattern does fit certain batterers: those who are chronically and intermittently abusive, but only in the family. Central to Dutton's conceptualization of an abusive personality is borderline personality disorder. Research findings show an association between borderline scores using the BPO scale (Oldham, Clarkin, Appelbaum, Carr, Kernberg, Letterman, & Hass, 1985) and "associated features" of abusiveness, including anger, jealousy, and blaming partner for negative events in the relationship (Dutton, in press). Surprisingly, higher BPO scores were also associated with higher trauma symptoms (depression, sleeplessness, anxiety attacks). Perhaps most importantly, high BPO scores were also associated with greater report by men of their use of both physical and psychological abuse toward their partners.

Men in treatment programs may appear clinically depressed or paranoid. These states may reflect, in part, reactions to the consequences of his battering—arrest, loss of family, and possibility of punishment. Batterers may even threaten suicide in response to the depression and in part as a means of manipulation—to get their wives or partners back.

Clinicians and researchers alike have characterized battering men as less communicative, more impulsive, lower in self-esteem, and more rigid in sex-role expectation (Maiuro, Cahn, & Vitaliano, 1986; see Dutton, 1992, for an overview). They are also more likely to have come from a violent home, as mentioned, and to be involved in substance abuse (see Hotaling & Sugarman, 1986). One shortcoming of profile data is that, to date, they do not substantially differentiate batterers from other sorts of offenders, such as rapists, robbers, and molesters.

The "characteristics" of batterers may represent merely an extension of a normative process that might be called the *failed macho complex* (Gondolf & Hanneken, 1987). A qualitative study of batterers suggests that their battering is an overcompensation for a distorted male ideal that they feel obliged to fulfill. Their distortions are in part the result of the role models of their fathers or of media heroes. Batterers are not so much super macho men as men who feel they fall short of what they are "supposed" to be as a man. Their low self-concept may be related to the abuse they witnessed or received while growing up.

Joan's husband, Ben, can be considered a chronic batterer. While some of his behavior might suggest a narcissistic/antisocial personality disorder, Ben's battering may be part of a larger continuum of normative male control and dominance. His psychological problems warrant attention, but they should be viewed more as compounding the battering rather than causing it. Primarily, the battering needs to be interrupted and addressed. Further, the batterer's distorted expectations for himself and for women need to be replaced with a more accepting and supportive self-image.

Treatment Options

Two specialized treatment options have been developed to deal with wife battering: battered women's shelters and batterer programs. These emerged in large part in response to the neglect or oversight of the professional social services to address the problem (Schechter, 1982). More recently, a variety of social services and family agencies have also developed treatment programs of their own for wife-abuse cases. Their philosophy and approach often differ from the domestic violence programs. They are more likely to adopt existing family systems practices or cognitive-behavioral therapy in the treatment of wife abuse (Adams, 1988; Gondolf, 1985).

The fundamental objective of treatment, in any case, should be to bring about a cessation of the battering. This means assuring interruption of the current battering and addressing the chronic nature of the battering. This generally is accomplished by separate group sessions for women, often convened at a shelter, and separate group sessions for batterers. Couples counseling, which has become a controversial format in this field, is generally discouraged at least until battering has been stopped for 6 months to a year, and after some period of separation (Bograd, 1984).

The counseling process for both men and women needs initially to confront denial and minimization where it exists (Gondolf, 1985). Helping the women and men to recognize the nature and dynamics of abuse in itself helps to develop precautions. This entails identifying the kinds of abuse that occur and their frequency, and establishing in this way that battering is not a series of isolated incidents but part of a controlling pattern of behavior. Several inventories are available to help identify emotional, financial, sexual, and child abuse accompanied by male privilege, intimidation, isolation, and threats (Pence, 1989; Tolman, 1989).

Treatment for Battered Women

A variety of counseling approaches have been proposed for battered women in recent years. A fundamental component of any intervention with battered women is safety planning (Davies, Lyon, & Monti-Catania, 1998; Dutton, 1992). Safety planning involves identifying both batterer-generated and life-generated risks and assisting the battered woman in developing strategies for responding to them. Fundamental to the counseling efforts should be a design to move the battered woman from status as a "victim" to that of a "survivor" (Reiker & Carmen, 1976). It is this shift in self-perception that is most associated with safety and recovery (Gondolf & Fisher, 1988).

Brown (1997) has applied a transtheoretical model of behavior change to the problems facing battered women in order to describe battered women's efforts to overcome abuse in their lives. The stages of change incorporated in this model move from precontemplation (no intention to change), contemplation (thinking about change), preparation (actively planning change), action (overly making changes), and finally, maintenance (solidifying change and resisting temptations to relapse). While this model has yet to be empirically tested with battered women, it shows promise as one approach to describing how battered women move from denying that the violent and abusive behavior is a problem to resisting the batterer's attempts to have her drop charges or return to the relationship, for example.

According to several victimization studies, battered women tend to move through several phases in response to abuse (Ferraro & Johnson, 1983; Mills, 1985). These phases are distinguished by an attributional shift on the woman's part. In essence, she begins to perceive that the battering was not "all her fault" but largely due to her husband. It is not up to her to change the batterer; in fact, it is not likely that he will change. She is capable of taking care of herself, with the support and assistance she deserves from others.

The objective in counseling, therefore, might be to reinforce and encourage this realization. Many shelters subscribe to an "empowerment" mode of counseling to achieve this end (Dutton, 1992). The feminist approach is directed toward helping the woman realize her options and choices and begin to make decisions that assure her worth, integrity, and determination (Bograd, 1984). As mentioned earlier, a study of formerly battered women rated this sort of counseling to be the most effective in stopping the violence (Bowker, 1983).

The study of Texas shelter women (Gondolf & Fisher, 1988) raises an additional objective: resource allocation. What seems to contribute most to a women's move toward safety is obtaining an income of her own, transportation, child care, and housing. Having mobility not only enables a woman to leave the violence but also helps "equalize" the relationship. These essential resources are, however, particularly problematic in wife-abuse cases. As mentioned, the majority of the Texas shelter women have little education, few job skills, and young children. Further, tangible support has been found to predict battered women's follow-through with criminal prosecution (Goodman, Bennett, & Dutton, in press).

For some battered women, treatment needs extend beyond safety and examining options for change. The effects of living in a violent relationship—exposed to chronic and often life-threatening acts, threats to family and friend, and loss of personal resources—can result in traumatic and associated symptoms such as posttraumatic stress disorder, dissociation, depression, and anxiety. These symptoms often remit once the battered woman is living in a safe environment free from continued violence and threats. However, in some cases, these symptoms continue, causing distress and interference with her ability to function. In such cases, trauma treatment (Dutton, 1992; Walker, 1994) can aide the battered woman in recovering from these negative effects of violence victimization.

Treatment for the Batterer

The treatment of batterers has seen a proliferation of approaches and with it increased debate (Adams, 1988). The leading programs are characterized by a group process that prompts men to take responsibility for their abuse, to exercise alternatives to the violence, and to restructure their sex-role perceptions (Gondolf, 1987a). There is a questionable trend, however, toward short-term anger-control treatment that unwittingly reinforces the batterer's penchant for control (Gondolf & Russell, 1986).

The research on cessation suggests that batterers who do reform their behavior pass through a series of developmental stages (Fagan, 1987; Gondolf, 1987a). The change process begins with *realization*. The egocentric batterer acknowledges the consequences of his abuse and that it may be in his own self-interest to contain it. Gradually, batterers become more *other-oriented* and begin to make some *behavioral changes* to improve relationships or at least avoid totally destroying them. Some men eventually begin to think more in terms of values and principles and integrate these into a change of self-concept. A number of the leading batterer programs consequently employ a phased approach that moves batterers from didactic sessions of accountability and consequence to social support groups with a focus on services (see Gondolf, 1985).

The most outstanding challenges for these programs, besides the high dropout rates, are collusion, self-pity, and self-congratulation. There is a tendency for batterers and even male counselors to "collude" with one another. They sometimes very subtly acknowledge one another's excuses or fail to challenge them. They begin to pity themselves for the consequences of their battering that add to bad experiences they had growing up. In simply attending a program, batterers feel some congratulations and trust are due them from their spouse and often cannot understand why she does not come running back. All these diversions from change can, of course, be challenged and turned into lessons about rationalization (Gondolf & Russell, 1986).

The most pressing question about batterer programs is how "successful" they are (Gondolf, 1987b). This is a difficult question to answer, given how one defines success. Shelter workers have noted that batterers after counseling may become "nonviolent terrorists." They cease their battering but heighten their psychological abuse and other controlling behaviors. Those who do stop their abuse and violence are likely to do so as a result of a constellation of interventions (Bowker, 1983). The counseling in and of
• itself does not stop the battering, but counseling, along with a coordinated community response such as police action, the woman's leaving, divorce suit, and Alcoholics Anonymous, may be an incentive (Steinman, 1988). It may be, as suggested previously, that certain types of batterers are poor candidates for counseling and need comprehensive residential psychiatric and substance-abuse treatment along with the batterer counseling (Gondolf, 1988a). It is important to emphasize, however, that there is good evidence that these treatments *alone* are not sufficient. Recent research supports the importance of court review, indicating evidence of compliance with referral to batterer counseling (Gondolf, 1998).

It is particularly important that batterer programs be carefully coordinated with, and accountable to, shelter services and women's counseling. Some shelter workers, in fact, have outlined a rationale and plan for monitoring batterer programs (Hart, 1987). This is critical for two immediate reasons: first, the variety and uncertain success of batterer counseling at this juncture, and second, the effect of batterer counseling on women. The batterer's participation in a counseling program is the most influential factor in a woman's returning to him and putting herself at risk (Gondolf, 1988a). It is the woman's separation that is the prime motivator for a man's attending counseling in the first place. Once batterers "get her back," they are much more likely to drop out of counseling—and batter again.

Summary

Increasingly, there is a call to recognize wife battering as a complex social problem that warrants decisive and comprehensive intervention. Single-issue treatment has historically been ineffective for the victims and frustrating for the practitioners. First, wife battering needs to be recognized as a chronic syndrome of control as well as violence. Second, decisive interruption of the violence and safety for the victims needs to be assured through legal and shelter options. Third, the survivor process in victims and cessation process in batterers may be reinforced by group counseling that establishes the responsibility for battering, its consequences, and alternatives to it. Fourth, battered women especially need substantial resources, as well as emotional support, to assure their mobility. Batterers contrarily need to be made accountable to a reference group that offers them an alternative role model and nonviolent values.

Model wife-abuse programs are distinguished by their integrated interventions (Brygger & Edleson, 1987; Edleson & Tolman, 1992; Pence, 1989; Saunders, 1996) and sensitivity to ethnic diversity (Williams, 1992). While this ideal is far from a reality in most common communities, as least better referral and coordination are possible. In sum, no professional should feel he or she can do it alone. The most valuable contribution may be to bring the wife-abuse case to a diversity of services. This makes the problem not just that of the battered woman but the community's problem as well.

References

Abbott, J., Johnson, R., Koziol-McLain, J., & Lowenstein, S. R. (1995). Domestic violence against women: Incidence and prevalence in an emergency department population. *Journal of the American Medical Association, 273*, 1763–1767.

Adams, D. (1988). Treatment models of men who batter: A profeminist analysis. In K. Yllo & M. Bograd (Eds.), *Feminist perspectives on wife abuse* (pp. 176–179). Newbury Park, CA: Sage.

Bograd, M. (1984). Feminist perspective on wife abuse: An introduction. In K. Yllo & M. Bograd (Eds.), *Feminist perspectives on the violent family*. Newbury Park, CA: Sage.

Bolton, F. G., & Bolton, S. R. (1987). *Working with violent families: A guide for clinical and legal practitioners*. Newbury Park, CA: Sage.

Bowker, L. (1983). *Beating wife beating*. Lexington, MA.

Bowker, L., & Maurer, L. (1985). The importance of sheltering in the lives of battered women. *Response, 8*, 2–8.

Brockner, J., & Rubin, J. (1985). *Entrapment in escalating conflicts: A social psychological analysis*. New York: Springer-Verlag.

Brown, J. (1997). Working toward freedom from violence: The process of change in battered women. *Violence Against Women, 3*, 5–26.

Brygger, M. P., & Edleson, J. (1987). The domestic abuse project: A multisystem intervention in woman battering. *Journal of Interpersonal Violence, 2*, 324–333.

Campbell, J. C., & Lewandowski, L. A. (1997). Mental and physical health effects of intimate partner violence on women and children. *Psychiatric Clinics of North America, 20*, 353–374.

Campbell, J. C., Miller, P., Cardwell, M. M., & Belknap, R. A. (1994). Relationship status of battered women over time. *Journal of Family Violence, 9*, 99–111.

Davidson, T. (1978). *Conjugal crime: Understanding and changing the wife-beating problem*. New York: Hawthorn.

Davies, J., Lyon, E., & Monti-Catania, D. (1998). *Safety planning with battered women: Complex lives/difficult choices*. Thousand Oaks, CA: Sage.

Dawson, J. M., & Langan, P. A. (1994). *Murder in families*. (NCJ-143498): Bureau of Justice Statistics, U.S. Department of Justice.

Dutton, D. G. (1995). Trauma symptoms and PTSD-like profiles in perpetrators of intimate abuse. *Journal of Traumatic Stress, 8*, 299–316.

Dutton, D. G. (in press). *Intimate abusiveness: A trauma model*. New York: Guilford Press.

Dutton, D. G., & Painter, S. L. (1993). Emotional attachments in abusive relationships: A test of traumatic bonding theory. *Violence and Victims, 8*, 105–120.

Dutton, M. A. (1992). *Empowering and healing the battered woman*. New York: Springer.

Dutton, M. A., Haywood, Y., & El-Bayoumi, G. (1997). Impact of violence on women's health. In S. J. Gallant, G. P. Keita, & R. Royak-Schaler (Ed.), *Health care for women: Psychological, social, and behavioral influences* (pp. 41–56). Washington, DC: American Psychological Association.

Dutton, M. A., Perrin, S., & Chrestman, K. (1995). *Differences among battered women's MMPI profiles: The role of context*. Paper presented at the fourth international family violence research conference, Durham, New Hampshire.

Edleson, J. L. (1996). *The overlap between child maltreatment and woman abuse*. Harrisburg, PA: National Resource Center on Domestic Violence, VAWnet.

Edleson, J. L., & Tolman, R. M. (1992). *Intervention for men who batter: An ecological approach*. Newbury Park, CA: Sage.

Fagan, J. (1987). Cessation of family violence: Deterrence and dissuasion. In L. Ohlin & M. Tonry (Eds.), *Crime and justice: An annual review of research* (pp. 377–425). Chicago: University of Chicago Press.

Fagan, J., & Browne, A. (1994). Violence between spouses and intimates: Physical aggression between women and men in intimate relationships. In A. J. Reiss, Jr. & J. A. Roth (Eds.), *Understanding and preventing violence: Vol. 3. Social influences* (pp. 115–292). Washington, DC: National Academy Press.

Ferraro, K., & Johnson, J. (1983). How women experience battering: The process of victimization. *Social Problems, 30*, 325–339.

Fisher, K., Vidmar, N., & Ellis, R. (1993). The culture of battering and the role of mediation in domestic violence cases. *Southern Methodist University Law Review, 46,* 2117.

Follingstad, D. R., Rutledge, L. L., Berg, B. J., Hause, E. S., & Polek, D. S. (1990). The role of emotional abuse in physically abusive relationships. *Journal of Family Violence, 5,* 107–120.

Gelles, R. J. (1974). *The violent home: A study of physical aggression between husbands and wives.* Beverly Hills, CA: Sage.

Goelman, D. M., Lehrman, F. L., & Valente, R. L. (1996). *The impact of domestic violence on your legal practice.* Washington, DC: American Bar Association, Commission on Domestic Violence.

Gondolf, E. W. (1985). *Men who batter: An integrated approach to stopping wife abuse.* Homes Beach, FL: Learning Publications.

Gondolf, E. W. (1987a). Changing men who batter: A developmental model of integrated interventions. *Journal of Family Violence, 2,* 345–369.

Gondolf, E. W. (1987b). Seeing through smoke and mirrors: A guide to batterer program evaluations. *Response, 10,* 16–19.

Gondolf, E. W. (1988a). The effect of batterer counseling on shelter outcome. *Journal of Interpersonal Violence, 3,* 275–289.

Gondolf, E. W. (1988b). Who are those guys? Toward a behavioral typology of batterers. *Violence and Victims, 3,* 187–204.

Gondolf, E. W. (1990). *Psychiatric response to family violence: Identifying and confronting neglected danger.* Lexington, MA: Lexington Books.

Gondolf, E. W. (1997). *Multisite evaluation of batterer intervention systems: A summary of findings for a 12-month follow-up* (Interim Report). Washington, DC: Centers for Disease Control and Prevention, U.S. Department of Health and Human Services.

Gondolf, E. W. (1998). *Program compliance: An evaluation of the Pittsburgh municipal courts and domestic abuse counseling center (DACC).* http://www.mincava.umn.edu/papers/gondolf/pccd.htm.

Gondolf, E. W., & Fisher, E. R. (1988). *Battered women as survivors: An alternative to treating learned helplessness.* Lexington, MA: Lexington Books.

Gondolf, E. W., & Hanneken, J. (1987). The gender warrior: Reformed barriers on treatment and change. *Journal of Family Violence, 2,* 177–191.

Gondolf, E. W., & Russell, D. M. (1986). The case against anger control treatment programs for batterers. *Response, 9,* 2–5.

Goodman, L. A., Rosenberg, S. D., Muesser, K. T., & Drake, R. E. (1997). Physical and sexual assault history in women with serious mental illness: Prevalence, correlates, treatment, and future research directions. *Schizophrenia Bulletin, 23,* 685–696.

Goodman, L., Bennett, L., & Dutton, M. A. (in press). *Obstacles women face in prosecuting their batterers: The role of social support.*

Gottman, J. M., Jacobson, N. S., Rushe, R. H., Shortt, J. W., Babcock, J., La Taillade, J. J., & Waltz, J. (1995). The relationship between heart rate reactivity, emotionally aggressive behavior, and general violence in batterers. *Journal of Family Psychology, 9,* 227–248.

Green, B. L. (1990). Defining trauma: Terminology and generic stressor dimensions. *Journal of Applied Social Psychology, 20,* 1632–1642.

Hamberger, K., & Hastings, J. (1986). Personality correlates of men who abuse their partners: A cross-validational study. *Journal of Family Violence, 1,* 323–341.

Hamberger, L. K., & Lohr, J. M. (1989). Proximal causes of spouse abuse: A theoretical analysis for cognitive–behavioral intervention. In P. L. Caesar & L. K. Hamberger (Eds.), *Treating men who batter: Theory, practice, and programs* (pp. 53–76). New York: Springer.

Hamberger, L. K., Saunders, D. G., & Hovey, M. (1992). Prevalence of domestic violence in community practice and rate of physician inquiry. *Family Medicine, 24,* 283–287.

Harrell, A., Smith, B., & Newmark, L. (1993). *Court processing and the effects of restraining orders for domestic violence victims*. Washington, DC: Urban Institute.

Hart, B. (1987). *Safety for women: Monitoring batterer's programs*. Harrisburg: Pennsylvania Coalition Against Domestic Violence.

Herman, J. (1992). *Trauma and recovery*. New York: Basic Books.

Holtzworth-Munroe, A., & Stuart, G. L. (1994). Typologies of batterers: Three subtypes and the differences among them. *Psychological Bulletin, 116*, 476–497.

Hotaling, G., & Sugarman, D. (1986). An analysis of risk makers in husband to wife violence: The current state of knowledge. *Violence and Victims, 1*, 101–124.

Jacobson, N., & Gottman, J. (1998). *When men batter women: New insights into ending abusive relationships*. New York: Simon & Schuster.

Jacobson, N. S., Gottman, J. M., & Shortt, J. W. (1995). The distinction between Type 1 and Type 2 batterers—Further considerations. *Journal of Family Psychology, 9*, 272–279.

Jaffe, P. G., Wolfe, D. A., & Wilson, S. K. (1990). *Children of battered women*. Thousand Oaks, CA: Sage.

Kantor, G. K., & Straus, M. A. (1987). The "drunken bum" theory of wife beating. *Social Problems, 34*, 213–230.

Keilitz, S. L., Hannaford, P. L., & Efkeman, H. S. (1997). *Civil protection orders: The benefits and limitations for victims of domestic violence*. Williamsburg, VA: National Center for State Courts.

Kemp, A., Green, B. L., Horowitz, C., & Rawlins, E., I. (1995). Incidence and correlates of PTSD in battered women: Shelter and community samples. *Journal of Interpersonal Violence, 10*, 43–55.

Kilpatrick, D. G., & Resnick, H. S. (1993). Posttraumatic stress disorder associated with exposure to criminal victimization in clinical and community populations. In J. R. T. Davidson & D. B. Foa (Eds.), *Posttraumatic stress disorder: DSM-IV and beyond* (pp. 113–143). Washington, DC: American Psychiatric Press.

Klein, E., Campbell, J., Soler, E., & Ghez, M. (1997). *Ending domestic violence: Changing public perceptions/halting the epidemic*. Thousand Oaks, CA: Sage.

Koss, M. P. (1994). The negative impact of crime victimization on women's health and medical use. In A. J. Dan (Ed.), *Reframing women's health: Multidisciplinary research and practice* (pp. 189–200). Thousand Oaks, CA: Sage.

Koss, M. P., Woodruff, W. J., & Koss, P. G. (1990). Relation of criminal victimization to health perceptions among women medical patients. *Journal of Consulting and Clinical Psychology, 58*, 147–152.

Kurz, D. (1987). Emergency department responses to battered women: Resistance to medicalization. *Social Problems, 34*, 69–81.

Launius, M. H., & Lindquist, C. U. (1988). Learned helplessness, external locus of control, and passivity in battered women. *Journal of Interpersonal Violence, 3*, 307–318.

Martin, D. (1976). *Battered wives*. New York: Pocket Books.

Maxfield, M. G., & Widom, C. S. (1996). The cycle of violence: Revisited six years later. *Archives of Pediatric and Adolescent Medicine, 150*, 390–395.

McFarlane, J. (1993). Abuse during pregnancy: The horror and the hope. *AWHONNS Clinical Issues in Perinatal and Women's Health Nursing, 4*, 350–362.

Meiuro, R. O., Chan, T. S., & Vitaliano, P. P. (1986). Assertiveness deficits and hostility in domestically violent men. *Violence and Victims, 1*, 279–289.

Mills, T. (1985). The assault on the self: Stages in coping with battering husbands. *Qualitative Sociology, 8*, 103–123.

Okum, L. (1988). Termination or resumption of cohabitation in woman battering relationships: A statistical study. In G. Hotaling, D. Finkelhor, J. Kirkpatrick, & M. Straus (Eds.), *Coping with family violence* (pp. 107–119). Newbury Park, CA: Sage.

Oldham, J., Clarkin, J., Appelbaum, A., Carr, A., Kernberg, P., Letterman, A., & Hass, G. (1985). A self-report instrument for Borderline Personality Organization. In T. H. McGlashan (Ed.), *The borderline: Current empirical research* (pp. 1–18). Washington, DC: American Psychiatric Press.

Pagelow, M. (1985). The battered husband syndrome: Social problem or much ado about little. In N. Johnson (Ed.), *Marital violence*. Boston: Routledge & Kegan Paul.

Parker, B., McFarlane, J. U., & Soeken, K. (1994). Abuse during pregnancy: Effects on maternal complications and birth weight in adult and teenage women. *Obstetrics and Gynecology, 84*, 323–328.

Peled, E., & Davis, D. (1995). *Groupwork for children of battered women*. Thousand Oaks, CA: Sage.

Peled, E., Jaffe, P., & Edleson, J. (1995). *Ending the cycle of violence: Community responses to children of battered women*. Thousand Oaks, CA: Sage.

Pence, E. (1989). Batterers programs: Shifting from community collusion to community confrontation. In P. L. Caesar & L. K. Hamberger (Eds.), *Therapeutic interventions with batterers* (pp. 24–50). New York: Springer.

Pleck, E. (1987). *Domestic tyranny: The making of American social policy against family violence from colonial times to the present*. New York: Oxford University Press.

Pleck, E., Pleck, J., Grossman, M., & Bart, P. (1978). The battered data syndrome: A reply to Steinmetz. *Victimology, 2*, 680–683.

Reiker, P., & Carmen, E. H. (1976). The victim-to-patient process: The disconfirmation and transformation of abuse. *Hospital and Community Psychiatry, 37*, 437–439.

Rich, R., & Burgess, A. W. (1986). NIMH report: Panel recommends comprehensive program for victims of violent crime. *Hospital and Community Psychiatry, 37*, 437–439.

Roberts, A. R. (1988). Substance abuse among men who batter their wives. *Journal of Substance Abuse Treatment, 5*, 83–87.

Rosenberg, M. S., & Rossman, B. B. R. (1990). The child witness to marital violence. In R. T. Ammerman & M. Hersen (Eds.), *Treatment of family violence: A sourcebook* (pp. 183–210). New York: Wiley.

Roy, M. (1988). *Children in the crossfire: Violence in the home—How does it affect our children?* Deerfield Beach, FL: Health Communications.

Saunders, D. G. (1986). When battered women use violence: Husband-abuse and self-defense. *Violence and Victims, 1*, 47–60.

Saunders, D. G. (1992). A typology of men who batter: Three types derived from cluster analysis. *American Journal of Orthopsychiatry, 62*, 264–275.

Saunders, D. G., Hamberger, K., & Hovey, M. (1993). Indicator of woman abuse based on a chart review at a family practice center. *Archives of Family Medicine, 2*, 537–543.

Saunders, D. G. (1996). Feminist-cognitive-behavioral and process-psychodynamic treatments for men who batter: Interaction of abuser traits and treatment models. *Violence and Victims, 11*, 393–414.

Schechter, S. (1982). *Women and male violence: The visions and struggles of the battered women's movement*. Boston: South End Press.

Schmidt, J. D., & Sherman, L. W. (1996). Does arrest deter domestic violence? In E. S. Buzawa & C. G. Buzawa (Eds.), *Do arrests and restraining orders work?* (pp. 43–53). Thousand Oaks, CA: Sage.

Sherman, L. W., & Berk, R. A. (1984). The specific deterrent effects of arrest for domestic assaults. *American Sociological Review, 49*, 261–272.

Steinman, M. (1988). Evaluating a systemwide response to domestic violence: Some initial findings. *Journal of Contemporary Criminal Justice, 4*, 172–186.

Stets, J. E., & Straus, M. A. (1990). Gender differences in reporting marital violence and its medical and psychological consequences. In M. A. Straus & R. J. Gelles (Eds.), *Physical violence in American families: Risk factors and adaptations to violence in 8,145 families.* New Brunswick: Transaction Publishers.

Straus, M., & Gelles, R. (1986). Societal change and change in family violence from 1975 to 1985 as revealed by two national surveys. *Journal of Marriage and the Family, 48,* 465–479.

Straus, M. A., & Gelles, R. (1990). *Violence in American families: Risk factors and adaptions to violence in 8,145 families.* New Brunswick: Transaction Publishers.

Straus, M. A. (1990). Ordinary violence, child abuse, and wife beating: What do they have in common? In M. A. Straus & R. J. Gelles (Eds.), *Physical violence in American families: Risk factors and adaptations to violence in 8,145 families* (pp. 403–424). New Brunswick: Transaction Publishers.

Strube, M. (1988). The decision to leave an abusive relationship: Empirical evidence and theoretical issues. *Psychological Bulletin, 104,* 236–250.

Tierney, K. J. (1982). The battered women movement and the creation of the wife-beating problem. *Social Problems, 29,* 207–220.

Tolman, R. (1989). The development of a measure of psychological maltreatment of women by their male partners. *Violence and Victims, 4,* 173–189.

Tweed, R., & Dutton, D. G. (1996). *Attachment style and personality disorder among clusters of domestically violent men.* Vancouver: University of British Columbia.

van der Kolk, B., McFarlane, A. C., & Weisaeth, L. (1996). *Traumatic stress.* New York: Guilford Press.

Van Hasselt, V. B., Morrison, R. L., & Bellack, A. S. (1985). Alcohol use in wife abusers and their spouses. *Addictive Behavior, 10,* 127–135.

Walker, L. (1984). *The battered woman syndrome.* New York: Springer.

Walker, L. E. A. (1994). *Abused women and survivor therapy: A practical guide for the psychotherapist.* Washington, DC: American Psychological Association.

Warshaw, C., & Ganley, A. L. (1995). *Improving the health care response to domestic violence: A resource manual for health care providers* (manual). San Francisco: Family Violence Prevention Fund.

Widom, C. (1989). The cycle of violence. *Science, 244,* 160–166.

Williams, O. J. (1992, December). Ethnically sensitive practice to enhance treatment participation of African American men who batter. *Families in Society: Journal of Contemporary Human Services,* 588–594.

Wingood, G. M., & DiClemente, R. J. (1997). The effects of an abusive primary partner on the condom use and sexual negotiation practices of African-American women. *American Journal of Journal of Public Health, 87,* 1016–1018.

16

Psychological Maltreatment of Partners

Amy H. Schwartz, Susan M. Andersen, Tracey J. Strasser, and Teresa Ramirez Boulette

Psychological Maltreatment of Partners

Abusive behavior in the context of intimate relationships can take many forms, ranging from intense psychological intimidation and threats of violence to life-threatening episodes of physical assault. In virtually all cases of physical violence, however, some form of psychological maltreatment is also present. Psychological maltreatment, in fact, can quite reasonably be considered a common denominator in ongoing interpersonal relationships that are violent.

In this chapter, we describe a particular constellation of patterns that are frequently involved in the psychological maltreatment of partners in the context of violent relationships. We focus much of our discussion on male violence against women, or wife battering, and we frequently apply the terms spouse, wife, husband, and marriage. However, the patterns of psychological maltreatment that we describe could occur in any intimate partnership, regardless of whether the members of the couple are heterosexual, homosexual, married, or unmarried. We focus on male violence

Amy H. Schwartz, Susan M. Andersen, and Tracey J. Strasser • Department of Psychology, New York University, New York, New York 10003.   Teresa Ramirez Boulette • Santa Barbara County Mental Health Care Services, Santa Barbara, California 93110.

Case Studies in Family Violence, Second Edition, edited by Ammerman and Hersen. Kluwer Academic / Plenum Publishers, New York, 2000.

against women because it is a startlingly prevalent problem that has come under increased empirical scrutiny in the past 10 years, and policy makers and legal, medical, and mental health professionals have begun to recognize the terrible human costs of this epidemic (Goodman, Koss, Fitzgerald, Russo, & Keita, 1993). Although we recognize that some serious husband battering does take place, it is not a social problem of the same proportions as is wife battering (Ptacek, 1988). It often emerges in self-defense, is usually not physical, and when it is physical, tends to be less severe (e.g., Ptacek, 1988; Saunders, 1986). It should be emphasized, however, that members of either sex could perpetrate the patterns of psychological maltreatment we describe and that maltreatment can occur in same-sex relationships as well as in heterosexual relationships. Although psychological abuse may be present in intimate relations when physical violence is not, psychological abuse may be construed as a risk factor for, and in many cases a precursor to, violent behavior in any couple.

The psychosocial climate within which such abuse takes place often involves subtle manipulation—a form of "mind control," or "brainwashing" even—perpetrated by the abuser, including the use of potent strategies of manipulation (Andersen, Boulette, & Schwartz, 1991; Boulette & Andersen, 1985). Elsewhere termed *the marital brainwashing syndrome* (Boulette, 1981) and *traumatic bonding* (Dutton & Painter, 1981), this pattern is characterized by many of the features of psychological coercion and deception found in religious or political cults and that distinguish cults from other tightly knit social systems in society (Andersen, 1985; Andersen & Zimbardo, 1980). Further research is necessary to determine the prevalence and limiting conditions of this form of psychological maltreatment in disturbed relationships, but it is of value to consider its dimensions when trying to understand distressed couples.

Description of the Problem

Mind Control and Battering

Over the last two decades increasing attention has been directed toward the phenomenon of wife battering, a syndrome that appears to transcend both social class and ethnicity (Berk, Berk, Loseke, & Rauma, 1983; Dobash & Dobash, 1979; Gelles, 1976, 1997; Goodman *et al.*, 1993; Hilberman, 1980; Steinmetz, 1977; although, see Snyder & Fruchtman, 1981). The hypothesized association between wife battering and mind control has been suggested (Andersen, 1985; Boulette, 1981; Boulette & Andersen, 1985; Dutton & Painter, 1981; Hilberman, 1980), focusing on the manipulative techniques battering men may use against their wives (Steinmetz, 1977; Walker, 1978, 1979). These include isolation and the provocation of fear; the alternation of kindness and threats, which produces disequilibrium; and the induction of guilt, self-blame, dependency, and learned helplessness (cf. Abramson, Seligman, & Teasdale, 1978; Abramson, Alloy, & Metalsky, 1988; Seligman, 1975). Members of extremist cults report similar experiences in the form of isolation from others and from familiar habits, prohibitions on free expression and dissent, the mobilization of fear and guilt, and the establishment of an omnipotent "master" who demands self-sacrifice (Andersen & Zimbardo, 1980; Enroth, 1977; Singer, 1979).

Interpersonal systems, whether they are two-person relationships or larger social groups, have the potential to become totalistic in that they may exercise exceptional control over the freedom of their individual members (Andersen, 1985). The presence of totalism can be identified based on the degree to which such hierarchical control is present in the system. All in all, the degree to which a relationship is totalistic can be assessed simply by counting the number and severity of the features of psychological coercion (e.g., extreme control, social isolation, threat of harm, confusion and guilt, love strictly contingent on self-sacrifice and self-denunciation) and deception (e.g., direct misrepresentation or lying, distortion by omission or by misrepresentation of the others apparent options) that are present in the system (Andersen, 1985). Taking all of these potential determinants into account, a given case may vary in terms of the number of these features it possesses as well as their individual severity and duration. Intimate relationships that involve psychological coercion or mind control typically possess a significant number of features of this kind (Boulette, 1981; Boulette & Andersen, 1985), with the overall list presented in Table 1, and described in more detail in the following paragraphs.

Table 1.   Features of a Prototypic Pattern of
Psychological Maltreatment (Termed Psychological
Coercion)

Early verbal and/or physical aggression and dominance
Isolation/imprisonment to various degrees
Guilt induction to promote victim self-blame
Hope-instilling behaviors via contingent expressions of love
Fear arousal, maintenance, and escalation to terror
Promotion of powerlessness and helplessness
Pathological expressions of jealousy
Required secrecy
Enforced loyalty and self-denunciation

Early Verbal and or Physical Aggression and Dominance

During the early phases of the relationship, the abuser typically establishes his role as "boss" and "master" by using acts of verbal aggression that communicate control and dominance and the "worthlessness" of the female. These early acts of verbal aggression have been found to predict subsequent physical violence and may be understood as a "prehistory" of wife battering (Hyden, 1995).

Isolation/Imprisonment to Various Degrees

The male frequently isolates the woman from her friends and relatives, both geographically and emotionally. In this way, he weakens her support system, produces a more malleable spouse, and prevents her escape (Barnett, Martinez, & Keyson, 1996). Cultural notions of male and female roles may be used to legitimize and reinforce the male's control. For example, a recent meta-analysis of 29 studies shows a significant relationship between the maintenance of patriarchal ideology and wife assault (Sugarman & Frankel, 1996).

Guilt Induction to Promote Victim Self-Blame

The battering male may induce guilt in his victim by blaming *her* for the abuse until she comes to blame herself. Blaming the victim is frequently used to justify the use of coercive power (Kipnis, 1976); self-blame is also found among rape victims (Janoff-Bulman, 1979; Libow & Doty, 1979). Recent research has indicated that male-to-female violence is negatively related to level of perceived social support and positively linked with levels of victim self-blame (Barnett *et al.*, 1996).

Hope-Instilling Behaviors via Contingent Expressions of Love

The battered woman is usually provided with periodic hope that somehow her mistreatment and abuse will end if she pleads, cries, prays, endures, or sacrifices long enough. The man offers occasional hope-instilling behaviors in the form of contingent expressions of love that provide powerful intermittent reinforcements, prompting further self-sacrifice (Dutton & Painter, 1981; Steinmetz, 1977; Walker, 1979).

Fear Arousal, Maintenance, and Escalation to Terror

The battering man arouses fear in his spouse by frightening verbalizations, including threats of abandonment and of physical violence, and by actual physical abuse of varying severity. Prevalence studies indicate that between 21% and 34% of women in the United States will be physically assaulted—slapped, kicked, beaten, choked, threatened, or attacked with a weapon—by a spouse or intimate partner (Goodman *et al.*, 1993). A full 50% of the female murder victims in the United States during the 1980s were the victims of partner homicide (Browne & Williams, 1989).

Promotion of Powerlessness and Helplessness

Unpredictable and pervasive abuse eventually debilitates the battered woman, promoting feelings of powerlessness and helplessness. Her failure to predict or control her abuse may engender learned helplessness (Seligman, 1975) and make her believe her situation is hopeless (Abramson *et al.*, 1978; Andersen, 1990; Andersen & Schwartz, 1992). Her husband's control over household finances impoverishes her, and the victim-blaming postures of helpers who often believe in a just-world hypothesis (e.g., she must have provoked it, it's a family matter; Lerner, 1970) further promote self-blame and powerlessness (Boulette & Andersen, 1985; Dutton & Painter, 1981; Walker, 1979).

Pathological Expressions of Jealousy

The abuser may express a pathological jealousy and may monitor his mate's every movement, yet simultaneously brag about his own infidelity while he accuses his spouse of infidelity. This emotionally abusive pattern of accusation and denunciation may contribute to reducing the woman's sense of agency, control, and self-esteem and may further ensnare her in the pathological dyad (Aguilar & Nightingale, 1994).

Required Secrecy

Secrecy is intimately a part of abusive relationships. The abused woman's support system is usually compromised by her spouse as part of his effort to control and contain her. Research on women's survival strategies in abusive relationships indicates that women may collude in helping to render the violence invisible due to shame or a kind of faulty "face-saving effort" to preserve a sense of social integrity (see Lempert, 1996). In fact, her secrecy protects the abuser, and she, the victim, thus contributes to perpetuating the pathological system.

Enforced Loyalty and Self-Denunciation

Living in a closed system and being isolated from other people's opinions debilitates the woman. Hence, she may come to believe in the

Table 2.   Amnesty International's
Definition of Psychological Torture[a]

Isolation
Induced debility (sleep and food deprivation)
Monopolizing of perceptions
Verbal degradation (denial of powers, humiliation)
Hypnosis
Drugs
Threats to kill
Occasional indulgences

---

[a]Adapted from Walker (1988).

worldview offered by the abuser, excusing his oppressiveness, romanticizing his desirable characteristics, and even showing a missionary zeal about being the only one who can rescue him from his vulnerability, temper, or alcoholism (Hilberman, 1980). Often she believes that only she can understand him. Interestingly, prisoners of war are debilitated in similar ways and come to feel intense loyalty to their captors (as in the Stockholm syndrome; Ochberg, 1971), expressing attachment based on the experience of terror and gratefulness for not being further damaged or killed (Boulette & Andersen, 1985; Dutton & Painter, 1981; Libow & Doty, 1979; Zimbardo, Ebbesen, & Maslach, 1977; see also Freire, 1984). The set of factors described in psychological maltreatment of partners is uncannily similar to the criteria for psychological torture applied by Amnesty International (cited by Walker, 1988), as shown in Table 2.

Case Histories

The following case histories demonstrate many of the prototypic features we have described as characteristic of psychological maltreatment in spouse abuse. Case 1 involves an unmarried Latino woman with four children who is ensnared in an abusive relationship with a violent, substance-abusing partner. Case 2 involves a married white woman from an affluent background, who struggles to disengage from a relationship marked by physical, psychological, and sexual abuse.

Case 1: Maria
Maria is a frail, 25-year-old Latino woman who presented at a shelter with her children seeking protection from her abusive boyfriend, Roberto, with whom she had been involved for the past 10 years. Roberto, 30, was the father

of Maria's four children, who ranged in age from 3 to 9 years. When she first met Roberto, Maria was flattered by his attention and impressed by his status in the neighborhood as a "cool" guy who always seemed to have money to spend on clothes, cars, and her. She became pregnant at 16 and dropped out of school, at Roberto's insistence, to have the baby. In the initial phase of the relationship, Maria was "crazy in love" with Roberto. He was generous, ardent, and made her feel "like a real woman." She recalls that he was always possessive of her and jealous of any time she spent with her friends or family. But initially she was flattered by his attention and by his passion for her.

After she become pregnant, she moved in with Roberto, and he began to show a different side of his personality to her. Specifically, he became "moody," alternating between adoring her and "snapping" at her for small things—not having food ready for him the moment he got home, not ironing his clothes well enough. Maria tried to please Roberto, believing that her duties were in the home taking care of him and preparing for the baby that would soon come.

Living with Roberto, Maria discovered that the money he had was earned through petty theft and drug dealing in the neighborhood. She was frightened and upset by the discovery and begged him to get a "regular job." She recalled that the confrontation about his work was the first violent incident between them. Roberto was enraged that "a little slut" like Maria dared to question him and he went after her, beating her badly in the face. Maria was so ashamed that she stayed inside for the next week, refusing to leave home or have contact with her family for fear they would see the bruises and blame her for provoking Roberto. After the initial incident, Roberto showered Maria with gifts, including an engagement ring, and promised to "marry her and take care of her for the rest of her life." By the time the baby arrived, Maria and Roberto had been together for almost a year and a half and a pattern of seduction and generosity, followed by arbitrary violence, jealousy, and rage, had been set in motion—which intensified over the years and finally culminated in Maria's fleeing to "save her life and her children."

Maria came from a family of five children. Her father worked sporadically as a handyman and was intermittently on public assistance. Her mother contributed with cleaning and baby-sitting when times were particularly tough, although Maria's father objected to his wife working and felt humiliated and angry at her attempts to bring in additional income. Maria's family life was stormy and dominated by her father and his anger at his plight in life. Although he never beat her mother, Maria's father was often verbally abusive toward her and cheated on her openly with women in the neighborhood. Her family, who believed that a woman's place was in the home with the babies, encouraged Maria's relationship with Roberto, although they wanted the two to marry. Throughout the relationship the issue of marriage was a source of conflict between Maria and Roberto. He dangled the prospect of marriage before her like a carrot, to bribe or control her. When she became frustrated with him and wanted to leave, he used her unmarried status to humiliate her, calling her a "slut" and a "whore" and assuring her that no other man would want "a used-up piece of shit" like Maria.

In spite of the intensifying cycles of abuse Maria stayed with Roberto. Over the years, he continued to deal drugs and to engage in petty crimes and he also began drinking heavily. Her decision to finally flee to the shelter came after a particular violent episode in which Roberto, while drunk, not only beat Maria but then turned on her oldest son, Robbie, 9, who was trying to protect his mother. The incident was provoked by a seemingly trivial event: Maria had not cleaned up the breakfast dishes by the time Roberto arrived home. When little Robbie attempted to intervene in Roberto beating Maria, Roberto punched his son and knocked him unconscious while the other children cowered in the corner of the kitchen, observing the scene. Roberto then punched Maria in the stomach, took the dirty dishes and broke them over her head, before slamming out of the small apartment.

Maria rushed her family to the emergency room where they were treated for bruises and injuries and then were referred by social workers to a shelter for battered women. By this time, Maria was well known in the emergency room, but this was the first time one of her children required medical attention because of Roberto's violence. Maria, who had presented on other occasions with injuries including a broken rib, a broken nose, and a fractured arm, always lied about the source of her injuries and refused to file a complaint against Roberto or seek assistance. This time, hospital social workers were able to facilitate an immediate placement in a shelter and also notified child welfare because of the injuries little Robbie sustained (bruising in the face and head, no concussion). When Maria arrived at the shelter she was depressed, confused, anxious, and afraid, worried about Roberto retaliating, and anguished at the idea of losing a man whom she still felt she loved and whom she believed loved her. She expressed feelings of hopelessness and suicidal ideation. She was referred to outpatient therapy for battered women (a group) and was counseled about her legal options. Maria felt overwhelmed at the idea of trying to live without Roberto. She had never supported herself or worked outside the home, and she had no skills or independent means.

Ultimately, she returned to Roberto and the cycle of violence and reconciliation continued. The children began to deteriorate in their functioning, developing symptoms that included enuresis and encopresis, conduct problems, and panic attacks. Child welfare eventually intervened and placed them in foster care. At that point, Maria gathered the resolve to leave Roberto permanently. She moved in with her sister (a single mother), retaining a court order to prevent Roberto from entering the property or approaching her or the children, and she petitioned to have the children returned to her custody. She then committed herself and her children to a course of outpatient psychiatric treatment for survivors of family abuse and violence.

Case 2: Anna

Anna was a 35-year-old white woman who worked as a bank teller. Her physician referred her for outpatient psychotherapy after he found no physical explanation for her recurrent panic attacks, dizziness, chest pain, cold numb hands and arms, and shortness of breath. She reported that she had experienced these symptoms 2 years ago when she left her husband. At that time, she had sought treatment with a psychiatrist who diagnosed her with an anxiety disorder and treated her with an anxiolytic. Her symptoms largely remitted after 10 months, and then recurred when she saw a man who looked like her ex-husband at the bank. She left work immediately and was unable to return to work due to her debilitating symptoms. In individual psychotherapy, she began to talk about her marriage and about the experiences that had culminated in her seeking treatment.

Anna reported that, 8 years prior, she had married an older man, Tom, who was a prominent and well-known attorney in the town where she lived in Texas. Anna remembered that she was initially struck by Tom's sensitivity, his generosity, and his desire for her. She had had a series of frustrating relationships with younger men who seemed "unable to commit," and she was moved and thrilled finally to meet a man who was able "to be close." Anna remembered early on in the relationship how Tom seemed endlessly interested in the details of her life, always wanting to know what she had done during the day, who she had seen, and what her schedule was like. At that time, Anna "appreciated Tom's caring so much." She later recognized these behaviors as precursors of the pathological jealousy and possessiveness that would develop.

Specifically, once the couple married, Tom insisted that Anna give up work and stay home. He bought a large house for his "princess" about an hour and a half away from her hometown. Tom always rejected any efforts to socialize with friends because he "just wanted to enjoy being together." He insisted on knowing Anna's whereabouts at all times and even checked the odometer on her car daily to make sure she had not left the house without reporting to him. He controlled all the finances and allotted her a small "allowance." She recalled an incident when they went shopping for groceries and she forgot an item. She turned down an aisle to get the item and Tom followed, seeing a man nearby. Tom flew into a rage and accused Anna of plotting to be unfaithful with this stranger. Anna was humiliated by Tom's behavior. When they returned home an angry fight ensued. Anna told him she could not "live this way" and threatened to leave him. Tom responded with tears, professing a great love for her, and promising to change. Instead, his jealousy, domination, and control only intensified.

Over time, Tom increasingly isolated and alienated Anna from her own personal network. He forbade her to visit her elderly parents as well as her friends. He called her repeatedly throughout the day to check on her. If she was not there, he would return home to find her. He came home at odd hours, parked the car blocks away from their house, and then snuck up to the house, spying on Anna, expecting to find her with another man. He accused her, insisted that she confess her infidelities, even begging and promising he would forgive her, and they could start over. In one encounter, exasperated by his insistence that she had been unfaithful, Anna jokingly "confessed" that she had had sex with the elderly non-English-speaking gardener. Tom became enraged. He punched her, dragged her into the bedroom by her hair, and raped her.

He told her he would never give her a divorce and that no one would ever believe her stories anyway, if she tried to tell everyone and to leave him. Shortly after this incident, Anna did leave Tom, returning to live with her parents, and she sought treatment for anxiety and panic attacks. She also began psychotherapy in which she sought to understand how this abusive relationship had developed, and why she still remained hesitant to divorce Tom. Although she recognized Tom's jealousy as excessive and irrational, she somehow believed she was to blame for the problems in the relationship and that it was her "job" to make the marriage work. It was very difficult for Anna to reconcile the coexistence of love and abuse in the marriage. Anna had come from an intact, middle-class background, with no family history of psychopathology, and no history of spousal abuse or battering. None of Anna's previous relationships had been abusive, and there were no clues in her past history or in her psychological profile to predict or account for her involvement in this abusive and dangerous relationship. The therapist focused on helping Anna to understand the danger she was in, to work through the trauma that she had experienced in the marriage, and to give up Tom.

Tom began stalking Anna and threatening her parents. Anna finally fled Texas, retained a restraining order, and filed for divorce. Eighteen months later, she was living independently and working as a bank teller when she saw the man who resembled Tom, and her symptoms were triggered once again. This time she returned to therapy and was able to work through the sequelae of the abuse.

Medical Issues

Certain types of injuries may be diagnostic of spousal abuse in particular, such as injuries to the head, neck, upper abdomen, and upper extremities (Goodstein, 1987; Goodstein & Page, 1981). In Case 1, the woman sustained a broken nose, a broken rib, and a fractured arm. Her son sustained injuries to his face and head. This victim's initial refusal to acknowledge the battering is also typical of first encounters with battered women (Hilberman, 1980). This poses a serious obstacle to appropriate psychological treatment, as well as to the recognition and reporting of abuse by medical professionals, who may be the providers of first resort.

Child abuse often co-occurs with spouse abuse, as illustrated in Case 1. A full evaluation of the physical and psychological well-being of the children in all families in which violence occurs should, of course, be performed. In Case 2, the victim was raped by her husband, but she did not press charges or present for medical treatment. Sexual abuse is a common concomitant of spousal abuse. As many as 58% of the battered women in one sample reported having been raped by their batterer (Walker, 1981).

Prevalence studies indicate that between 22% and 35% of women who present at emergency rooms are there because of symptoms related to ongoing abuse—either an injury directly resulting from abuse or secondary manifestations of the stress of living under abuse (Warshaw, 1989). Recent research on domestic violence, performed by confidentially sampling the case histories of 648 women who presented in an emergency room or walk-in clinic for any reason, indicated that 52.2% of the subjects reported having been assaulted, threatened, or made to feel afraid by partners at some time in their lives, and 11.9% of the sample reported having experienced domestic violence in the last month (Abbott, Johnson, Koziol-McLain, & Lowenstein, 1995). It has been reported that as many as 64% of hospitalized female psychiatric patients have histories of physical abuse as adults and 37% of all obstetric patients are at risk for abuse during pregnancy (cf. Warshaw, 1989).

Research has suggested that the staff in hospital emergency rooms rarely ask patients about the cause of their injuries and readily accept seemingly plausible stories of accidental misfortunes (Dutton, 1983; Kurz, 1987; Stark, Flitcraft, & Frazier, 1979). In fact, one survey of 1,000 battered women (solicited by advertisement) indicated that they sought help from medical professionals more frequently than from other professionals, and yet were less satisfied with the physician's response (Bowker & Maurer, 1987).

It should be noted that psychological abuse is likely to be even more difficult for primary care physicians and nurses to detect than the causes of their multiple injuries. The woman's psychological damage can vary dramatically in symptom presentation and in severity. In Case 1, the victim manifested both anxiety and depressive symptomatology, while the victim in Case 2 manifested more prominent anxiety symptomatology, including full-blown panic attacks. In recent years, the diagnosis of posttraumatic stress disorder has been applied to conceptualizing the constellation of symptoms that abused women may manifest, including anxiety, depression, suicidality, depersonalization, autonomic arousal, and dissociation (Browne, 1993; Koss, 1993; Goodman et al., 1993). It is also essential to evaluate and treat children who have witnessed or been the object of abuse and family violence. The children in Case 2 manifested some of the common and prevalent childhood disorders associated with stress and trauma, including enuresis and encopresis, acting-out behavior, and childhood depression, the latter of which may present in masked form and require careful assessment and treatment.

Legal Issues

It has been suggested that if physical assault between a man and a woman in an intimate relationship were simply treated in the same manner as physical assault between strangers, more progress would be made in the justice system response to battering (Emery, 1989). Research on the efficacy of using the criminal justice system to respond to cases of wife assault supports the notion that arrest, prosecution, and treatment of offenders may be effective in reducing recidivism (Dutton, 1987). In one study, for example, police officers were randomly assigned to respond to domestic calls either by attempting to mediate the dispute informally, by ordering the assailant to leave the premises, or by arresting him. A 6-month follow-up indicated that only 10% of the men in the arrest group repeated the violence, in contrast to 19% in the informal mediation group and 24% in the leave-the-premises group (Sherman & Berk, 1984).

Unfortunately, many factors other than the requirement to sign a complaint and press charges seem to conspire to make the criminal justice system ineffectual in cases of spousal abuse. One factor has to do with the attitudes of medical and mental health professionals who often appear to believe that spousal assault is best dealt with within the family (Saunders & Size, 1986) and that efforts should be made to keep the family together (Emery, 1989). Hence, law enforcement and legal professionals often fail to make appropriate referrals. Not surprisingly, when police officers have made it a policy to bring criminal charges against husbands who beat their wives, surveys of battered wives indicate a higher level of satisfaction with police services. However, police officers themselves report more negative attitudes about the policy (Jaffe, Wolfe, Telford, & Austin, 1986). Similarly, when battered women have been compared with police officers, the majority of the victims preferred arrest, while very few of the police officers viewed arrest as the best solution (Saunders & Size, 1986; see also Bowker, 1983). Even in the mid-1990s, research examining the role of patriarchal attitudes in police enforcement of protective orders for battered women indicated that protective orders are rarely treated seriously by the police or the courts (Rigakos, 1995). That is, the occupational culture of police forces may lead to exaggerated patriarchal notions of male roles and to blaming the victim by fostering images of women as manipulative and histrionic. Victim blaming among police officers was also found to be positively correlated with traditional attitudes about women's roles (Saunders & Size, 1986).

Social and Family Issues

It has been suggested that battering is not only a societal problem but also one that is largely social in origin (Davis, 1987; Ferraro, 1988; Walker, 1979). Historically, husbands in Western society were legally and morally responsible for their wives' actions, and the use of physical force was acceptable for certain offenses, so long as it did not cause serious physical injuries (Walker, 1979, 1981). In fact, it was legal for a man to physically chastise his wife less than 100 years ago (Davidson, 1978; Ptacek, 1988). Recent data from a national sample of over 5,000 families suggests, in fact, that men who agree with the normative question, "Are there situations you can imagine in which you would approve of a husband slugging his wife?" are more likely to abuse their wives (Kantor & Straus, 1987). Furthermore, within the context of sex-role socialization, a man may be taught that his role is to be intelligent, strong, and the economic provider in a marriage and that his wife's role is to take care of his emotional needs. He may also learn that "controlling" his wife, making her adhere to his desires, is his "right," a belief that may serve to legitimize violence (Ponzetti, Cate, & Koval, 1982). When his wife fails to meet his emotional needs, he may then act out aggressively, at which point "the difference between a slap in the name of discipline and one occurring out of frustration may become an issue of semantics" (Walker, 1981, p. 82; see also Ferraro, 1988).

In Case 1, the battered woman, her partner, and her family shared common patriarchal notions about the subservient role of women in marriage. In both Case 1 and Case 2 the women were nearly powerless in their relationships, were socially isolated, and were burdened with the belief that it was their responsibility to make the relationship work. Sex-role socialization, in general, tends to support the notion that the success or failure of intimate relationships is the woman's responsibility, and this may lead some women to make great efforts to stay in intimate relationships, even after episodes of abuse, to show their commitment to their partner and to weathering the "difficult times" together (Dutton & Painter, 1981; Strube, 1988). In addition, when an abusive event occurs, the woman may presume it will not recur, and so "try to make the relationship work under the belief that if she tries hard enough her efforts will succeed" (Strube, 1988, p. 24).

Traumatic Bonding

In cases of wife assault, the aggressor usually uses violence in part to create and sustain a power advantage in the relationship (Dutton & Painter, 1981). Creating a power advantage that bonds the victim to her abuser can be accomplished using various forms of psychological abuse which include complete control of a woman's use of her time, her social contacts, and her capacity to view herself as a worthwhile person. It need not be (and usually is not) limited to physical violence. *Traumatic bonding*, which refers to the tenacious attachment that develops between a victim and her abuser, is illustrated in both of the case histories.

Psychological Entrapment/Investment Models

It has been argued that a kind of psychological entrapment exists in battering relationships (Strube, 1988). The woman begins the relationship with her partner with the goal of making it work and later encounters obstacles that she tries to disregard, making a greater investment (trying harder) to reach her goal of relationship harmony (cf. Brockner & Rubin, 1985). As further incidents of abuse occurs, she is likely to feel conflicted about staying as she may feel there is still some chance that she can make the relationship work. In this view, it is the woman's choice to stay or leave the relationship, but the extent of initial investment militates against her leaving because she feels personally responsible for the success of the relationship (Strube, 1988). An investment model of commitment to explain women's "stay/leave" behaviors in abusive relationships has been proposed (Rusbult & Martz, 1995). Analyses of data from 100 interviews at a battered women's shelter suggested that women did not stay in or return to abusive relationship because they were satisfied with those relationships. Rather, they stayed because they felt they had poorer-quality economic alternatives and were more heavily invested (e.g., had children or were married). On another level, the baffling simultaneity of love and violence for abused women doubtless contributes to the tenacity of their bond to the aggressor in these pathological dyads (Lempert, 1996).

Economic Stress

People in battering relationships are often financially burdened, usually owing to unemployment (Straus, Gelles, & Steimetz, 1980). When a woman has few personal resources, this is associated with greater severity in violence (Mitchell & Hodson, 1983), and it is much more difficult to leave the relationship (Kalmuss & Straus, 1982; Walker, 1979). Interestingly, recent research on correlates of battered women's decisions to return home to the abuser showed that women were more likely to return home when (1) family income was relatively high, (2) they were unemployed, (3) they had been victims of severe abuse, and (4) they had negative perceptions of themselves (Johnson, 1992).

Alcohol Abuse

As illustrated in Case 1, the literature clearly indicates a strong relationship between alcohol use and marital violence (Eisenberg & Micklow, 1977; Gayford, 1975; Gelles, 1975, 1998a; Kantor & Straus, 1987; Leonard, 1999; Ponzetti et al., 1982; Rosenbaum & O'Leary, 1981; Roy, 1977; Walker, 1979, 1988). Battering husbands often abuse alcohol, and this may have a disinhibiting effect on their violent behavior. Abusive men are significantly more alcoholic than are nonabusive men, even when both are in discordant marriages (Van Hasselt, Morrison, & Bellack, 1985). Recent research has shown that male alcoholics who physically abuse their partners differ in important ways from alcoholics who do not (Murphy & O'Farrell, 1996). Specifically, alcoholic abusers have a more severe, early onset form of alcoholism, are more likely to binge-drink, have more negative styles of communicating, and maintain strong beliefs about the negative influences of alcohol on marriage.

Power Imbalance in the Relationship

Power-imbalanced relationships are associated with spousal abuse, especially when the imbalance threatens the male's power (Babcock, Waltz, Jacobson, & Gottman, 1993). Research based on a random sample of over 1,000 married women (Harris and Associates, 1979) showed a greater risk for wife battering, including both life-threatening violence (i.e., with a weapon) and psychological abuse, in couples in which the woman's occupational status exceeded her education to a greater degree than did her husband's (i.e., when she was, relatively speaking, an overachiever) (Hornung, McCullough, & Sugimoto, 1981). Furthermore, egalitarian couples have a lower rate of conflict and violence than do couples in which one partner is dominant, among whom conflict is more positively correlated with violent behavior (Coleman & Straus, 1986).

Intergenerational Transmission of Violence

A cycle of violence hypothesis has been proposed that states that men who experience childhood abuse become more likely to abuse others as adults, probably due to vicarious learning through exposure to violent models. Numerous studies have shown evidence for long-term, specific effects of childhood abuse and neglect on subsequent abusive and criminal behavior in men (see Dutton & Hart, 1992, for review). The empirical literature on wife battering demonstrates that it does tend to be learned in the home and to be passed down between generations (Choice, Lamke, & Pittman, 1995; Doumas, Margolin, & Richard, 1994; Gayford, 1975; Gelles, 1975, 1998b; Giles-Sims, 1998; Hilberman & Munson, 1978; Roy, 1977; Straus *et al.*, 1980). In particular, a large percentage of battering men sampled either observed or experienced violence as children (Rosenbaum & O'Leary, 1981). Hence, the importance in spousal abuse of the perpetrator's own familial upbringing has been stressed (e.g., Belsky, 1980; Kalmuss, 1984).

Assessment of Psychopathology

The Battering Male

While the two men in the cases described in this chapter differ widely in terms of their socioeconomic backgrounds and occupations, they share certain characteristics, including their need for excessive control, their inability to tolerate any threat to their domination, and marked problems managing anger. In characterizing the battering male, mounting empirical evidence debunks the notion of a single "prototypic" batterer, although certain common characteristics or clusters of characteristics may distinguish men who batter from those who do not (Walker, 1995). Specifically, typologies have been described around the dimension of severity of abuse, as well as around the dimension of target of abuse—distinguishing men who batter exclusively within their families from men who are also violent outside the family (see Walker, 1995, for review). Recently, a third typology has evolved, leading to the identification of three distinct groups of batterers: (1) men who batter at home and are motivated by abnormal power and control needs, who may be helped with psychological work and education about anger management and gender role attitudes; (2) men who have significant psychological problems (including depression, obsessive-compulsive behavior, paranoid disorders, and borderline traits); and (3) men who have committed other crimes outside the home and who meet criteria for antisocial personality disorder, who are quite treatment resistant (Dutton & Starzomski, 1993; Saunders, 1992).

Research has shown that battering men often meet criteria for various personality disorders, the most prominent being borderline and antisocial (Dutton & Starzomski, 1993; Hamberger & Hastings, 1986). Recent research on a sample of 75 dyads in which wife abuse had occurred showed that borderline personality organization and anger (in the male partners) accounted for 50% of the variance in women's reports of domination and isolation and for 35% of the women's reports of emotional abuse by their spouses (Dutton & Starzomski, 1993).

As noted, it has been suggested that abusive men have more traditional views of women relative to nonabusive men (Rosenbaum & O'Leary, 1981; Walker, 1979, 1988) and that they may be particularly sensitive to threats to their masculinity (Gondolf & Hanneken, 1987). Research indicates that batterers may have low self-esteem and use violence to compensate for these feelings (Johnston, 1988). In addition, battering men have been shown to lack assertiveness (i.e., the skills to communicate their emotions and needs in interpersonal relationships; Rosenbaum & O'Leary, 1981) and also show deficits in interpersonal problem-solving skills (Van Hasselt, Morrison, & Bellack, 1987). Similarly, men who lack communication skills have been found to be more likely to respond to their own anger as a cue to aggression (Dutton & Browning, 1988; Rule & Nesdale, 1976).

From a physiological perspective, studies of arousal responses among abusive males have shown that these men respond with more arousal and anger than do nonabusive males to an argument between a man and a woman (Dutton & Browning, 1988). It has been suggested that, for battering men, the argument signifies threat of abandonment and loss of power over the woman (Dutton & Browning, 1988; Walker, 1988), and hence any hint of this in the woman may serve as a situational trigger for violence.

The Battered Woman

It is difficult to identify the battered woman and to separate longstanding personality characteristics from the psychosocial responses to the pathological system in which she is ensnared. While research supports the existence of a common symptomatic presentation that develops as a result of psychological and physical abuse, there is little evidence to suggest a prototypic premorbid portrait of the battered woman (Goodman et al., 1993). Rather, the current literature on spousal abuse suggests that women who have endured abusive relationships frequently develop a distinguishable pattern of symptoms, termed the *battered woman syndrome*, which may be conceptualized as a version of posttraumatic stress disorder (PTSD) (Walker, 1988). The symptoms overlap with both affective and anxiety disorders, but they contain other features as well, such as dissociation, memory loss, reexperiencing of the traumatic event, disruption of interpersonal relationships, and associated psychophysiological responses. The use of the PTSD diagnosis to describe abused women has important conceptual and political implications, as it suggests that the psychological sequelae of spouse abuse (or "aftereffects") are normal reactions to external trauma rather than manifestations of individual psychopathology (Goodman *et al.*, 1993).

The sequalae of psychological coercion and battering can be described in terms of three aversive psychological states: debility, dependency, and dread, all of which typically are suffered by victims of brainwashing (Hilberman & Munson, 1978; West, 1963). Battered women experience paralyzing terror, constant anxiety, apprehension, vigilance, and feelings of impending doom (Walker, 1988). As the oppression and fear continue and perhaps escalate, these women may also come to feel fatigued, passive, and unable to act, exhibiting concrete thinking and poor memory (Dutton & Painter, 1981; Strube, 1988; Walker, 1979; see also West, 1963).

Clinically, these victimized women often appear detached and often smile when describing their frightening experiences, separating their affective responses (e.g., terror, humiliation) from their description. They rarely express anger over their plight and typically report multiple somatic and other symptoms that fit within the diagnostic categories of panic disorder, recurrent major depression, dysthymic disorder, or somatization disorder (American Psychiatric Association, 1994).

Research has shown that the frequency of personally experienced violence in a woman's family of origin is associated with increased violence in her own marriage (Dutton, 1983; Schulman, 1979; Straus, 1977). However, battered and nonbattered women do not always differ in whether or not they witnessed parental spousal abuse or experienced child abuse in their families of origin (Rosenbaum & O'Leary, 1981). Hence, neither witnessing violence in one's own parents nor being the target of it is a necessary or sufficient condition for being a battered woman later in life. Even if the abuse in the child's home is mainly psychological, however, she may learn important victim characteristics, such as passivity, self-sacrifice, and tolerance for psychological abuse and may ultimately be attracted to abusive men. It is important to note that, from a social-psychological standpoint, it is quite possible that a marital situation could be constructed in which the features of psychological coercion and mind control were of sufficient magnitude (cf. Andersen, 1985; Boulette & Andersen, 1985) that women from any number of different backgrounds might be retained within it.

Treatment Options

One major challenge in the treatment of spousal abuse is that the intervention for either partner is unlikely to be successful while the couple remains together, because in this case the abuse is unlikely to end. Although some have argued for a family systems approach, most interventions in spousal abuse focus on individual family members (Emery, 1989). Treatments directed at the abuser may be most appropriate, especially as an initial intervention, because changing the individual changes the cycle of abuse (Emery, 1989).

Unfortunately, helping to effect a separation is, perhaps, the most difficult challenge. The husband's psychological coercion may have rendered the wife too helpless to escape, and the husband remains inaccessible to treatment because he denies any problems and projects all blame onto his wife (Boulette & Andersen, 1985; Steinmetz, 1977; Straus *et al.*, 1980; Walker, 1979, 1988). The irony for the battered woman is that separation is necessary for treatment and ultimately for survival, and yet when she leaves her husband she exposes herself to an ever-increasing risk of violent retaliation for this abandonment.

Treating the Battering Man

Consistent with the notion that there does not exist a single, "prototypic" abuser (Walker, 1995), the most relevant treatment issues for the battering male can be identified only on the basis of a comprehensive assessment. If the individual has an antisocial personality or borderline personality disorder, the prognosis is poor. If he has a severe identity disorder characterized by low self-esteem and easily threatened masculinity, treatment is likely to be long-term. If he is abusing alcohol or other substances, proper referral is obviously needed. For an intermittent impulse control disorder, referral to a psychiatrist may be appropriate as medication can be helpful. With relatively minor disorders characterized by poor anger management and interpersonal skills, as well as with the more severe disorders, the individual may benefit (within the limitations of his pathology) from learning how to (a) control anger and physical aggression, (b) handle separation/abandonment, (c) treat his partner with respect rather than trying to control her, (d) value relationships built on equal partnership, (e) admit mistakes and personal foibles, and (f) become more empathic with others (Walker, 1981).

Treatment programs for spousal abuse are often based on cognitive-behavioral approaches to stress management, parenting, and controlling anger and aggression (Ptacek, 1988). Both researchers and clinicians have noted that violent men may have trouble distinguishing anger from sexual arousal cues (cf. Malamuth, Feshback, & Jaffee, 1977, for rapists), suggesting the importance of developing treatment techniques that focus on this problem (Walker, 1981). Interestingly, one study of abusive men who had reformed in treatment indicated that they attributed their successful treatment to learning to accept responsibility for their problems, learning to become more empathetic, and learning to redefine their conceptions of their own manhood (Gondolf & Hanneken, 1987). Other interventions have also focused on the reduction of stereotypic sex-role expectations among abusive males and on teaching effective interpersonal skills as an alternative to explosive, violent outbursts (Ponzetti *et al.*, 1982). Even though there is debate about the effectiveness of court-mandated treatment program for offenders, recent research has begun to suggest that mandated cognitive-behavioral intervention strategies can be effective (Emery, 1989).

Treating the Battered Woman

In dealing with the female in a battering relationship, it is critical to assess not only her symptoms and the level of her impairment but also her potential for being hurt or killed. In addition, battered, debilitated, helpless women have been known to kill their aggressors. This risk *must* be evaluated. If the woman remains in the home, her treatment may need to be kept hidden from her partner because of the danger of treatment sabotage and danger to the therapist. At the outset, the biggest problem in treating the battered woman is that she may minimize her psychological and physical abuse. She may even succeed in convincing the therapist that she has the situation under control. That is, she may believe that if she just does everything the batterer wants, she will have nothing to fear (Walker, 1981).

Once the denial and minimization has been overcome, treatment should focus on reducing risk of harm, facilitating escape and resettlement, ultimately dealing with any posttraumatic stress sequelae, helping her to work through the loss of the relationship, and helping her to recognize her own worth and value. Ultimately, the battered woman's own conflicts about vulnerability, power, and control must also be explored so as to discourage her from repeating the same pattern with other abusive men. As she improves, social support groups may be helpful to the battered woman in reinforcing her role as rescuer rather than victim and by reducing her sense of alienation and shame through sharing common experiences with other women who have survived abuse. Community, family-system, and individual interventions that empower women and encourage both men and women to value equal partnership in marital relationships are important in reducing spousal abuse and in preventing the development of marital conflict and pathological family ties (Coleman & Straus, 1986).

Summary

Although the precise methodology for identifying psychological maltreatment in relationships, especially in battering relationships, awaits further empirical research, any relationship that involves covert strategies of psychological coercion or regulation over individual freedoms is maladaptive (Andersen et al., 1991; Andersen, 1985; Boulette & Andersen, 1985). By definition, the batterer in such relationships makes use of psychological coercion, oppression, and degradation to get his partner to adhere to his needs (Boulette & Andersen, 1985; Dutton & Painter, 1981; Walker, 1979). If physicians, nurses, police officers, legal professionals, community workers, and mental health professionals can learn to identify this syndrome with its developing signs and to make the appropriate referrals when such abuse is suspected, further progress might be made in ending the human tragedy of spousal abuse.

References

Abbott, J., Johnson, R., Koziol-McLain, J., & Lowenstein, Sr. (1995). *Journal of the American Medical Association, 273,* 1763–1767.

Abramson, L. Y., Seligman, M. E. P., & Teasdale, J. D. (1978). Learned helplessness in humans: Critique and reformulation. *Journal of Abnormal Psychology, 87,* 40–47.

Abramson, L. Y., Alloy, L. B., & Metalsky, G. I. (1988). The cognitive diathesis-stress theories of depression: Towards an adequate evaluation of the theories' validities. In L. B. Alloy (Ed.) *Cognitive processes in depression* (pp. 3–30). New York: Guilford Press.

Aguilar, R. J., & Nightingale, N. N. (1994). The impact of specific battering experiences on the self-esteem of abused women. *Journal of Family Violence, 9,* 35–45.

American Psychiatric Association. (1994). *Diagnostic and statistical manual of mental disorders* (4th ed.). Washington, DC: Author.

Andersen, S. M. (1985). Identifying coercion and deception in social systems. In B. Kilbourne (Ed.), *Divergent perspectives on the new religions* (pp. 12–23). Washington, DC: American Association for the Advancement of Science.

Andersen, S. M. (1990). The inevitability of future suffering: The role of depressive predictive certainty in depression. *Social Cognition, 8,* 203–228.

Andersen, S. M., & Schwartz, A. H. (1992). Intolerance of ambiguity and depression: A cognitive vulnerability factor linked to hopelessness. *Social Cognition, 10,* 271–298.

Andersen, S. M., & Zimbardo, P. G. (1980). Resisting mind control. *USA Today, 109,* 44–47.

Andersen, S. M., Boulette, T. R., & Schwartz, A. H. (1991). Psychological maltreatment of spouses. In R. T. Ammerman & M. Hersen (Eds.), *Case studies in family violence* (pp. 293–327). New York: Plenum Press.

Babcock, J. C., Waltz, J., Jacobson, N. S., & Gottman, J. M. (1993). Power and violence: The relation between communication patterns, power discrepancies, and domestic violence [Special section: Couples and couples therapy]. *Journal of Consulting and Clinical Psychology, 61,* 40–50.

Barnett, O., Martinez, T. E., & Keyson, M. (1996). The relationship between violence, social support and self-blame in battered women. *Journal of Interpersonal Violence, 11,* 221–233.

Belsky, J. (1980). Child maltreatment: An ecological integration. *American Psychologist, 35,* 320–335.

Berk, R. A., Berk, S. F., Loseke, D. R., & Rauma, D. (1983). Mutual combat and other family violence myths. In D. Finkelhor, R. J. Gelles, G. Hotaling, & M. A. Straus (Eds.), *The dark side of families* (pp. 197–212). Beverly Hills, CA: Sage.

Boulette, T. R. (1981, August). *The marital brainwashing syndrome.* Paper presented at the American Psychological Association Convention, Los Angeles.

Boulette, T. R., & Andersen, S. M. (1985). "Mind control" and the battering of women. *Community Mental Health Journal, 21,* 109–117.

Bowker, L. H. (1983). Battered wives, lawyers, and district attorneys: An examination of law in action. *Journal of Criminal Justice, 11,* 403–412.

Bowker, L. H., & Maurer, L. (1987). The medical treatment of battered wives. *Women and Health, 12,* 25–45.

Brockner, J., & Rubin, J. Z. (1985). *Entrapment in escalating conflicts: A social psychological analysis.* New York: Springer-Verlag.

Browne, A. (1993). Violence against women by male partners: Prevalence, outcomes, and policy implications. *American Psychologist, 48,* 1077–1087.

Browne, A., & Williams, K. R. (1989). Exploring the effect of resource availability and the likelihood of female-perpetrated homicides. *Law and Society Review, 23,* 75–94.

Choice, P., Lamke, L. K., & Pittman, J. F. (1995). Conflict resolution strategies and marital distress as mediating factors in the link between witnessing interparental violence and wife battering. *Violence and Victims, 10,* 107–119.

Coleman, D. H., & Straus, M. A. (1986). Marital power, conflict, and violence in a nationally representative sample of American couples. *Violence and Victims, 12,* 141–157.

Davidson, T. (1978). *Conjugal crime: Understanding and changing the wife beating pattern.* New York: Hawthorn.

Davis, L. V. (1987). Battered women: The transformation of a social problem. *Social Work, 32,* 306–311.

Dobash, R. E., & Dobash, R. (1979). *Violence against wives.* New York: Free Press.

Doumas, D., Margolin, G., & John, R. (1994). The intergenerational transmission of aggression across three generations. *Journal of Family Violence, 9,* 157–175.

Dutton, D. G. (1983, April). *Masochism as an explanation for traumatic bonding: An example of the "fundamental attribution error."* Paper presented at the American Orthopsychiatric Convention, Boston.

Dutton, D. G. (1987). Wife assault: Social psychological contributions to criminal justice policy. *Applied Social Psychology Annual, 7,* 238–261.

Dutton, D. G., & Browning, J. J. (1988). Concern for power, fear of intimacy, and aversive stimuli for wife assault. In G. T. Hotaling, D. Finkelhor, J. T. Kirkpatrick, & M. A. Straus (Eds.), *Family abuse and its consequences* (pp. 163–175). Beverly Hills, CA: Sage.

Dutton, D. G., & Hart, S. D. (1992). Evidence for long-term, specific effects of childhood abuse and neglect on criminal behavior in men. *International Journal of Offender Therapy and Comparative Criminology, 36,* 129–137.

Dutton, D. G., & Painter, S. L. (1981). Traumatic bonding: The development of emotional attachments in battered women and other relationships of intermittent abuse. *Victimology: An International Journal, 1,* 139–145.

Dutton, D. G., & Starzomski, A. J. (1993). Borderline personality in perpetrators of psychological and physical abuse. *Violence and Victims, 8,* 327–337.

Eisenberg, S. E., & Micklow, P. L. (1977). The assaulted wife: Catch-22 revisited. *Women's Rights Law Reporter, 58,* 138–161.

Emery, R. E. (1989). Family violence. *American Psychologist, 44*, 321–328.

Enroth, R. (1977). *Youth, brainwashing, and the extremist cults.* Ann Arbor, MI: Zondervan.

Ferraro, K. J. (1988). An existential approach to battering. In G. T. Hotaling, D. Finkelhor, J. T. Kirkpatrick, & M. A. Straus (Eds.), *Family abuse and its consequences* (pp. 126–138). Newbury Park, CA: Sage.

Freire, P. (1984). *Pedagogy of the oppressed.* New York: Continuum.

Gayford, J. J. (1975). Wife battering: A preliminary study of 100 cases. *British Medical Journal, 1*, 194–197.

Gelles, R. J. (1975). *The violent home: A study of physical aggression between husbands and wives.* Beverly Hills, CA: Sage.

Gelles, R. J. (1976). Abused wives: Why do they stay? *Journal of Marriage and the Family, 38*, 659–668.

Gelles, R. J. (1997). *Intimate violence in families* (3rd ed.). Thousand Oaks, CA: Sage.

Gelles, R. J. (1998a). Family violence: In M. H. Tonry (Ed.), *The handbook of crime and punishment* (pp. 178–206). New York: Oxford University Press.

Gelles, R. J. (1998b). The youngest victims: Violence towards children. In R. K. Bergen (Ed.), *Issues in intimate violence* (pp. 5–24). Thousand Oaks, CA: Sage.

Giles-Sims, J. (1998). The aftermath of partner violence. In J. L. Jasinski & L. M. Williams (Eds.), *Partner violence: A comprehensive review of 20 years of research* (pp. 44–72). Thousand Oaks, CA: Sage.

Gondolf, E. W., & Hanneken, J. (1987). The gender warrior: Reformed batterers on abusers, treatment, and change. *Journal of Family Violence, 2*, 177–191.

Goodman, L. A., Koss, M. P., Fitzgerald, L. F., Russo, N. F., & Keita, G. P. (1993). Male violence against women: Current research and future directions. *American Psychologist, 48*, 1054–1058.

Goodstein, R. K. (1987). Violence in the home: The battered spouse syndrome. *Carrier Foundation Letter, 125*, 1–4.

Goodstein, R. K., & Page, A. W. (1981). Battered wife syndrome: Overview of dynamics and treatment. *American Journal of Psychiatry, 138*, 1036–1044.

Hamberger, L. K., & Hastings, J. E. (1986). Personality correlates of men who abuse their partners: A cross-validation study. *Journal of Family Violence, 1*, 323–341.

Harris, L. & Associates (1979). *A survey of spousal violence against women in Kentucky.* Report prepared for the Kentucky Commission on Women.

Hilberman, E. (1980). Overview: The wife beater's wife considered. *American Journal of Psychiatry, 137*, 1336–1347.

Hilberman, E., & Munson, M. (1978). Sixty battered women. *Victimology: An International Journal, 2*, 460–471.

Hornung, C. A., McCullough, B. C., & Sugimoto, T. (1981). Status relationships in marriage: Risk factors in spouse abuse. *Journal of Marriage and the Family, 43*, 675–692.

Hyden, M. (1995). Verbal aggression as prehistory of woman battering. *Journal of Family Violence, 10*, 55–71.

Jaffe, P., Wolfe, D. A., Telford, D. A., & Austin, G. (1986). The impact of police charges in incidents of wife abuse. *Journal of Family Violence, 1*, 37–49.

Janoff-Bulman, R. (1979). Characterological versus behavioral self-blame: Inquiries into depression and rape. *Journal of Personality and Social Psychology, 37*, 1798–1809.

Johnson, I. M. (1992). Economic, situational, and psychological correlates of the decision-making process of battered women. *Families in Society, 73*, 168–176.

Johnston, M. E. (1988). Correlates of early violence experience among men who are abusive toward female mates. In G. T. Hotaling, D. Finkelhor, J. T. Kirkpatrick, & M. A. Straus (Eds.), *Family abuse and its consequences* (pp. 192–202). Beverly Hills, CA: Sage.

Kalmuss, D. (1984). The intergenerational transmission of marital aggression. *Journal of Marriage and Family, 47*, 11–19.

Kalmuss, D., & Straus, M. A. (1982). Wife's marital dependency and wife abuse. *Journal of Marriage and the Family, 44,* 277–286.

Kantor, G. K., & Straus, M. A. (1987). The "drunken bum" theory of wife beating. *Social Problems, 34,* 213–230.

Kipnis, D. (1976). *The powerholders.* Chicago: University of Chicago Press.

Koss, M. P. (1993). Rape: Scope, impact, intervention and public policy response. *American Psychologist, 48,* 1062–1069.

Kurz, D. (1987). Emergency department responses to battered women: Resistance to medicalization. *Social Problems, 34,* 69–81.

Lempert, L. B. (1996). Women's strategies for survival: Developing agency in abusive relationships. *Journal of Family Violence, 11,* 269–289.

Leonard, K. E. (1999). Alcohol use and husband marital aggression among newlywed couples. In X. B. Arriaga & S. Oskamp (Eds.), *Violence in intimate relationships* (pp. 113–135). Thousand Oaks, CA: Sage.

Lerner, M. J. (1970). The desire for justice and reactions to victims. In J. McCauley & L. Berkowitz (Eds.), *Altruism and helping behaviors: Social psychological studies of some antecedents and consequences.* New York: Academic Press.

Libow, J., & Doty, D. (1979). An exploratory approach to self-blame and self-derogation by rape victims. *American Journal of Orthopsychiatry, 49,* 670–679.

Malamuth, N., Feshback, S., & Jaffee, Y. (1977). Sexual arousal and aggression: Recent experiments and theoretical issues. *Journal of Social Issues, 22,* 110–113.

Mitchell, R. E., & Hodson, C. A. (1983). Coping with domestic violence: Social support and psychological health among battered women. *American Journal of Community Psychology, 11,* 629–654.

Murphy, C. M., & O'Farrell, T. J. (1996). Marital violence among alcoholics. *Current Directions in Psychological Science, 5,* 183–186.

Ochberg, F. M. (1971). Victims of terrorism. *Journal of Clinical Psychiatry, 41,* 73–74.

Ponzetti, J. J., Cate, R. M., & Koval, J. E. (1982). Violence between couples: Profiling the male abuser. *Personnel and Guidance Journal, 61,* 222–224.

Ptacek, J. (1988). The clinical literature on men who batter: A review and critique. In G. T. Hotaling, D. Finkelhor, J. T. Kirkpatrick, & M. A. Straus (Eds.), *Family abuse and its consequences* (pp. 149–162). Beverly Hills, CA: Sage.

Rigakos, G. S. (1995). Constructing the symbolic complainant: Police subculture and the nonenforcement of protection orders for battered women. *Violence and Victims, 10,* 227–246.

Rosenbaum, A., & O'Leary, K. D. (1981). Marital violence: Characteristics of abusive couples. *Journal of Consulting and Clinical Psychology, 41,* 63–71.

Roy, M. (Ed.). (1977). *Battered women: A psychosocial study of domestic violence.* New York: Van Nostrand Reinhold.

Rule, B. G., & Nesdale, A. R. (1976). Emotional arousal and aggressive behavior. *Psychological Bulletin, 83,* 851–863.

Rusbult, C. E., & Martz, J. M. (1995). Remaining in abusive relationships: An investment model analysis of nonvoluntary dependency. *Personality and Social Psychology Bulletin, 21,* 558–571.

Saunders, D. G. (1986). When battered women use violence: Husband-abuse or self-defense? *Violence and Victims, 1,* 47–60.

Saunders, D. G. (1992). A typology of men who batter women: Three types derived from cluster analysis. *American Orthopsychiatry, 62,* 264–265.

Saunders, D. G., & Size, P. B. (1986). Attitudes about woman abuse among police officers, victims, and victim advocates. *Journal of Interpersonal Violence, 1,* 25–42.

Schulman, M. (1979). *A survey of spousal violence against women in Kentucky*. Washington, DC: U.S. Department of Justice, Law Enforcement Assistance Administration.

Seligman, M. E. P. (1975). *Helplessness: On depression, development and death*. San Francisco: W. H. Freeman.

Sherman, L. W., & Berk, R. A. (1984). *The Minneapolis domestic violence experiment*. Washington, DC: Police Foundation.

Singer, T. (1979, January). Coming out of cults. *Psychology Today*, 72–82.

Snyder, D. K., & Fruchtman, L. A. (1981). Differential patterns of wife abuse: A data-based typology. *Journal of Consulting and Clinical Psychology, 49*, 878–885.

Stark, E., Flitcraft, A., & Frazier, W. (1979). Medicine and patriarchal violence: The social construction of a private event. *International Journal of Health and Services, 9*, 461–493.

Steinmetz, S. K. (1977). *The cycle of violence: Assertive, aggressive, and violent family interaction*. New York: Praeger.

Straus, M. A. (1977). Sociological perspective on the prevention and treatment of wife beating. In M. Roy (Ed.), *Battered women: A psychosocial study of domestic violence*. New York: Van Nostrand Reinhold.

Straus, M. A., Gelles, R. J., & Steinmetz, S. K. (1980). *Behind closed doors: Violence in the American family*. Garden City, NY: Anchor Books.

Strube, M. J. (1988). The decision to leave an abusive relationship: Empirical evidence and theoretical issues. *Psychological Bulletin, 104*, 236–250.

Sugarman, D. B., & Frankel, S. L. (1996). Patriarchal ideology and wife assault: A meta-analytic review. *Journal of Family Violence, 11*, 13–40.

Van Hasselt, V. B., Morrison, R. L., & Bellack, A. S. (1985). Alcohol use in wife abusers and their spouses. *Addictive Behaviors, 10*, 127–135.

Van Hasselt, V. B., Morrison, R. L., & Bellack, A. S. (1987). Assessment of assertion and problem-solving skills in wife abusers and their spouses. *Journal of Family Violence, 2*, 227–238.

Walker, L. E. (1978). Battered women and learned helplessness. *Victimology, 2*, 525–534.

Walker, L. E. (1979). *The battered woman*. New York: Harper & Row.

Walker, L. E. (1981). Battered women: Sex roles and clinical issues. *Professional Psychology, 12*, 81–91.

Walker, L. E. (1988). The battered woman syndrome. In G. T. Hotaling, D. Finkelhor, J. T. Kirkpatrick, & M. A. Straus (Eds.), *Family abuse and its consequences* (pp. 139–148). Beverly Hills, CA: Sage.

Walker, L. E. (1995). Current perspectives on men who batter women: Implications for intervention and treatment to stop violence against women. *Journal of Family Psychology, 3*, 264–271.

Warshaw, C. (1989). Limitations of the medical model in the care of battered women. *Gender and Society, 4*, 506–517.

West, L. J. (1963). Brainwashing. In A. Deutsch (Ed.), *The encyclopedia of mental health* (Vol. 1). New York: Franklin Watts.

Zimbardo, P. G., Ebbesen, E. B., & Maslach, C. (1977). *Influencing attitudes and changing behavior*. Reading, MA: Addison-Wesley.

17

Marital Rape

Heidi S. Resnick, Sherry A. Falsetti, and Shawn P. Cahill

Description of the Problem

In the past 10 years, there has been increased recognition of the magnitude of the problems of sexual assault-related violence, domestic violence, and marital rape. It has been shown across a range of studies that completed rape is a potentially traumatic event that is associated with the greatest risk of posttraumatic stress disorder (PTSD) among women (Kessler, Sonnega, Bromet, Hughes, & Nelson, 1995; Kilpatrick *et al.*, 1987; Resnick, Dansky, Saunders, & Best, 1993). Data also indicate that marital rapes constitute a significant proportion of all rape incidents, are more prevalent in the context of other physical violence, and may be associated with more severe physical violence (Browne, 1993). Rapes by romantic partners are characterized by similar rates of injury and fear of death as incidents perpetrated by strangers (Kilpatrick, Best, Saunders, & Veronen, 1988), and rapes in marriage and dating relationships are associated with negative mental health outcomes at rates that are comparable to or higher than those associated with rapes perpetrated by strangers (Kilpatrick *et al.*, 1988; Riggs, Kilpatrick, & Resnick, 1992; Shields & Hanneke, 1987).

Heidi S. Resnick, Sherry A. Falsetti, and Shawn P. Cahill • Department of Psychiatry and Behavioral Sciences, National Crime Victims Research and Treatment Center, Medical University of South Carolina, Charleston, South Carolina 29425-0742.

Case Studies in Family Violence, Second Edition, edited by Ammerman and Hersen. Kluwer Academic / Plenum Publishers, New York, 2000.

It is also now recognized that one in five women seen in emergency room settings has symptoms related to sexual or physical assault-related violence (American Medical Association Council on Scientific Affairs, 1992). The physical health impacts of domestic violence include acute injuries (Goodman, Koss, & Russo, 1993) as well as longer-term negative health outcomes and inappropriate medical care utilization (Koss & Heslet, 1992). Thus, rape and domestic violence in general, and marital rape in particular, exact a great toll from its victims. This chapter reviews what is known about marital rape, and where existing literature is deficient, draws from the larger literatures on rape and domestic violence in an attempt to provide suggestions to assist therapists in the treatment of victims of marital rape. Two case studies that illustrate several points related to the assessment and treatment of the psychological sequelae of marital rape are presented at the end of this section.

Prevalence

Greater sophistication in methods used to assess completed rape has led to a better understanding of the *extent* of rape in the United States. Studies that have employed specific behavioral definitions to identify instances of vaginal, anal, or oral penetration occurring as a result of force or threat of force, rather than legal terminology such as the word "rape," have led to more reliable and valid general population estimates of rape (Kilpatrick, 1993; Koss, 1993). General population rates of rape across several well-conducted studies indicate that prevalence rates range from 13% (Kilpatrick, Edmunds, & Seymour, 1992) to as high as 24% (Koss, 1993). Based on the findings from a series of studies, Koss has estimated the prevalence of completed rape at 20%. Even the lower prevalence rate observed by Kilpatrick *et al.* (1992) among a representative sample of 4,008 adult women in the United States indicates that at least 1 in 8 adult American women has been raped during her lifetime. Based on a population estimate of 96,056,000 adult women in 1989, when the study was conducted, and the 13% sample prevalence of rape, Kilpatrick *et al.* (1992) estimated that 12.1 million American women had experienced a completed rape.

As noted in several sources, sexual assaults and rapes by intimate partners represent a significant subset of all rapes committed (Kilpatrick *et al.*, 1992) and may exceed rates of rape perpetrated by strangers (Browne, 1993; Finkelhor & Yllo, 1983; Kilpatrick *et al.*, 1988; Russell, 1982). In her study, Russell found that 14% of women who had ever been married experienced a rape perpetrated by a husband or ex-husband. Only half of this percentage (7%) reported rapes by a stranger. Similarly, in a sample of

326 women who had been married or lived with a romantic partner, Finkelhor and Yllo (1983) found that 10% reported having experienced a rape by a partner compared with 3% reporting rape perpetrated by a stranger. Within a national sample of 4,008 women, Kilpatrick et al. (1992) found that 9% of all *rape cases* were perpetrated by husbands or ex-husbands. Based on the total prevalence of rape of 13% and the rate of marital rape of 9%, it can be estimated that approximately 1% of all adult women have experienced marital rape. This estimated prevalence of marital rape is similar to rates ranging from 1% to 4% identified in groups of women who were not exposed to other forms of physical violence or battering (Frieze, 1983; Hanneke, Shields, & McCall, 1986).

Rates of marital rape are much higher in groups of women exposed to other forms of domestic violence (e.g., battery; Browne, 1993). Rates of marital rape range from one-third to one-half of women identified from shelter populations or identified as being exposed to nonsexual violence within their relationships (Frieze, 1983; Hanneke et al., 1986). Other data indicate that more severe levels of physical violence occur in cases where sexual violence is also present (Shields & Hanneke, 1983). Hanneke et al. (1986) suggested that strong associations between sexual and other forms of partner violence may indicate that similar processes underlie both types of behavior. For example, both may be expressions of violence or control. Alternatively the low frequencies of rape observed apart from other violence may reflect perceptual biases. In reference to victims of rape in general, Koss (1983) has suggested that presence of higher levels of physical force may be a stereotype about rape that affects the victims' conceptualizations. A related issue raised by Finkelhor and Yllo (1983) is that, thus far, only the use or threat of physical force has been included to formulate the definitions of rape. However, there may be other very real threats aside from physical force involved in marital rape, including threats of the loss of social or financial support, and memories of past instances of physical force following resistance. Finally, as Hanneke and Shields (1985) noted, because of their relationship and continued contact with the perpetrator, victims of marital rape may have difficulty disclosing the rape for fear of retribution from the partner.

Two studies examined characteristics of marital rape cases versus stranger rape. Importantly, the term *rape* was not used to assess such incidents. Instead, rape was behaviorally defined as nonconsensual completed vaginal, oral, or anal penetration that involved force or threat of force. Kilpatrick et al. (1988) assessed rape incidents in a community sample of 391 women. A total of 91 women (23%) had been victims of at least one completed rape and 10 had experienced two rapes. Data on prevalence of different types of rape indicated that marital rape occurred as frequently as stranger rape, occurring in 24 (24%) of the 101 rape cases, versus 21 cases (22%) in which the perpetrator was a stranger. Date rape occurred in 17% of cases. Comparisons among the three groups of rape victims in terms of sustained physical injury and the presence of perceived life threat or serious injury indicated there were no significant differences on these measures of objective and subjective aspects of dangerousness. Physical injuries were sustained in 46%, 47%, and 38% of marital, date, and stranger rapes, respectively. Perceived life threat or fear of serious injury was reportedly present during 42%, 53%, and 38% of the marital, date, and stranger rapes. In addition, marital rape victims did not differ from the other groups of rape victims in terms of rates of a variety of mental health disorders. Kilpatrick *et al.* (1988) concluded that these data on the prevalence, level of dangerousness, and effects of marital rape directly contradict major assumptions that are the foundation of the previous lack of societal and legal recognition of the significance of the problem of marital rape.

In an attempt to describe characteristics of cases of sexual versus nonsexual violence as a function of relationship to the perpetrator, Riggs *et al.* (1992) studied four groups of women from the original Kilpatrick *et al.* (1988) sample. To control for exposure to multiple types of violence, groups were restricted to women who experienced only completed rape or only physical assault incidents. Thus, Riggs identified a group of women who reported a completed rape by a stranger ($n = 10$); a group who reported a completed rape by a husband ($n = 14$); a group who reported an aggravated assault by a stranger ($n = 11$); and a group who reported an aggravated assault by a husband ($n = 12$). Results indicated that marital rape and marital aggravated assault victims were more likely than stranger rape and stranger assault victims to report that their assaults were part of a series of incidents in which the same person attacked them over a period of days, weeks, or months. Specifically, 64% of marital rape victims and 58% of marital aggravated assault victims reported a series of assaults versus 0% of stranger rape victims and 9% of stranger aggravated assault victims. Both groups of aggravated assault victims were more likely to report that they feared death or injury during the incidents (100% and 82%, for marital and stranger assaults, respectively) than the groups of rape victims (36% and 50%, for marital and stranger rapes, respectively). This latter finding is not surprising given that the definition of aggravated assault *required* the report of an assault in which either a weapon was used or the victim perceived the assailant intended to kill or seriously injure her. Rates of reported injury did not differ across groups.

In summary, data on prevalence rates of marital rape may be considered to be conservative, given the likelihood that such incidents do not fit women's stereotypic views of rape and would thus be less likely to be acknowledged as rape (Koss, 1983). Consistent with this idea, Frieze (1983) reported that although more than a third of women acknowledged having been pressured to have sex by their partners, only a small percentage reported experiencing marital rape incidents. Despite this, prevalence estimates indicate that marital rape may be the most frequently occurring type of rape. The data also indicate that marital rape occurs more frequently, or is reported at a higher rate, in cases where nonsexual battering is also present. In addition, marital rape incidents are characterized by similar rates of injury and fear of death or serious injury as cases of stranger rape (Kilpatrick et al., 1988). However, marital rape incidents are more likely to be described as part of a pattern or series of assaults by the same perpetrator than are stranger rapes (Riggs et al., 1992).

Victim Characteristics

Data from representative samples of marital rape victims are too limited to draw conclusions about victim characteristics. Instead, data from studies evaluating risk factors for domestic violence in general may be more informative. Hotaling and Sugarman (1986) reviewed case-comparison studies for potential correlates of husband-to-wife violence. Across studies, 16 variables were identified that could be considered to be victim characteristics and had been examined in at least three independent investigations. These variables included witnessing violence as a child, age, race, assertiveness, education, income, alcohol use, housewife status, self-esteem, and traditional sex-role expectations. "Consistent risk markers" were defined as those variables significantly associated with husband-to-wife violence in at least 70% of the cases studied. Results indicated that only one variable could be classified as a consistent risk marker: women who experienced partner violence were more likely to have witnessed violence between their parents while growing up. Variables found to be consistently *unrelated* to partner violence (positively associated with violence in 30% or less of the cases studied) included victim alcohol abuse, housewife status, and income. The authors concluded that their findings were not consistent with notions that victim personality characteristics or behaviors were associated with husband-to-wife violence.

Psychological and Behavioral Indices Associated with Marital Rape

Hanneke and Shields (1985) suggested that, because study of reactions to marital rape is a relatively new and small area, it would be beneficial to examine findings related to the effects of spouse abuse and rape in general. Their summary of psychological and behavioral variables associated with battery included decreased self-esteem, increased rates of suicide attempts, alcohol use, psychosomatic symptoms, social isolation, physically abusive behavior toward children, help seeking, divorce or separation, and initiation of other legal actions. Negative attitudes toward men, sex, marriage in general, and specifically toward their spouses were also associated with nonsexual violence.

Results from the rape literature indicate that victims report increased levels of general psychological distress, including depression and anxiety, as well as problems associated with later sexual functioning. A longitudinal study of psychological functioning among rape victims and nonvictimized women by Kilpatrick, Veronen, and Resick (1979) indicated that rape victims displayed significantly higher levels of distress than nonvictims on virtually all standardized measures included to evaluate psychological distress at assessment periods immediately following assault. By 3 months postassault, however, indices of general distress had decreased in the rape victim group, while indices of specific and general fear and anxiety remained at significantly higher levels than those observed in the control group. These differences were maintained at the 6-month assessment period.

Kilpatrick, Veronen, and Best (1985) were among the first to describe the responses of rape victims as consistent with the diagnostic category of PTSD (American Psychiatric Association, 1994), noting that the most frequently observed symptoms among rape victims included fear and anxiety, intrusive cognitions, avoidance behavior, and sleep disturbance. Kilpatrick, Saunders, Amick-McMullan, Best, Veronen, and Resnick (1989) later found that PTSD was associated with the crime of rape at a higher rate than those observed for other crimes. In that study, 57% of victims of completed rape met criteria for PTSD. Significant predictors of PTSD in a subgroup of 295 women who had experienced a variety of crimes included the fear of death or serious injury during the crime, actual injury sustained during crime, and the crime of rape itself. Rape was the only type of crime that was associated with the PTSD after controlling for perceived life threat and injury. Kilpatrick et al. (1989) concluded from these findings that there must be additional elements involved in rape associated with the increased risk of PTSD. Data from national samples of women have also observed high rates of PTSD associated with history of rape, ranging from 32% (Resnick et al., 1993) to 46% (Kessler et al., 1995). Even higher rates of PTSD have been observed in more select samples, such as women who have reported the rape to police or other authorities (Rothbaum, Foa, Riggs, Murdock, & Walsh, 1992).

The study of PTSD associated with physical battery has also developed over the past several years (Brown, 1993). Given the nature of battery, which can include repeated threats to life or physical integrity over a number of years, it is not surprising that high rates of PTSD have also been found in this population. For example, Kemp, Rawlings, and Green (1991) found that 84% of women in a shelter sample met diagnostic criteria for PTSD. They also found that frequency and severity of battering were significantly correlated with PTSD, as was the degree of self-reported distress during or immediately following battery. Other studies of shelter populations have identified rates of PTSD ranging from 45% to 58% of the women studied (Housekamp & Foy, 1991; Astin, Ogland-Hand, Foy, & Coleman, 1995).

Given high rates of PTSD among women who have experienced rape or battery, it would be expected that marital rape victims might display even higher rates of PTSD. This is based on the data reviewed here that indicate a high rate of co-occurrence of physical battery, violence severity, and marital rape. In addition, recall that Kilpatrick *et al.* (1989) found that rape may include unique factors that increase risk for PTSD beyond fear of death or actual injury. Unfortunately, the data relevant to this question are limited. Only one study to date (Kilpatrick *et al.*, 1988) assessed current frequency of major psychiatric disorders among a group of rape victims that included a marital rape subgroup. Although rates of disorders were not reported separately for the marital rape subgroup, it was previously noted that the marital rape subgroup did not differ significantly from the subgroups of date and stranger rape victims on any of the disorders assessed. As a whole, the rape victim group displayed significantly higher rates of all disorders, except obsessive-compulsive disorder, than women who were not crime victims. Specifically, the current rates of sexual dysfunction, social phobia, and major depressive episode were 30%, 14%, and 12%, respectively, within the rape victim group. Rape victims were 11 times more likely to be clinically depressed, 6 times more likely to display criteria for social phobia, and 2.5 times more likely to currently meet criteria for sexual dysfunction than were nonvictims.

The previously mentioned study by Riggs *et al.* (1992) utilized the same Kilpatrick *et al.* (1988) community sample described earlier to evaluate the potential differential mental health correlates of rape and physical battery. They compared scores on the Impact of Event Scale (IES; Horowitz, Wilner, & Alvarez, 1979) and the Symptom Checklist 90-R (SCL-90-R; Derogatis, 1983) from 47 women who were distributed into four mutually exclusive groups based on the following event history patterns: (a) rape by husband; (b) rape by stranger; (c) physical assault by husband; (d) physical assault by stranger. Results indicated there were no group differences on any measures of current psychological distress. These findings extend those reported by Kilpatrick *et al.* (1988) to indicate similar patterns of distress among women who experienced rape or physical battery, regardless of whether their assailants were husbands or strangers. It must be cautioned that groups were carefully selected to identify only those women who experienced a single type of assault. Thus, generalizability to representative groups of marital rape victims may be limited.

Frieze (1983) examined specific emotional and behavioral factors associated with marital rape in her group of 137 women who experienced marital violence and control groups of battered and nonbattered women. To examine associated emotional and behavioral indices (acknowledging the problem of order of occurrence, which is not controlled for in the methodology of the study), she conducted a regression analysis using marital rape as the predicted variable with the other indices as predictors. Results indicated that trying to leave the husband, filing legal charges, having lesbian affairs, having a husband who would not seek emotional or psychological treatment, and wanting to leave the husband were significantly associated with marital rape, in that order. A second regression analysis with marital rape as one of the predictor variables and leaving the husband as the predicted variable was conducted. Results indicated that marital rape was not significantly associated with leaving the husband, although the wife's finding sex unpleasant because of force or pressure was predictive of leaving, second only to presence of violence. Frieze concluded that behavioral reactions were more common than emotional reactions in association with marital rape. She raised the issue that studies of effects associated with marital rape need also to examine and attempt to control for the effects of violence in general.

Shields and Hanneke (1983) attempted to examine factors that might be uniquely associated with marital rape after controlling for levels of violence. Their sample of women included a group that had experienced rape and battery and a group that had experienced only battery. Initial analyses indicated that women who had experienced rape had been exposed to higher levels of violence, which, in turn, was significantly associated with several psychological and behavioral indices. Within the subgroup that had experienced marital rape, correlational analyses were conducted between frequency of marital rape and other variables while controlling for level of violence. These analyses indicated significant relationships between frequency of marital rape and lower self-esteem, psychosomatic reactions, and suicide attempts. Results of analyses of variance that included a third, nonbattered group indicated the group that experienced rape and battery had significantly lower ratings of self-esteem than the battered-only and nonbattered controls, which were not significantly different on this measure. Use of retaliatory violence and alcohol were significantly more frequent in both battery groups. The authors noted that, without a separate rape-only group, the effects of marital rape alone remain unclear because there may be interactive effects of rape and battery.

A final study by Shields and Hanneke (1987) was an attempt to test the hypothesis that marital rape victims experience *less* serious psychological reactions than stranger rape victims. The groups consisted of 44 women who had experienced rape and battery, 48 who had experienced battery only, and 45 nonvictimized women. In this study, standardized measures of general psychological distress, anxiety, and questions about sexual functioning that had previously been used with general rape samples were administered. Scores on these measures were compared across the three groups. They were also compared with scores obtained with general rape victims from previously published reports in the rape literature. The authors noted that results of any differences between their sample and the previously conducted studies need to be interpreted cautiously, because there were significant demographic differences between the samples that could relate to other findings. Similarly, they acknowledged that in the cases of rape and battery, there may be an ongoing problematic marital relationship that may include chronic rather than acute victimization, which might account for differences on symptom measures across groups.

Within these limitations, results generally indicated that marital rape victims reported significantly *higher* levels of distress than stranger rape victims on several indices, including some measures of anxiety, paranoid ideation, psychoticism, and impaired sexual functioning. In addition, the battery-only group also reported high levels of distress on several measures, in some cases as high as or greater than those observed in the stranger rape samples. The authors concluded that, contrary to their hypotheses, occurrence of marital rape and battery is associated with serious mental health effects, as is battery alone. They suggested that these results highlight the need to be aware of the possible separate and interactive effects of battery in association with marital rape.

In summary, the area of assessment of psychological distress and behavioral reactions associated with marital rape is still fairly limited. Few studies have been conducted to date that have used standardized assessment instruments or structured diagnostic interviews. Results of the studies reviewed here indicate that marital rape is associated with low self-esteem, elevated levels of psychological distress on standardized psychological assessment measures, and increased rates of major psychiatric disorder. Results also indicate that marital rape is associated with the presence of nonsexual violence and that both marital rape and nonsexual violence may have separate as well as interactive effects. Perhaps one useful paradigm for examining these effects would be to compare groups of subjects who have experienced rape only, battery only, and rape plus battery, while controlling for relationship with assailant and chronicity of exposure (i.e., serial versus single-incident assaults). Studies of PTSD associated with marital rape specifically would also be useful in order to tailor relevant psychological interventions.

Partner and Relationship Characteristics

The major focus of research within the marital rape area has been the reaction of the victim. To date, no study has utilized a methodology of partner/perpetrator as respondent in the research. What is known about the partner-as-perpetrator in marital rape has been acquired from studies of the marital rape victim. More data are available about partner and relationship characteristics related to the broader category of domestic violence. These latter studies have also included studies of perpetrators as respondents.

Frieze (1980) investigated the causes and consequences of marital rape. A sample of 137 women who reported physical violence were interviewed about the violence and about marital rape. A matched control group was also interviewed. Analyses were conducted to determine whether there were differences in "battering" men versus those who were "battering" and "raping" men. "Raping" men were reported as having more children, being more dominant in the marital relationship, and more likely to have greater drinking problems. "Raping" husbands were more violent generally and experienced fights outside the home as well. Violence included sexual abuse (often associated with injuries resulting from forced anal intercourse) as well as rape and violence toward their wives when they were pregnant. They were also more often drunk when violent. This investigation has several strengths, including use of comparison groups that strengthen the interpretations and the use of appropriate data analyses.

Hotaling and Sugarman (1986) reviewed extant studies of partner and relationship characteristics as risk factors for more general domestic violence. All the studies evaluated in their review included comparison samples. An attempt was made to evaluate findings carefully according to whether comparison samples included couples experiencing marital discord or no violence or marital discord. Hotaling and Sugarman found that of 38 potential risk markers, 9 were associated with consistent findings across at least 70% of studies in which they were assessed. Among the most consistent partner risk factors for marital violence were use of violence toward children, sexual aggression toward the wife, witnessing interparental violence during childhood or adolescence, and alcohol use. Hotaling and Sugarman also noted that education level, occupation, and income were inversely related to partner violence across several studies. However, they cautioned that these patterns were not consistently found within the subset of studies that included the most representative population samples. Across studies, abusive men were found to be less assertive than nonabusive men. Finally, traditional sex-role expectations were identified as a consistent *nonrisk* factor, such that higher rates of traditional attitudes were observed among batterers in only 2 of 8 studies that had been conducted. Partner characteristic variables identified as risk factors in at least 66% of studies that assessed them included experiencing violence as a child or adolescent, unemployment, and criminal arrest record.

Hotaling and Sugarman (1986) also reviewed studies that included assessment of relationship characteristics that might be associated with domestic violence. Variables that were consistently found to be present at significantly higher rates among violent relationships were increased frequency of verbal arguments, marital conflict, and religious incompatibility. Being currently married, as opposed to any other marital status, was associated with lower rates of violence and there was an inverse relationship between family income/social class with violence.

More recently, Saunders (1992) studied responses on standardized measures of psychological functioning and self-reported historical variables in a sample of 165 men referred for evaluation and treatment of partner violence behaviors. Cluster analysis indicated possible heterogeneity within this group, as reflected by the identification of three distinct profiles. Type 1 was defined as "family-only aggressors." This group was least likely to have been abused as children. They were also least likely to be violent outside of the home, reported highest marital satisfaction, least marital conflict, and lowest rates of psychological abuse compared to other men in the sample. Saunders noted that alcohol use was reportedly involved in half the incidents reported by Type 1 men. Type 2 was labeled "generally violent." These men were most likely to be violent outside the home, were most likely to have experienced childhood abuse themselves, and engaged in more severe violence than the men in the other two groups. They reported that alcohol use was typical of their incidents of partner violence and they reported more rigid sex-role attitudes. Rates of arrest for violence and drunk driving were relatively higher in this group than in the other two groups. Type 3 men were labeled "emotionally volatile" and were found to report higher rates of anger, depression, and jealousy. They also reported infrequent alcohol use in association with violence. Saunders suggested that these profiles, if established as reliable and valid, might serve to guide treatment approaches tailored to the particular problems indicated. For example, he suggested that Type 2 (generally violent) men would require more long-term treatment and that, in addition to cognitive restructuring related to anger management or altering violence, they might benefit from treatment related to their own early violence experiences.

Findings from studies consistently indicate a positive relationship between sexual aggression and other forms of physical violence in marital relationships. It is clear that more risk indicators of partner violence have been identified that are characteristics of the male partner or the relationship than for characteristics of the victim. Consistent findings indicate that witnessing parental violence during childhood or adolescence is associated with risk of victimization by and perpetration of partner violence. In addition, alcohol use by the male partner is a factor associated with partner violence across studies, although this finding may be stronger within some subsets of men than others. These data have important implications for treatment and prevention. Interventions must be directed at the male partner and the relationship, rather than have a restricted focus on the victim. Such interventions might serve to prevent partner violence in the next generation.

The following case descriptions illustrate many of the medical, legal, and social issues related to marital rape, and to the assessment of psychopathology and available treatment options discussed in subsequent sections of the chapter.

Case 1: Treatment of PTSD Resulting from Marital Rape

C.A. was a 34-year-old white female who worked full time and had two children. Her first husband, to whom she had been married from ages 23 to 29, had been physically and sexually abusive. She also experienced childhood sexual assault by her brother from ages 7 to 9. She sought treatment because she was having problems in her second marriage and believed that the traumatic events she experienced contributed to mistrust of her current husband and lack of sexual desire. She also reported having difficulty concentrating, difficulty sleeping, loss of interest in activities, unpleasant memories about the abusive incidents in her marriage, and feeling very anxious and on guard.

C.A. was assessed using the Trauma Assessment for Adults (TAA) Interview (Stamm, 1996), which assesses traumatic events history and other stressful life events. Posttraumatic stress disorder was assessed using a modified version of the Diagnostic Interview Schedule (DIS; Robins, Helzer, Croughan, & Ratcliff, 1981). A family history interview was also completed. In addition the following self report measures were collected: Impact of

Event Scale (IES; Horowitz *et al.*, 1979), Beck Depression Inventory (BDI; Beck, Ward, Mendelsohn, Mock, & Erbaugh, 1961), PTSD Symptom Assessment for DSM-IV-Self-Report Version, an updated version of the Modified PTSD Symptom Scale-Self-Report (MPSS-SR; Falsetti, Resnick, Resick, & Kilpatrick, 1993), Physical Reactions Scale (Falsetti & Resnick, 1997), and the Symptom Checklist 90-Revised (SCL-90-R; Derogatis, 1977).

The trauma history interview revealed that C.A. considered physical and sexual abuse in her first marriage to be causing her the most problems. Many of her intrusive thoughts were about specific incidences of sexual abuse by the first husband. She described her first husband as an alcoholic and said he would often come home drunk, and then beat and rape her. She was embarrassed and ashamed of these incidents and did not disclose the abuse to anyone. She described one of the worst incidents of marital rape as including anal penetration and being gagged with her underwear. She reported that her husband tied her to the bed with fishing line, which cut into her wrists and legs. He refused to untie her, even when she asked to use the bathroom, and then beat her with a belt for urinating on the bed after she had been tied up for over 12 hours. During this period, he anally raped her several times. She found this incident particularly humiliating and had great difficulty disclosing it in session. Shortly after this incident, she moved out and filed for divorce. Results of the initial evaluation indicated that C.A. met criteria for posttraumatic stress disorder. C.A. completed the Diagnostic Interview Schedule for PTSD pretreatment and posttreatment. She also completed the PTSD Symptom Assessment for DSM-IV to assess the frequency and severity of her PTSD symptoms throughout the course of treatment. C.A. completed the SCL-90-R and the Beck Depression Inventory pre- and posttreatment (see Table 1 and Figure 1).

After completion of the initial evaluation, C.A. was seen for 15 therapy sessions. She was treated using cognitive processing therapy (Resick & Schnicke, 1993). Session 1 included psychoeducation about PTSD. During this session C.A. revealed anger toward her brother and her first husband. For homework, she was asked to write about the meaning of these events in terms of how they affected her belief systems about herself, others, and the world.

Table 1. Case 1 Pre- and Postassessment Measures

Measure	Preassessment	Postassessment
Diagnostic Interview Schedule for PTSD	PTSD positive	PTSD negative
Impact of Events Scale	3.4	1.8
PTSD Symptom Assessment for DSM-IV	47	15
SCL-90-R Global Severity Index	73	46
Beck Depression Inventory	12	4
Physical Reactions Scale	7	3

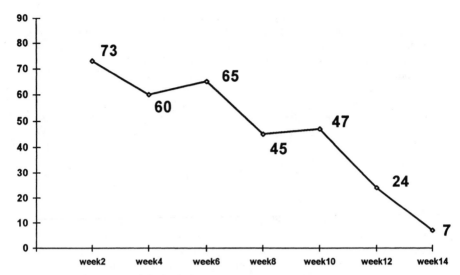

Figure 1.   Case 1: Modified PTSD symptom scale scores over course of treatment.

In session 2 the homework was reviewed. C.A. was tearful in the session and unsure if she could read the assignment. With some encouragement she was able to do so. In this assignment she reported "growing up afraid and alone" and "feeling dirty and ashamed." She did not disclose the abuse by her brother because she was afraid her parents would think she was bad and would not love her anymore. She disclosed how the early abuse affected her later relationships: "When I got old enough to have boyfriends, I used to run off all the good ones because I thought I did not deserve them. When I was 23, I married a man that was very possessive and violent. He was an alcoholic, very strong and abusive, but between his outbursts things were OK. When I left my husband, I began to realize that I did deserve better and that I did matter and deserve to be happy, and nobody should live in fear all their life. And that is why I left." During this session we discussed the connections among events, thoughts, and feelings, with an emphasis on how thoughts or interpretations of events can affect how we feel. How traumatic events can affect thoughts was also discussed. Homework to complete A-B-C sheets, which asked to specify an event, the associated thought, and her feelings, was assigned.

Session 3 began with a review of the homework. She had completed several worksheets and was able to understand how certain things she said to herself caused her to feel bad in situations that reminded her of the abuse. She was very upset that her husband had disclosed her abuse history to his brother. She felt very betrayed and out of control. We discussed other possible explanations for his disclosure, other than her original interpretation which was, "He's trying to make me the scapegoat of our marriage problems." She was able to also see that perhaps he was seeking support and did not intend to betray her. Her homework for the next session was to write about an abusive incident in as much detail as possible and in the present tense.

In session 4, C.A. disclosed a molestation incident by her father of which she had never told anyone. She viewed this incident as "different" than the abuse by her brother and the abuse by her first husband. She reported that her father had touched her breasts and kissed her one time. She thought she was 5 or 6 years old when this event occurred. She did not complete the writing assignment given for homework in the previous session; thus, she was asked to do this assignment for the next session.

C.A. called and canceled the next session, but came in the following week. She had completed the writing assignment. She read it in session, which was very difficult for her. She stopped and cried while reading particularly painful parts, including when her husband was tieing her to the bed, when he anally raped her, and when she urinated on herself. The remainder of the session was spent processing this event. She raised issues about why she waited so long to leave this relationship and why she did not disclose the abuse sooner. She reported feeling a lot of shame for her experiences and did not think she deserved anything better, something her first husband had often told her. She was asked to write about the same incident a second time, to provide further exposure and reduction in anxiety.

In session 6 we reviewed C.A.'s second writing assignment about the same event. She was less distressed when reading the account this session. She also reported feeling less upset when writing the account. In this assignment, she wrote more about the anger she now feels regarding what had happened to her. The Challenging Questions Worksheet, a worksheet designed to help challenge distorted cognitions, was introduced for homework.

Session 7 focused on challenging distorted thinking about the physical and sexual abuse in her first marriage and by her brother. Her homework was reviewed and she reported having a more objective perspective of the abuse. Her self-blame about her body responding to the sexual abuse as a child decreased significantly. The Faulty Thinking Patterns Worksheet, a worksheet designed to challenge more global cognitive distortion patterns, was introduced for homework.

C.A. did not complete homework for session 8, so this session was devoted to completing the Faulty Thinking Patterns Worksheets homework in session. For session 9 she completed further cognitive work using this worksheet. During this session we also focused on safety issues. For C.A. much of this revolved around nighttime and sleeping, as these were cues for the abuse by both her brother and her first husband. The final cognitive processing worksheet, the Challenging Beliefs Worksheet, was introduced this session and assigned for homework. This worksheet combines aspects of the previous cognitive worksheets to help clients effectively challenge distorted thinking.

In session 10 C.A. reported a particularly difficult week. She and her current husband had mutually decided to separate. Much of this session was focused on helping her to process this event. Homework on safety issues was also reviewed. How traumatic events can affect trust was discussed and she was asked to complete several Challenging Beliefs Worksheets on events pertaining to trust issues for homework.

Session 11 focused on the homework related to trust issues. C.A. revealed in this session that the word "rape" really bothered her. She said this made the traumatic events she experienced real and very serious, rather than just some strange things that had happened in her first marriage. One of the worksheets she completed was on thoughts about not being able to trust her current husband because he had disclosed her abuse history to a relative. Although she had worked on this earlier in therapy, she continued to struggle with this. She was able to use the worksheet to come up with alternative thoughts, instead of saying to herself that he did not care about her. How trauma affects power and competence issues was introduced and she was asked to complete Challenging Beliefs Worksheets on events regarding power and competence issues.

C.A. did not bring homework to session 12, so this session was used to review her progress in therapy and discuss what else she wanted to work on in therapy. She felt she was doing much better, despite the separation with her husband, and she thought she would be ready to end therapy after completing the Cognitive Processing Therapy Protocol. When asked what behavior would indicate to her that she was ready to end therapy, she said when she would be able to disclose the abuse to a close friend.

For session 13, C.A. also failed to complete the previously assigned homework. She said she had left the worksheets at the therapist's office during the previous session. She completed several worksheets in session. She reported still struggling with labeling her experience in her first marriage as rape because it took place while she was married. She processed her ambivalence about this and what it would mean to her to have been raped by her husband. She was asked to write about this for homework and also to consider the effects of the traumatic events on her self-esteem.

Session 14 focused on processing the homework assignments that C.A. had completed. She reported feeling a lot of anger toward her first husband when she labeled her experience in the marriage as rape. She said that although she knew what he had done was wrong, labeling it as rape made it a crime, and then she would not have to feel responsible. However, the downside of this for her was that it made her feel helpless and a "victim." We processed these thoughts further until she was able to focus her anger on her husband and not at herself. In her cognitive worksheets she challenged thoughts about not feeling worthy of good things happening in her life and thinking she had to do better than other people to prove her worth. She was asked to focus on intimacy issues for her homework for the next week.

Session 15 was C.A.'s final therapy session. Her homework was reviewed as well as the progress she had made in therapy. She reported that she had disclosed her abuse history to her best friend and felt very good about doing so. Her friend had been supportive and C.A. reported feeling like "a huge weight was lifted from my shoulders." She completed several assessment measures, which indicated that C.A. no longer met criteria for PTSD (see again Table 1 and Figure 1). She was encouraged to continue work on her own, and call to schedule a booster session if needed.

Case 2: Treatment of Comorbid PTSD and Panic Attacks

T.J. was a 30-year-old twice-divorced white female. She had no children and was working part time as a graphic arts designer. She had a previous history of alcohol abuse and had been sober for 3 months. She sought treatment because, since she had quit using alcohol, she was having intrusive memories about physical and sexual abuse perpetrated by both of her former husbands. She was also suffering from panic attacks and reported that her upstairs neighbors had a violent relationship, which often triggered thoughts of the violence that had been perpetrated against her.

T.J. was assessed using the Trauma Assessment for Adults Interview (Stamm, 1996), the Clinician Administered PTSD Scale (CAPS; Blake, Weathers, Nagy, Kaloupek, Klauminzer, Charney, & Kedne, 1990), the Modified PTSD Symptom Scale, the Beck Depression Inventory, the Structured Clinical Interview for DSM-III-R Personality Disorders (SCID II; Spitzer, Williams, Gibbon, & First, 1990), and the Anxiety Disorder Interview Schedule—Revised Panic Module (ADIS-R; DiNardo & Barlow, 1988).

The trauma assessment indicated that T.J. had experienced several events in her lifetime that she considered traumatic. She reported that from ages 5 to 9 she witnessed violence against her mother by her father. Her father was a Vietnam veteran and most likely had PTSD himself, in addition to an alcohol problem. She reported that he was very explosive when he drank and frequently hit her mother. Her parents divorced when T.J. was 9 years old and she lived with her mother. She reported that she is still fearful of her father, although he was never physically abusive to her.

T.J. first married at age 19 and divorced at age 20 because her first husband was physically abusive. She remarried at age 23 and divorced again at age 27. Her second husband was both physically and sexually abusive. She reported that her second husband was very jealous of other men and would force her to have sex, telling her that he "would keep her sore, so she wouldn't want to sleep with anybody else." She had not labeled these experiences as rape until several years after her divorce. Her second husband also hit her once, when he thought she was looking at another man, and choked her when he thought she was going to leave him. Results of the diagnostic evaluation indicated that T.J. was suffering from PTSD with comorbid panic disorder. She also experienced symptoms of depression. See Table 2 for pretreatment and posttreatment scores on all assessment measures. T.J. was treated using multichannel exposure therapy (M-CET), a treatment that combines elements of CPT with cognitive-behavioral therapy for panic disorder, and completed 12 sessions of individual therapy using this approach.

Table 2.   Case 2 Pre- and Postassessment Measures

Measure	Preassessment	Postassessment
Clinician Administered PTSD Scale	PTSD positive	PTSD negative
ADIS Panic Module	Panic Disorder +	Panic Disorder −
Modified PTSD Symptom Scale	66	6
Beck Depression Inventory	22	9
Physical Reactions Scale	57	9

Sessions 1 and 2 of treatment focused on psychoeducation about PTSD and panic symptoms. T.J. was asked to complete monitoring forms on a daily basis for PTSD symptoms and to complete a panic attack record each time she had a panic attack. These symptoms were assessed over the course of treatment (see Figure 2). She was also asked to write about the meaning of the traumatic events she had experienced and was taught diaphragmatic breathing and asked to practice this on a daily basis for homework.

In sessions 3 and 4, the cognitive component of panic and PTSD was the main focus. Education about overestimating the probability of negative events and catastrophizing about the consequences of panic attacks was emphasized. T.J. was taught how to challenge distorted thinking using a worksheet that was modified from CPT.

Session 5 was a difficult session for T.J. She disclosed that she was considering dropping out of treatment because she found it so painful. We

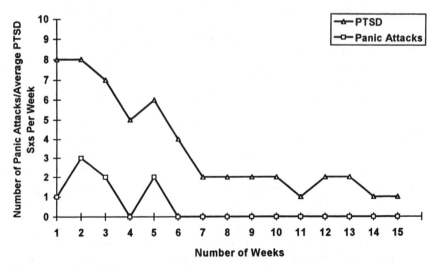

Figure 2.   Case 2: Progress record over course of treatment.

discussed this and she committed to continuing with treatment. The interoceptive exercises from the *Mastery of Your Anxiety and Panic* (Barlow & Craske, 1988) treatment were introduced. These are exercises that bring on sensations similar to those experienced during panic attacks. Exercises include spinning in a chair, hyperventilating, breath holding, and head shaking, among others. Each exercise was assessed for similarity to feeing of panic and for fear and anxiety resulting from the exercise. A hierarchy for practicing the exercises for homework was developed from these ratings.

Sessions 6, 7, and 8 focused on cognitive exposure through writing about the traumatic events. T.J. chose to write about one of the rapes in her second marriage that also included physical abuse. This was a particularly painful incident about which she previously avoided thinking. During this incident, her husband had become jealous of a friendship she had developed with a male co-worker and was convinced she was having an affair. One day after she had worked late, he accused her of having sex with the co-worker and began hitting her in the face, telling her, "I'll fix you so no man will ever want you." She reported trying to leave the house, but he would not let her leave, saying he had something planned "to fix her good." She reported that he dragged her in their bedroom and threw her on the bed, ordering her to take off her clothes. He then penetrated her with his penis and, after ejaculating, went into the bathroom and came out with a hot curling iron, which he used to penetrate her vagina, saying he was "branding her for being wicked." She thinks that she passed out and does not remember what happened after this. She did not tell anyone or seek any medical assistance. She was forced to quit her job after this incident, and left her second husband about 8 months later. She was very tearful when reading this incident in session and had to stop several times. She was able to continue with encouragement. For homework, she continued to practice the diaphragmatic breathing and the interoceptive exposure exercises in addition to writing about the event. The effects of trauma on her sense of safety was also introduced and she was asked to complete cognitive worksheets on this.

In session 9, the homework on safety issues was reviewed and the topic of trust was introduced and discussed. *In vivo* exposure was also introduced. T.J. identified three target fears: bike riding, going to a movie or dinner alone, and going to the mall. She had been avoiding these situations because of her fear of having a panic attack. Hierarchies for each of these fears were developed and she was asked to begin at the bottom of the hierarchy for riding a bike, which included riding only short distances in her neighborhood. She was also asked to complete cognitive worksheets about trust issues.

Session 10 focused on reviewing the homework assigned the previous session as well as introducing the issue of power/competence. On one of her cognitive worksheets about trust, she challenged the following thoughts, "Every man in my life has been a disappointment to me. They leave my life, they are unfaithful, and have been abusive. It is difficult to trust men." She was able to challenge these thoughts and say to herself, "Men can be disappointing, but that doesn't mean they all will be unfaithful or abusive. They are only human, too." She was asked to practice going to stores and going to movies for exposure homework and to complete Events–Thoughts–Feelings worksheets on power and competence issues.

There was a 3-week lapse between sessions 10 and 11; one week the therapist was on vacation and the other week T.J. had transportation difficulties. Despite the lapse, T.J. kept up with homework and monitoring of panic attacks and PTSD symptoms. She made significant progress on her *in vivo* exposure exercises and was beginning to feel comfortable going to movies and restaurants by herself. The issue of esteem was introduced and T.J. was asked to complete worksheets to challenge any distorted thinking in this area. It was decided to meet again in 2 weeks for her final therapy session to give her more time to complete other *in vivo* exposure exercises.

Session 12 was the final therapy session. T.J. was doing quite well and felt ready to terminate treatment. She had no panic attacks since 6 weeks into treatment and experienced only occasional symptoms of PTSD. She was scheduled for a posttreatment evaluation for the following week.

The posttreatment evaluation indicated T.J. no longer met criteria for PTSD or panic disorder. In addition, scores on the Beck Depression Inventory had decreased to a nondepressed level. Her scores on the Modified PTSD Symptom Scale and the Physical Reactions Scale, continuous measures of PTSD and panic attacks for the 2 weeks prior to assessment, indicated a dramatic decrease in current symptoms (see again Table 2). T.J.'s panic attacks and PTSD symptoms were assessed throughout treatment. Her monitoring records indicated that she had her last panic attack during the fifth week of treatment and remained panic free throughout the remainder of treatment. Her average number of PTSD symptoms per day dropped from an average of eight per day to an average of one per day by the end of treatment (see again Figure 2).

Discussion

These two cases demonstrate the effectiveness of cognitive behavioral therapy for treatment of PTSD and other symptoms associated with marital rape. In both cases, however, other types of traumatic events had been experienced, and while treatment focused on the physical and sexual violence that took place in a marital relationship, it was also necessary to acknowledge and process the cumulative effects of many traumas. Both of these women had terminated the violent marriages and no longer felt they were in danger. This allowed them to be able to process the events as memories rather than as current realities. In many cases, women may seek treatment while still involved in a violent relationship. In these cases it is important to assess the current level of safety and to devise a safety plan.

Initial work in these cases may focus on safety issues and how to leave the relationship rather than on processing traumatic memories. In other cases that may be relatively less violent and in which the marital partners are both seeking treatment to reduce violence or marital conflict, conjoint treatment programs may be recommended (Schlee, Heyman, & O'Leary, 1998). Additional research is needed to evaluate the conditions under which such conjoint treatment approaches or those that include separate perpetrator treatment components are most useful.

Medical Issues

Marital rape occurs at a high rate in subgroups of women who experience nonsexual battery, and rape in marriage has been found to be positively associated with high levels of nonsexual violence (Frieze, 1983; Shields & Hanneke, 1983). Such co-occurrence of sexual assault and battery was reported by both women described in the cases. For example, T.J. reported incidents of being hit and choked by her husband that were separate from sexual assault incidents. In addition, both women reported particularly violent sexual assaults by their spouses. Such incidents of violence can clearly be associated with acute physical injuries. Women who are physically assaulted by their partners are especially likely to be injured in the areas of their breasts, chest, or abdomen (Browne, 1993). As noted by Browne, studies indicate that one-fifth of women seen in emergency or surgical departments may have experienced partner violence. In the cases described here, both women reported incidents that were likely to be associated with acute injury that may have ranged in severity. Both women should have received medical care for acute injuries and potential exposure to sexually transmitted diseases. However, neither woman reported the assault to police, medical personnel, or anyone else. Hence they received no medical treatment. This failure to receive acute medical care is consistent with findings by Kilpatrick, Resnick, Saunders, and Best (1998) indicating that the vast majority of rape victims (84%) do not report the rape to police or other authorities and do not receive medical care for rape-related injuries or medical concerns.

Rape and physical assault incidents have also been found to be associated with increased rates of chronic physical health problems and high rates of medical utilization (Acierno, Resnick, & Kilpatrick, 1997; Browne, 1993; Goodman et al., 1993; Koss, Koss, & Woodruff, 1991; Resnick, Acierno, & Kilpatrick, 1997). Koss et al. (1991) found that women with histories of *both* physical assault and rape had the highest rates of medical utilization. Other data indicate the increased rates of medical utilization are mediated by actual impairments in health or increased health complaints observed within victimized, as opposed to nonvictimized, groups (Golding, 1996).

A variety of factors have been hypothesized to explain increased rates of negative health outcomes or complaints among women who have experienced physical assault or rape. Proposed mechanisms include actual health changes that may be a result of stress-related changes in immune or other hormonal systems; resultant effects of long-term physiological arousal as a function of exposure to trauma-related cues; misinterpretation of physiological arousal as a sign of physical illness; illness that is secondary to poor health behaviors, such as smoking or alcohol abuse; and failure to seek routine preventive medical care (Koss & Heslet, 1992; Resnick et al., 1997). The magnitude of the physical health problems associated with crime victimization is currently recognized by the American Medical Association (AMA Council on Scientific Affairs, 1992), and routine screening for a history of physical and sexual assault is recommended within healthcare settings (Browne, 1993; Cutton, Mitchell, & Haywood, 1996; Kilpatrick, Resnick, & Acierno, 1997; Koss et al., 1991). Such screening can help identify women who may benefit from treatment focused on the mental-health impact of past traumatic experiences as well as assist women who remain in potentially dangerous situations to develop an appropriate safety plan. These findings also highlight the importance of thorough assessment of victimization history with female clients by mental health professionals. They may need to address medical referral issues with these women, who may not have received medical care for their injuries.

Legal and Social Issues

The Marital Exemption

Legal Status

The two women in the case studies described here did not report their assaults to police or other authorities, so their alleged assailants suffered no legal consequences for their actions. The legal status of marital rape in the United States has undergone change in the past 20 years. For the majority of U.S. history, marital rape was not recognized as a crime. The first state to eliminate these so-called marital exemption laws was Nebraska in 1976 (Caringella-MacDonald, 1988). By 1991, 18 other states had followed suit and completely eliminated the marital exemption from their rape laws (Whatley, 1993), while only two states retained absolute exemption laws that prevented a husband from being prosecuted for rape under any circumstances. The remaining states enacted partial exemptions that would permit rape charges to be brought against a husband under limited circumstances, such as when partners are not cohabiting or are legally separated. Alternatively, partial exemptions in some states permit husbands accused of marital rape to be charged with a lesser degree of offense or to receive a lesser sentence. Currently, no states retain absolute exemptions for husbands, although many continue to provide for partial exemptions (National Clearinghouse on Marital and Date Rape, March 1996). Further, some states extend the marital exemption to unmarried cohabitants.

For a historical review of legal issues related to the marital rape exemption, including legal arguments in favor of and against retention of the exclusion law, the reader is referred to Barshis (1983). For more updated discussions of the status of marital rape exemptions, see Small and Tetreault (1990) and Whatley (1993), while Caringella-MacDonald (1988) provides a useful discussion of the consequences of legal reform for marital rape victims. Two resources for obtaining information in regard to marital rape laws on a state-by-state basis are the National Clearinghouse on Marital and Date Rape[1] and the National Organization for Women Legal Defense and Education Fund.[2]

Barshis (1983) argues for abolition of marital exemptions on the grounds that they violate a married woman's right to equal protection under the law by distinguishing between spousal and nonspousal assailants. She also discusses arguments that have been made for retaining marital exemptions. One particular argument that is worthy of comment here is the fear that repeal of the marital exemption would result in an "ensuing flood of litigation [that] would prove to be unbearably heavy on our already overburdened system" (p. 387). This fear has not materialized. Although rape in general is a highly underreported crime, marital rape is apparently even less likely to be reported. Caringella-MacDonald (1988) further discusses data indicating that actual prosecution is rare indeed. However, Whatley (1993) reviews data indicating that when marital rape is prosecuted, convictions are obtained in approximately 50% of cases and that rates do not differ as a function of whether or not the spouses were living together.

Societal Bias

Barshis (1983) argued that the traditional marital rape exemptions reflect more general societal attitudes. Although it is difficult to determine whether laws simply reflect or rather influence societal attitudes, there is

[1]National Clearinghouse on Marital and Date Rape, 2325 Oak Street, Berkeley, CA 94708; (510) 524-1582. http://members.aol.com/ncmdr/index/html
[2]National Organization for Women (NOW) Legal Defense and Education Fund, 99 Hudson Street, 12th Floor, New York, NY 13313; (212) 925-6635.

dence that individuals may view spousal and nonspousal rape differ-
tly. For example, in a poll of 1,300 people in the state of Texas, Jeffords
d Dull (1984) found that two-thirds of their sample *supported* marital-
pe exemption laws. Experimental paradigms have also been used to
vestigate this issue. Monson, Byrd, and Langhinrichsen-Rohling (1996)
ovided undergraduates with a written vignette describing a heterosex-
l interaction in which the man forced himself on top of the woman and
mpleted the act of intercourse, despite the woman's repeated resistance.
udents were less certain the act constituted rape and viewed it as less of a
olation of the woman's rights when he was identified as the woman's
usband than when he was identified as a stranger. Students rated the
sault as involving less violence, being less psychologically damaging to
e woman, and more likely to be a communication failure when the
erpetrator was a husband. Yet the groups did not differ in the degree to
hich they perceived the woman's sexual interest, enjoyment, or obliga-
on to engage in intercourse, which were uniformly low. On two measures—
ertainty of rape and violation of the woman's rights—the magnitude of
his effect was larger for men than for women.

Shotland and Goodstein (1992) obtained a similar effect for a history of
rior consensual intercourse on perceptions of a sexual assault between
onmarried partners. In their study, students read a vignette about a date
n which a man forced a woman into intercourse in the face of repeated
verbal and physical resistance. Respondents were less likely to view the
assault as rape and rated it as less violent when they were told the couple
had engaged in intercourse on 10 prior occasions in comparison to either 1
or no previous occasions. In addition, respondents inferred a greater level
of intent to have sex on the woman's part and greater obligation to have
sex when the couple shared a history of 10 prior intercourse experiences.

Summary

Due to changes in marital exemption laws in the past 20 years, a
greater number of women now have legal recourse to deal with spousal
rapists. However, conditions under which women can press rape charges
still varies as a function of state. Further, few women actually press
charges, although when they have done so convictions have been obtained
in approximately 50% of cases. To better assist victims of marital rape,
therapists should be familiar with local laws so that victims are fully aware
of their legal rights and can make informed decisions regarding participation in the criminal justice system. Therapists should also be prepared to
help educate clients that marital rape is a crime.

Members of our society at large, perhaps men in particular, and even victims themselves, appear to share this bias of distinguishing between spousal and nonspousal rape in a manner that views marital rape as a less serious offense. This bias may be related to a history of previous consensual sexual experiences, and therefore may extend beyond legal marriages to other sexually involved relationships. It was clear in the case of C.A. described earlier that she did not initially consider her rape a crime. This has important therapeutic implications in that a victim's social network, as well as the victim herself, may share similar attitudes. This may foster guilt and confusion in the victim, and reduce social support from those around her.

Family Issues

It has been noted that because of the nature of the relationship between victim and perpetrator, marital rape contains a number of components not present in stranger rape (including betrayal of intimacy and trust, and the victim's continued contact with her assailant) that warrant special attention. Thus, Kilpatrick et al. (1988) stressed the importance of assessing the victim's attitudes rather than ignoring or making assumptions about the relationship in a judgmental way. In addition, Kilpatrick (1983) urged that therapists take into consideration the impact that rape may have on significant others in the victim's life, including children and parents. Data cited earlier indicated that witnessing interpersonal violence between parents may increase risk of partner violence in the next generation. Thus, it is important to assess possible witnessing of marital rape or other violence by children in the family and provide appropriate intervention. Assessment of family functioning and family therapy, as well as individual treatment targeting specific problems and behaviors of individual family members, may be warranted in addition to individual treatment of the marital rape victim. Lystad (1982) recommended the assessment of the physical, psychological, social, and legal needs of family members subsequent to disclosure of sexual abuse in the family.

Assessment of Psychopathology

General Considerations

As previously noted, Hanneke and Shields (1985) suggested that reactions to marital rape may be similar to reactions to battering and stranger rape. Thus, assessment and treatment approaches derived from work with battered women and those used to assess and treat reactions following stranger rape may be useful tools in dealing with victims of marital rape. However, major differences between marital rape and stranger rape victims are the chronicity of exposure to stress and the possibility that the victim may still be living with her assailant at the time assessment and treatment are sought. Therefore, as with battering, the first issues that should be addressed are those related to physical safety. At this stage in assessment or treatment, therapists may have to help the woman develop a safety plan (Dutton *et al.*, 1996; Neufeld, 1996) and gain access to community resources for social, material, and financial support.

Beyond issues of immediate safety, Kilpatrick (1983) has noted several issues related to therapist interactions with rape victims in general that may also apply to marital rape victims. These include the need for the therapist to guard against displaying a judgmental attitude toward the victim, owing to possible personal biases, or allowing inconsistent or disorganized behavior on the victim's part to cause frustration and anger. Similarly, in terms of possible attitudinal biases that may affect the therapeutic interaction, Hanneke and Shields (1985) suggested that the ambiguous legal and social atmosphere in which marital rape occurs may cause some therapists to doubt the validity of the victims' claims and problems. Also contributing to this is a tendency in our society to blame the victim (Weingourt, 1985).

Finally, suggestions made by Douglas (1982), based on her work with domestic violence victims, argue for the importance of empowering the victim and modeling a more balanced relationship with the client (including facilitation of autonomous decision making and acquisition of more adaptive responses to stress). As in the case studies described earlier, this would include providing feedback and education to the client about results of assessment and related treatment recommendations, getting feedback from the client indicating what she would consider to be significant indicators of progress in treatment (e.g., being able to disclose the assaults to a friend), and emphasizing the importance of the client's active role in completing and practicing treatment homework assignments for treatment efficacy.

Assessment of Victimization History

Major issues in assessment include the importance of conducting a thorough victimization history as well as use of standardized assessment instruments to assess psychological distress and functioning. As was noted in both of the case studies described earlier, the experience of marital rape occurred in the context of a history of multiple exposures to traumatic events, including childhood sexual assault. In addition, both women reported the experience of physical assaults by their partners that were separate from the rape experiences. As part of our structured assessment for lifetime history of traumatic event exposure we identified the history of marital rape and other violent experiences. These marital rape incidents may not have been disclosed by the client without careful assessment by the therapists. Many rape victims may not seek psychological treatment immediately after their assault (Kilpatrick, 1983), and when they do, the focus may be on presenting symptoms such as anxiety or depression, rather than the rape incident *per se*. In addition to possible failure to associate an assault with later symptoms, many victims may not label or acknowledge the incident as rape. Hanneke and Shields (1985) suggested that women who experience both marital rape and battering may define the rape as simply another instance of violence and may not specifically report the occurrence of rape. Also, these women may be more likely to focus on nonsexual violence or general marital problems in treatment, rather than marital rape specifically.

To address these issues, Kilpatrick (1983) recommended that a thorough assault history of female clients be done routinely by mental health providers. In addition, use of specific operational language in questions about the occurrence of concrete behaviors, versus labels such as "rape," "sexual abuse," or "battery," is recommended to avoid biases about what actually constitutes rape (Kilpatrick, 1983; Weingourt, 1985). Kilpatrick also recommended obtaining a careful assessment of chronological sequencing of victimization incidents and psychological distress to formulate hypotheses about the association between specific traumatic events and symptoms. This may be particularly important for cases of marital rape in which the abuse has been chronic and involved both sexual and nonsexual violence and in cases in which previous or extramarital sexual assaults or other types of victimization have also occurred. One self-report instrument that may be of particular help in obtaining a thorough history of interpersonal violence in a particular relationship is the Revised Conflict Tactics Scales (CTS2; Straus, Hamby, Boney-McCoy, & Sugarman, 1996), which now includes a new sexual coercion scale. This series of questions about force and pressure to make a partner have sexual activity is an important addition that will allow for assessment of marital rape. Other measures for the assessment of a variety of traumatic events are reviewed in greater detail elsewhere (Norris & Riad, 1996; Resnick, Falsetti, Kilpatrick, & Freedy, 1996; Stamm, 1996).

The traumatic event history assessment that was conducted in the case studies described earlier was conducted following a structured interview designed for clinicians called the Trauma Assessment for Adults

(Stamm, 1996). This interview guides the assessment of lifetime incidents of potentially traumatic events including combat, serious accidents, and sexual and physical assaults. Follow-up questions are asked for each type of event endorsed to determine age at occurrence and whether the individual feared that she would be seriously injured or killed during any incidents of that type.

Assessment of Symptomatology

It is important to conduct a thorough interview to assess potential emergent issues prior to conducting additional symptom assessment. Douglas (1982), in light of her work with victims of domestic violence, recommended that a mental status examination be done if the victim was recently assaulted by her husband, with particular attention paid to risk of suicide, homicidal intent toward the assailant, and assessment of capacity to care for herself and her children. As noted earlier, we also assess whether the victim received needed medical care for possible injuries secondary to assault and try to facilitate clients' accessing appropriate medical care.

We recommend use of standardized instruments to assess psychological functioning, such as those in the Shields and Hanneke (1987) study. Included are several standardized measures of general psychological distress and social adjustment, as well as measures of specific fears that have previously been used with rape victim samples. A variety of such measures were used to assess psychological functioning in the two case studies described. These included measures of general psychological distress such as the Symptom Checklist 90–Revised (Derogatis, 1977) and measures of distress related to specific disorders such as depression using the Beck Depression Inventory (Beck et al., 1961) or PTSD using the Modified PTSD Symptom Severity Self-Report (Falsetti et al., 1993). Other useful self-report measures of PTSD include the PTSD Symptom Scale (PSS-Self Report; Foa, Riggs, Dancu, & Rothbaum, 1993) and the Impact of Event Scale (Horowitz et al., 1979). As noted in Case Study 1, we routinely administer the Physical reactions Scale (developed by Falsetti and Resnick and cited in Falsetti & Resnick, 1997) to assess whether clients are experiencing panic attack symptoms that are causing them distress and anticipatory anxiety, regardless of whether the client perceives the panic attacks to be cued by reminders of a traumatic event. Thorough descriptions of other PTSD symptom assessment measures are included in Norris and Riad (1996).

We also recommend using structured diagnostic interviews in assessment. Currently, we conduct assessments of lifetime and current major depression, lifetime and current panic attacks and panic disorder, and agoraphobia, and lifetime and current PTSD following the Structured Clinical Interview for DSM-IV (SCID-I; First, Spitzer, Gibbon, & Williams, 1997). This allows us to assess longer-term functioning and to assess for multiple mental health outcomes that may be associated with exposure to traumatic events. Additional diagnostic assessment can be conducted as indicated by self-report screening. The Diagnostic Interview Schedule (DIS-IV; Robins, Cottler, Bucholz, & Compton, 1996) also allows for assessment of PTSD and a range of other Axis I diagnoses. There are additional interviews that focus specifically on anxiety disorders, such as the Anxiety Disorders Interview Schedule—Revised (DiNardo & Barlow, 1988) and the Clinician Administered PTSD Scale (CAPS; Blake *et al.*, 1990) for the clinical interview assessment of PTSD symptom frequency and severity.

Treatment Options

The literature on marital rape has focused mainly on assessment issues rather than specific techniques to be used in treatment, and there are no controlled outcome studies of effectiveness of different treatment approaches with this particular population. This section, therefore, contains a summary of suggestions for treatment based primarily on the literature related to treatment of posttraumatic stress disorder and other outcomes associated with traumatic events and rape in general.

In this section, we briefly summarize three cognitive–behavior treatments that have accumulated some evidence for their efficacy in the treatment of posttraumatic stress reactions among rape victims. A fourth treatment that is currently being developed at the Medical University of South Carolina by two of the authors (S.A.F. and H.S.R.) specifically to address PTSD with comorbid panic attacks is also described.

Stress Inoculation Training (SIT)

SIT is a comprehensive coping skills training approach, developed at the Medical University of South Carolina, to treat anxiety-related symptoms following rape (Veronen & Kilpatrick, 1983). The treatment, which was patterned after Meichenbaum's stress inoculation procedures, includes instruction in coping skills for management of anxiety in physiological, cognitive, and behavioral response channels. It is to be applied to rape-related fears as well as to anxiety related to other stressful situations. SIT includes an initial educational phase in which clients are provided with information about typical reactions to rape, as well as a learning theory formulation of the development of rape-related fears that may be expressed in the three response channels. Clients actively participate in the process of identifying fear-eliciting cues related to the rape (target fears), as well as identification of their own unique responses experienced in each of the three channels. The rationale for application of various component skills are outlined, and treatment is presented as an active strategy for the management of anxiety in a variety of situations. This phase of treatment may serve to normalize reactions and promote a sense of control by assisting clients to discriminate particular situations that are more or less anxiety provoking.

In the next phase of treatment, a variety of strategies are taught to the client for each of the three channels in which anxiety is expressed. Clients are encouraged to select those techniques they find most useful.

Physiological Channels

For application in the physiological channel, muscle relaxation and controlled breathing techniques are taught. Clients are instructed to practice relaxation techniques at home and to apply them with both rape-related (target) and nontarget fear stimuli. For example, a target fear might be staying home alone at night; a nontarget fear might be a job interview.

Cognitive Channel

The techniques of thought stopping and guided self-dialogue are taught to address the cognitive expressions of anxiety. Self-dialogue is a cognitive restructuring technique that includes identification of irrational or dysfunctional cognitions and adoption and use of more adaptive cognitions to cope with a stressor.

Behavioral Channel

Finally, role-playing, covert modeling, imaginal progression through anxiety-producing situations, and assertion techniques are applied to decrease behavioral avoidance.

Veronen and Kilpatrick (1983) reported improvement on measures of anxiety and mood in a small group of rape victims following SIT treatment. Kilpatrick and Amick (1985) also reported positive results in a single case study, in which cognitive, physiological, and behavioral assessment measures were used pre- and posttreatment. Resick, Jordan, Girelli, Huter, and Marhoeger-Dvorak (1988) found that SIT was associated with significantly greater reduction in anxiety-related symptoms, compared with a waiting list control group, but results indicated that there were no significant differences between SIT and assertion training or supportive/ educational psychotherapy group treatments. Finally, Foa, Rothbaum, Riggs, and Murdock (1991) reported results of a comparative treatment study that evaluated SIT and prolonged exposure against supportive counseling and no treatment. Both active treatments resulted in significant improvements. Although SIT appeared somewhat more effective than prolonged exposure immediately after treatment, this pattern was reversed at follow-up.

Prolonged Exposure (PE)

A number of different exposure therapies have been developed to reduce anxiety reactions and behavioral avoidance, such as systematic desensitization, imaginal flooding, and participant modeling. Although each treatment has its own unique features, what they have in common is repeated exposure to stimuli that elicit strong feelings of fear and avoidance tendencies under conditions of safety. The goal of such therapies is the extinction of conditioned fear acquired during the traumatic event. Foa and Rothbaum (1998), along with their colleagues (e.g., Foa et al., 1991), have been involved in developing evaluating, and manualizing this approach for use with rape victims. Treatment consists of four major components: (1) education about PTSD symptoms and provision of a treatment rationale based on emotional processing theory (Foa & Kozak, 1986); (2) training in diaphragmatic breathing; (3) development of a fear hierarchy for *in vivo* exposure assignments to be carried out as homework; and (4) imaginal exposure to the rape memory conducted in sessions and repeated as homework. During imaginal exposure, clients are instructed to close their eyes, recall the memory of the assault in as much detail as possible, and to "describe the assault in the present tense, as if it were happening right now" (Foa & Rothbaum, 1998, p. 162). Ideally, this reliving process continues until the client experiences a decline in anxiety within the session. Although research into the use of prolonged exposure with other anxiety reactions suggests that within-session fear reduction is not *necessary* to achieving long-term fear reduction (Chaplin & Levine, 1981), within-session fear reduction does appear to facilitate between-session fear reduction and is generally predictive of better outcome (Foa, Grayson, Steketee, Doppelt, Turner, & Latimer, 1983).

In addition to the study by Foa et al. (1991) that found PE and SIT to generally be of comparable effectiveness, a recent study by Foa, Hearst-Ikeda, and Perry (1995) found that a brief (4-week) intervention that combined PE with cognitive restructuring applied within a month of the index assault prevented the development of PTSD in 9 of the 10 women who received the treatment. In contrast, 7 of the 10 women in a matched assessment only condition developed PTSD over a comparable period of time. In a randomized controlled study, Echeburua, deCocral, Zubizarreta, & Sarasua (1997) found PE to be more effective than relaxation training among a group of female sexual assault victims. Approximately half of their sample were adult victims of rape, while the remaining participants had been victims of childhood sexual abuse. Comparisons between these two subgroups indicated that treatment was equally effective. For a more detailed review of PE in the treatment of PTSD, see Foa and Meadows (1997).

Cognitive Processing Therapy (CPT)

CPT (Resick & Schnicke, 1993) is based on the concepts of *assimilation*, altering the representation of new information to fit an existing schema, and *accommodation*, altering an existing schema to accept the new, otherwise discrepant, information. It is believed that the experience of a traumatic event, such as rape, violates existing schemas about safety, trust, intimacy, esteem, and power (McCann, Sakheim, & Abrahamson, 1988). It is further assumed that posttraumatic stress symptoms, such as PTSD, guilt, anger, and shame, are caused by the conflict between existing schemas and the new schema-discrepant information. In the attempt to process the new information, a woman may try to assimilate the new information (e.g., "Maybe it really wasn't rape, maybe I wanted it to happen") or she may *overaccommodate* the information (e.g., "Since the assault, I will never be safe," "I will never trust anyone ever again"). The goal of CPT is to assist in the integration of the event, with complete processing of the emotions and accommodation of the schema, while helping the client to maintain a healthy, balanced outlook on the world (i.e., prevention of overaccommodation).

To accomplish these goals, CPT provides information about PTSD and a treatment rationale in terms of an information processing model; exposure to the traumatic memory through writing about the event and reading the narrative; and training in the identification and challenging of maladaptive cognitions. An important focus of treatment is to identify and challenge "stuck points," inadequately processed conflicts between prior schema and new information. These skills of learning to identify, challenge, and modify distorted cognitions are then applied to each of the domains of safety, trust, intimacy, esteem, and power. Further details of the application of CPT to a case of marital rape were discussed in the first case study earlier in this chapter.

Resick and Schnicke (1993) reported significant improvements on symptoms of PTSD and depression following CPT among a group of 19 rape victims. Prior to treatment, 17 of the women met full criteria for PTSD and 12 met criteria for major depression. At posttreatment, none of the women met criteria for PTSD while only 5 continued to meet criteria for major depression. These positive results were maintained at six month follow-up. At present, Resick, Nishith, & Astin (1996) are in the process of comparing CPT with PE.

Multiple Channel Exposure Therapy (M-CET) for PTSD with Comorbid Panic

M-CET is a treatment currently undergoing development and evaluation specifically for individuals suffering from PTSD with comorbid panic attacks. It was adapted from a combination of SIT, CPT, and Barlow and Craske's (1988) *Mastery of Your Anxiety and Panic.* As with the preceding treatments, M-CET begins with information about PTSD and a cognitive-behavioral rationale for the remaining components of treatment, which consist of writing about the traumatic event and reading the narrative, *in vivo* exposure to feared situations that are otherwise objectively safe, and cognitive restructuring exercises. Worksheets addressing disruptions in beliefs about safety, trust, esteem, and power have also been adopted from CPT. What is unique about M-CET is the provision of exposure to the sensations of physiological arousal prior to the cognitive (i.e., writing) and behavioral (i.e., *in vivo*) exposure exercises. This is based on the rationale that individuals who are fearful of panic attacks may not be willing or able to tolerate the high levels of physiological arousal that can occur during cognitive and behavioral exposure. Therefore, by first targeting the "fear of fear," clients may be able to derive greater benefit from the later cognitive and behavioral exposure assignments. This is accomplished through having participants engage in a variety of interoceptive exposure exercises developed by Barlow and Craske (1988) (e.g., intentional hyperventilation, spinning in a chair, stair-stepping) designed to induce symptoms of panic attacks, such as light-headedness, dizziness, and tachycardia.

A second reason for incorporating exposure to the physiological sensations of panic is based on the observation that panic symptoms are frequently present during a violent assault such as a rape (Resnick, 1997). A panic attack that occurs during a traumatic event is conceptualized as an unconditioned response (a "true alarm") to the trauma that becomes a conditioned response to reminders of the trauma. Thus interoceptive exposure exercises also serve to provide exposure to the physiological component of fear directly associated with the trauma. Preliminary data on a small group of participants ($n = 13$) are encouraging (Falsetti & Resnick,

1998). All patients who completed treatment no longer experienced panic attacks and displayed a significant reduction in symptoms of PTSD. Currently, the effectiveness of M-CET is being formally evaluated in a controlled study. Further details of the application of M-CET to a case of marital rape were presented in the second case study described earlier in this chapter.

Selecting a Treatment

Given the availability of a number of promising treatments for rape-related PTSD but absence of relevant comparative-treatment or client-treatment matching data, clinicians must look elsewhere for guidance in selecting among available treatments. Falsetti (1997) has discussed this issue in terms of Nezu and Nezu's (1995) problem-solving approach to making treatment decisions. To further assist decision making, she organized components of the various treatments for PTSD into six phases of treatment and provides guidelines to help select among treatment options at each phase. All treatments begin with an *education* phase that provides information about PTSD and a general cognitive–behavioral orientation. The primary decision at this point is in regard to whether the client requires additional education related to comorbid conditions (e.g., panic disorder, depression).

Following client education, the therapist should assess the client's *coping skills*, and where appropriate, provide training in specific skills (e.g., diaphragmatic breathing, relaxation). An initial *exposure* phase is then implemented focusing on symbolic exposure to the rape memory. Here, the therapist may select between imaginal exposure (as in the PE protocol) or writing about the trauma (as in CPT and M-CET protocols), based on such considerations as the client's ability to engage in vivid imagery and preference of imagery or writing. In cases where the client experiences comorbid panic attacks, interoceptive exposure exercises are introduced prior to initiating symbolic exposure to the assault memory. Because symbolic exposure often elicits distorted beliefs and faulty thinking patterns, this naturally leads into a *cognitive* phase. Clients receive education about the interconnections among thoughts, feelings, and behaviors, and learn skills to identify and challenge dysfunctional beliefs. The various CPT modules related to safety, trust, intimacy, esteem, and power may serve as a useful guide to important domains in which the client may have developed dysfunctional beliefs.

The final active phase of treatment targets behavioral avoidance of situations and activities that serve to cue panic attacks or are trauma-related through *in vivo* exposure exercises. An important consideration in the development of a fear hierarchy for such exercises is the objective safety of the various situations, as some assaults may have occurred in dangerous situations and their continued avoidance would be adaptive. Following treatment is an *evaluation* phase in which the course of treatment is reviewed and the client's level of functioning is reevaluated. The goals for such a review are to identify those aspects of treatment viewed by the client and therapist as having been helpful and make decisions about continued treatment or termination.

The two case studies described in this chapter illustrate the selection of manualized treatment approaches designed to be implemented with patients with PTSD (Cognitive Processing Therapy) or PTSD with comorbid panic attacks (Multiple Channel Exposure Therapy). Each treatment approach contains an integration of skills training and exposure components. The treatments differ in that the role of physiological arousal and exposure to physiological arousal cues is an important component of M-CET. M-CET also includes an emphasis on behavioral avoidance in the etiology of PTSD and panic symptoms and includes directed *in vivo* exposure exercises. In addition, M-CET includes both behavioral learning theory and cognitive theoretical rationales.

Summary

The two cases included in this chapter are good examples of the characteristics of marital rape that are described in the extant literature. As such, they consisted of extremely violent assaults, they co-occurred with other physical violence in the relationship, and they were associated with significant mental health outcomes reflected by diagnoses for PTSD as well as PTSD with comorbid panic disorder. Also, as is true in the majority of rape cases, the crimes were not reported to the police and the victims did not receive timely medical care for potential injuries suffered. Although further legal reforms have been enacted since the first edition of this book, social attitudes may not have changed significantly about marital rape. Thus, it is important to emphasize that this type of rape can be the most violent type of incident, including injuries or physical restraint as well as fear on the part of the victim that she might be killed or seriously injured.

In other cases, threatening or pressuring may be less overtly violent, victims may not acknowledge or identify the incident as rape, and the victims may not be at a decision point with regard to their relationships. These factors highlight the need for clinicians and researchers to conduct epidemiological research to understand the prevalence, characteristics, and impacts of marital rape within representative samples of women. It is clear that from the extant research with marital rape victims, who often experience multiple forms of violence, that marital rape is associated with increased levels of psychological distress, with rates of major psychiatric disorder (including PTSD or symptoms consistent with PTSD) comparable to those observed in stranger rape victims.

It appears that currently available manualized treatments such as SIT, PE, and CPT may be highly effective in treatment of mental health sequelae associated with marital rape. In addition, a treatment in development, M-CET also has demonstrated efficacy in several case studies in which it has been used. Preliminary data indicate effectiveness of this treatment relative to a minimal attention comparison group (Falsetti & Resnick, 1998). In addition to such treatment approaches, it may also be important to develop or include treatment components to further address economic and vocational resource needs of victims of marital rape. In all such cases, it is essential to identify and address any immediate safety concerns as a first step in treatment.

References

Acierno, R., Resnick, H. S., & Kilpatrick, D. G. (1997). Health impact of interpersonal violence 1: Prevalence rates for sexual assault, physical assault, and domestic violence in men and women. *Behavioral Medicine, 23*, 53–64.

American Medical Association Council on Scientific Affairs. (1992). Violence against women: Relevance for medical practitioners. *Journal of the American Medical Association, 267*, 3184–3189.

American Psychiatric Association. (1994). *Diagnostic and statistical manual of mental disorders* (4th ed.). Washington, DC: Author.

Astin, M. C., Ogland-Hand, S. M., Coleman, E. M., & Foy, D. W. (1995). Posttraumatic stress disorder and childhood abuse in battered women: Comparisons with maritally distressed women. *Journal of Consulting and Clinical Psychology, 63*, 308–312.

Barlow, D. H., & Craske, M. G. (1988). *Mastery of your anxiety and panic* [manual]. Albany, NY: Center for Stress and Anxiety Disorder.

Barshis, V. R. G. (1983). The question of marital rape. *Women's Studies International Forum, 6*, 383–393.

Beck, A. T., Ward, C. H., Mendelsohn, M., Mock, J., & Erbaugh, J. (1961). An inventory for measuring depression. *Archives of General Psychiatry, 4*, 561–571.

Blake, D. D., Weathers, F. W., Nagy, L. M., Kaloupek, D. G., Klauminzer, G., Charney, D. S., & Keane, T. M. (1990). A clinician rating scale for assessing current and lifetime PTSD: The CAPS-1. *The Behavior Therapist, 18*, 187–188.

Browne, A. (1993). Violence against women by male partners: Prevalence, outcomes, and policy implications. *American Psychologist, 48*, 1077–1087.

Caringella-MacDonald, S. (1988). Parallels and pitfalls: The aftermath of legal reform for sexual assault, marital rape, and domestic violence. *Journal of Interpersonal Violence, 3*, 174–189.

Chaplin, E. W., & Levine, B. A. (1981). The effects of total exposure duration and interrupted versus continuous exposure in flooding therapy. *Behavior Therapy, 12*, 360–368.

Derogatis, L. R. (1977). *SCL-90: Administration, scoring and procedure manual I for the R (revised) version*. Baltimore: Johns Hopkins University School of Medicine.

DiNardo, P. A., & Barlow, D. H. (1988). *Anxiety Disorders Interview Schedule—Revised (ADIS-R)*. Albany, NY: Graywind Publications.

Douglas, M. A. (1982, August). *Behavioral assessment with battered women*. Paper presented at the 90th annual convention of the American Psychological Association, Washington, DC.

Dutton, M. A., Mitchell, B., & Haywood, Y. (1996). The emergency department as a violence prevention center. *JAMWA, 51*, 92–95, 117.

Echeburua, E., de Corral, P., Zubizarreta, I., & Sarasua, B. (1997). Psychological treatment of chronic posttraumatic stress disorder in victims of sexual aggression. *Behavior Modification, 21*, 433–456.

Falsetti, S. A. (1997). The decision-making process of choosing a treatment for patients with civilian trauma-related PTSD. *Cognitive and Behavioral Practice, 4*, 99–121.

Falsetti, S. A., & Resnick, H. S. (1997). Frequency and severity of panic attack symptoms in a treatment seeking sample of trauma victims. *Journal of Traumatic Stress, 10*, 683–689.

Falsetti, S. A., & Resnick, H. S. (1998, March). *Preliminary results of a manualized group treatment: Cognitive behavioral therapy for PTSD with comorbid panic attacks*. Presented at the 18th annual national conference of the Anxiety Disorders Association of America, Boston.

Falsetti, S. A., Resnick, H. S., Resick, P. A., & Kilpatrick, D. G. (1993). The modified PTSD symptom scale: A brief self-report of posttraumatic stress disorder. *The Behavior Therapist, 16*, 161–162.

Finkelhor, D., & Yllo, K. (1983). Rape in marriage: A sociological view. In D. Finkelhor, R. J. Gelles, G. T. Hotaling, & M. A. Straus (Eds.), *The dark side of families* (pp. 119–130). Beverly Hills, CA: Sage.

First, M. B., Spitzer, R. L., Gibbon, M., & Williams, J. B. W. (1997). *Structured Clinical Interview for DSM-IV Axis I Disorders (SCID-I)*. Washington, DC: American Psychiatric Press.

Foa, E. B., & Kozak, M. J. (1986). Emotional processing of fear: Exposure to corrective information. *Psychological Bulletin, 99*, 20–35.

Foa, E. B., & Meadows, E. A. (1997). Psychosocial treatments for posttraumatic stress disorder: A critical review. *Annual Review of Psychology, 48*, 449–480.

Foa, E. B., & Rothbaum, B. O. (1998). *Treating the trauma of rape: Cognitive-behavior therapy for PTSD*. New York: Guilford Press.

Foa, E. B, Grayson, J. B., Steketee, G. S., Doppelt, H. G., Turner, R. M., & Latimer, P. R. (1983). Successes and failure in the behavioral treatment of obsessive-compulsives. *Journal of Consulting and Clinical Psychology, 51*, 287–297.

Foa, E. B., Rothbaum, B. O., Rigs, D. S., & Murdock T. B. (1991). Treatment of posttraumatic stress disorder in rape victims: A comparison between cognitive-behavior procedures and counseling. *Journal of Consulting and Clinical Psychology, 59*, 715–723.

Foa, E. B., Riggs, D. S., Dancu, C. V., & Rothbaum, B. O. (1993). Reliability and validity of a brief instrument for assessing posttraumatic stress disorder. *Journal of Traumatic Stress, 6*, 459–473.

Foa, E. B., Hearst-Ikeda, D., & Perry, K. J. (1995). Evaluation of a brief program for the prevention of chronic PTSD in recent assault victims. *Journal of Consulting and Clinical Psychology, 63*, 948–955.

Frieze, I. H. (1980, September). *Causes and consequences of marital rape*. Paper presented at the annual meeting of the American Psychological Association, Montreal, Canada.

Frieze, I. H. (1983). Investigating the causes and consequences of marital rape. *Signs, 8*, 532–533.

Golding, J. M. (1996). Sexual assault history and limitations in physical functioning in two general population samples. *Research in Nursing and Health, 19,* 33–44.

Goodman, L. A., Koss, M. P., & Russo, N. F. (1993). Violence against women: Physical and mental health effects. Part I: Research findings. *Applied and Preventative Psychology, 2,* 79–89.

Hanneke, C. R., & Shields, N. M. (1985). Marital rape: Implications for the helping professions. *Social Casework, October,* 451–458.

Hanneke, C. A., Shields, N. M., & McCall, G. J. (1986). Assessing the prevalence of marital rape. *Journal of Interpersonal Violence, 1,* 350–362.

Horowitz, M., Wilner, N., & Alvarez, W. (1979). Impact of Event Scale: A measure of subjective stress. *Psychosomatic Medicine, 41,* 209–218.

Hotaling, G. T., & Sugarman, D. B. (1986). An analysis of risk markers in husband to wife violence: The current state of knowledge. *Violence and Victims, 1,* 101–124.

Housekamp, B. M., & Foy, D. W. (1991). The assessment of posttraumatic stress disorder in battered women. *Journal of Interpersonal Violence, 6,* 367–375.

Jeffords, C. R., & Dull, R. T. (1982). Demographic variations in attitudes toward marital rape immunity. *Journal of Marriage and the Family, 44,* 755–762.

Kemp, A., Rawlings, E. I., & Green, B. L. (1991). Posttraumatic stress disorder (PTSD) in battered women: A shelter sample. *Journal of Traumatic Stress, 4,* 137–148.

Kessler, R. C., Sonnega, A., Bromet, E., Hughes, M., & Nelson, C. B. (1995). Posttraumatic stress disorders in the National Comorbidity Survey. *Archives of General Psychiatry, 52,* 1048–1060.

Kilpatrick, D. G. (1983). Rape victims: Detection, assessment, and treatment. *Clinical Psychologist, 36,* 92–95.

Kilpatrick, D. G. (1993). Introduction [Special section on rape]. *Journal of Interpersonal Violence, 8,* 193–197.

Kilpatrick, D. G., & Amick, A. E. (1985). Rape trauma. In M. Hersen & C. G. Last (Eds.), *Behavior therapy casebook* (pp. 87–103). New York: Springer.

Kilpatrick, D. G., Best, C. L., Saunders, B. E., & Veronen, L. J. (1988). Rape in marriage and in dating relationships: How bad is it for mental health? *Annals of the New York Academy of Sciences, 528,* 335–344.

Kilpatrick, D. G., Edmunds, C. S., & Seymour, A. K. (1992). *Rape in America: A report to the nation.* Arlington, VA: National Victims Center and Medical University of South Carolina.

Kilpatrick, D. G., Resnick, H. S., & Acierno, R. (1997). Health impact of interpersonal violence 3: Implications for public policy. *Behavioral Medicine, 23,* 79–85.

Kilpatrick, D. G., Resnick, H. S., Saunders, B. E., & Best, C. L. (1998). Rape, other violence against women, and posttraumatic stress disorder: Critical issues in assessing the adversity-stress-psychopathology relationship. In B. P. Dohrenwend (Ed.), *Adversity, stress, and psychopathology* (pp. 161–176). New York: Oxford University Press.

Kilpatrick, D. G., Saunders, B. E., Amick-McMullan, A., Best, C. L., Veronen, L. J., & Resnick, H. S. (1989). Victim and crime factors with the development of crime-related disorder. *Behavior Therapy, 20,* 199–214.

Kilpatrick, D. G., Saunders, B. E., Veronen, L. J., Best, C. L., & Von, J. M. (1987). Criminal victimization: Lifetime prevalence, reporting to police and psychological impact. *Crime and Delinquency, 33,* 479–489.

Kilpatrick, D. G., Veronen, L. J., & Best, C. L. (1985). Factors predicting psychological distress among rape victims. In C. R. Figley (Ed.), *Trauma and its wake* (pp. 113–141). New York: Brunner/Mazel.

Kilpatrick, D. G., Veronen, L. J., & Resick, P. A. (1979). The aftermath of rape: Recent empirical findings. *American Journal of Orthopsychiatry, 49,* 658–699.

Koss, M. P. (1983). The scope of rape: Implications for the clinical treatment of reactions. *Clinical Psychologist, 36,* 88–91.

Koss, M. P. (1993). Detecting the scope of rape: A review of prevalence research methods. *Journal of Interpersonal Violence, 8,* 198–222.

Koss, M. P., & Heslet, L. (1992). The somatic consequences of violence against women. *Archives of Family Medicine, 1,* 53–59.

Koss, M. P., Koss, P. G., & Woodruff, J. (1991). Deleterious effects of criminal victimization on women's health and medical utilization. *Archives of Internal Medicine, 151,* 342–347.

Lystad, M. H. (1982). Sexual abuse in the home: A review of the literature. *International Journal of Family Psychiatry, 3,* 3–31.

McCann, I. L., Sakheim, D. K., & Abrahamson, D. J. (1988). Trauma and victimization: A model of psychological adaptation. *The Counseling Psychologist, 16,* 531–594.

Monson, C. M., Byrd, G. R., & Langhinrichsen-Rohling, J. (1996). To have and to hold: Perceptions of marital rape. *Journal of Interpersonal Violence, 11,* 410–424.

National Clearinghouse on Marital and Date Rape: http://members.aol.com.ncmdr/index.html

Neufeld, B. (1996). SAFE questions: Overcoming barriers to the detection of domestic violence. *American Family Physicians, 53,* 2575–2580.

Nezu, C. M., & Nezu, A. M. (1995). Critical decision making in everyday practice: The science in the art. *Cognitive and Behavioral Practice, 2,* 5–25.

Norris, F. H., & Riad, J. K. (1996). Standardized self-report measures of civilian trauma and PTSD. In J. Wilson & T. Keane (Eds.), *Assessing psychological trauma and PTSD: A practitioner's handbook.* New York: Guilford Press.

Resick, P. A., & Schnicke, M. K. (1993). *Cognitive processing therapy for rape victims: A treatment manual.* Newbury Park, CA: Sage.

Resick, P. A., Jordan, D. G., Girelli, S. A., Hutter, C. K., & Marhoefer-Dvorak, S. (1988). A comparative outcome study of behavioral group therapy for sexual assault victims. *Behavior Therapy, 19,* 385–401.

Resick, P. A., Nishith, P., & Astin, M. C. (1996, November). Preliminary results of an outcome study comparing cognitive processing therapy and prolonged exposure. In P. Resick (Chair), *Treating sexual assault/sexual abuse pathology: Recent findings.* Symposium conducted at the meeting of the Association for Advancement of Behavior Therapy, New York.

Resnick, H. S. (1997). Acute panic reactions among rape victims: Implications for prevention of post-rape psychopathology. *National Center for PTSD Clinical Quarterly, 7,* 41, 43–45.

Resnick, H. S., Acierno, R., & Kilpatrick, D. G. (1997). Health impact of interpersonal violence 2: Medical and mental health outcomes. *Behavioral Medicine, 23,* 65–78.

Resnick, H. S., Falsetti, S. A., Kilpatrick, D. G., & Freedy, J. R. (1996). Assessment of rape and other civilian trauma-related PTSD: Emphasis on assessment of potentially traumatic events. In T. W. Miller (Ed.), *Theory and assessment of stressful life events.* Madison, CT: International Universities Press.

Resnick, H. S., Kilpatrick, D. G., Dansky, B. S., Saunders, B. E., & Best, C. L. (1993). Prevalence of civilian trauma and posttraumatic stress disorder in a representative national sample of women. *Journal of Consulting and Clinical Psychology, 61,* 984–991.

Riggs, D. S., Kilpatrick, D. G., & Resnick, H. S. (1992). Long-term psychological distress associated with marital rape and aggravated assault: A comparison to other crimes. *Journal of Family Violence, 7,* 283–296.

Robins, L. N., Cottler, L., Bucholz, K., & Comptom, W. (1996). *Diagnostic Interview Schedule for DSM-IV (DIS-IV).* St. Louis, MO: Washington University School of Medicine.

Robins, L. N., Helzer, J. E., Croughan, J., & Ratcliff, K. S. (1981). National institute of mental health diagnostic interview schedule. *Archives of General Psychiatry, 38*, 381–389.

Rothbaum, B. O., Foa, E. B., Riggs, D. S., Murdock, T., & Walsh, W. (1992). A prospective examination of posttraumatic stress disorder in rape victims. *Journal of Traumatic Stress, 5*, 455–475.

Russell, D. E. H. (1982). *Rape in marriage*. New York: Macmillan.

Saunders, D. G. (1992). A typology of men who batter women: Three types derived from cluster analysis. *American Orthopsychiatry, 62*, 264–275.

Schlee, K. A, Heyman, R. E., & O'Leary, K. D. (1998). Group treatment for spouse abuse: Are women with PTSD appropriate participants? *Journal of Family Violence, 13*, 1–20.

Shields, N. M., & Hanneke, C. R. (1983). Battered wives' reactions to marital rape. In D. Finkelhor, R. J. Gelles, G. I. Hotaling, & M. A. Strauss (Eds.), *The dark side of families* (pp. 131–148). Beverly Hills, CA: Sage.

Shields, N. M., & Hanneke, C. R. (1987, July). *Comparing the psychological impact of marital and stranger rape*. Paper presented at the National Conference on Family Violence Research, Durham, NH.

Shotland, R. L., & Goodstein, L. (1992). Sexual precedence reduces the perceived legitimacy of sexual refusal: An examination of attributions concerning date rape and consensual sex. *Personality and Social Psychology Bulletin, 18*, 756–764.

Small, M. A., & Tetreault, P. A. (1990). Social psychological, "marital rape exemptions," and privacy. *Behavioral Science and the Law, 8*, 141–149.

Spitzer, R. L., Williams, J. B. W., Gibbon, M., & First, M. B. (1990). *Structured clinical interview for DSM-III-R-personality disorders (SCID-II, Version 1.0)*. Washington, DC: American Psychiatric Press.

Stamm, B. H. (1996). *Measurement of stress, trauma, and adaptation*. Lutherville, MD: Sidran Press.

Strauss, M. A., Hamby, S. L., Boney-McCoy, S., & Sugarman, D. B. (1996). The Revised Conflict Tactics Scale (CTS2): Development and preliminary psychometric data. *Journal of Family Issues, 17*, 283–316.

Veronen, L. J., & Kilpatrick, D. G. (1983). Stress management for rape victims. In D. Meichenbaum & M. E. Jarenko (Eds.), *Stress reduction and prevention* (pp. 341–373). New York: Plenum Press.

Weingourt, R. (1985). Wife rape: Barriers to identification and treatment. *American Journal of Psychotherapy, 39*, 187–192.

Whatley, M. A. (1993). For better or worse: The case for marital rape. *Violence and Victims, 8*, 29–39.

18

Intimate Partner Homicide

Daniel G. Saunders and Angela Browne

Introduction

> Despite her pregnancy, LaQuana decided that she must leave her boyfriend, Blakely. He had been physically assaulting her for over a year, and she believed she had to leave him for the safety of herself and her child. One night, Blakely found her at her family's home with her mother and brother. He insisted that she come back to him. When he tried to force her to go with him, LaQuana threatened to call the police. Blakely then announced his intention to kill everyone in the house. He shot and killed LaQuana, and also shot and wounded her mother as she tried to shield LaQuana. In court, Blakely claimed that he accidentally shot LaQuana while struggling with her brother, who had reached for the gun. (adapted from Michigan Domestic Homicides, 1995–1996)

Could anything have prevented this tragedy? Professionals and the public alike ask such questions when they hear about homicides in families. Attempts to understand homicides between husbands and wives and boyfriends and girlfriends raise a number of additional questions. Are rates of homicide between intimate partners increasing or decreasing? How do partner homicides differ from other kinds of homicide? What are the motives? Are there risk factors we can identify? In hindsight, it often seems that there were clear signs that a tragedy might occur, but how useful are these signs for predicting future tragedies?

Daniel G. Saunders • School of Social Work, University of Michigan, Ann Arbor, Michigan 48109. **Angela Browne** • Harvard Injury Control Center, Harvard School of Public Health, Boston, Massachusetts 02115.

Case Studies in Family Violence, Second Edition, edited by Ammerman and Hersen. Kluwer Academic / Plenum Publishers, New York, 2000.

In this chapter, we describe the extent of and trends in homicide between intimate partners and synthesize the empirical evidence available on motives and risk factors. We then present two case studies that illustrate some common dynamics of partner homicide and discuss society's responses to the problem. A major emphasis will be on differences in rates, trends over time, and motives for homicides by women and men perpetrators. We use the terms *partner* or *intimate partner* homicide throughout to mean *homicides occurring between current or former dating, cohabiting, common-law, and married heterosexual couples.* An enhanced understanding of the dynamics of homicide between intimate partners may prove useful for preventing it in future generations. Prevention may also occur in current relationships by identifying persons and situations at greatest risk. Although the prediction of rare events like homicide is always difficult, many in the mental health and criminal justice fields are now asked to attempt such predictions, and the seriousness of the problem alone means that we should take advantage of our growing—if imprecise—knowledge (Monahan, 1996).

Until recently, homicide between partners was relatively ignored as an area of study. Most research focused on stranger and acquaintance killings, with only brief statistical descriptions of other categories. Clinical case studies existed on homicide between partners, but these created the impression that such homicides were rare and idiosyncratic events. Existing empirical studies often failed to identify trends over time or to explore differences in partner homicides by gender of the perpetrators and type of intimate relationships (e.g., partner versus ex-partner; married versus unmarried; Browne & Williams, 1993). Unfortunately, without these analyses, important differences in intimate partner homicide remained hidden.

Homicide in general is a serious problem in the United States. The rate of homicide just within *families* in this country is higher than the *total* homicide rates in most other Western industrialized nations (Browne, Williams, & Dutton, 1999). These unusually high levels of lethal aggression are not new; a multicountry comparison of homicide rates for all victims over 14 years of age between the years of 1950 and 1980 found that U.S. rates were nearly three times as high as the next highest country (Gartner, 1990). Homicides between intimate partners are the most common type of homicide occurring within families (e.g., Dawson & Langan, 1994; Kellerman & Mercy, 1992).[1] From 1976 through 1996, approximately 52,000 men and women were killed by an intimate partner in the United States (Green-

---

[1] Compared with nonlethal forms of violence between intimate partners, however, partner homicide is still a relatively rare event. Over 12 million husbands and wives admit to using aggression every year (Straus & Gelles, 1990), making it over 5,400 times as likely as partner homicide. This does not mean that 1 out of 5,400 intimate violence cases ends in homicide, because homicide may not always be preceded by other marital violence (cf. Campbell, 1981; Scott, 1974).

field, Rand, Craven, Klaus, Perkins, Ringel, Warchol, Maston, & Fox, 1998). These homicides represented 14% of all homicides in 1976 (about 3,000 per year) and 9% of all homicides in 1996 (about 2,000 per year).

National statistics on homicide are drawn from the Supplementary Homicide Reports (SHR), filed by the police at the time a homicide is investigated and collected by the FBI as a part of its Uniform Crime Reporting program. These reports include only brief descriptions of the context of the incident (e.g., domestic argument, drug-related), the means used to kill, and the relationship between victim(s) and perpetrator(s) if known to the police. Almost all police jurisdictions participate in filing Supplementary Homicide Reports, although data are based on those suspected to be perpetrators at the time of the investigation, and approximately 31% of homicides may still be under investigation when an SHR is filed; the identity of those offenders is often listed as "unknown" (Kellerman & Mercy, 1992). Despite these problems with the SHR, there appears to be a significant decline in intimate homicides over the past 20 years in this country. In one analysis for 1976 through 1996, the rate for homicides of marital partners fell 52% and the rate for total partner homicides fell 36% (Greenfield et al., 1998). Another SHR analysis of trends in partner homicide for the years of 1980 through 1995 that adjusted for missing data in the SHR also noted a decline (Browne, Williams & Dutton, 1999). However, changes in homicide rates over time varied sharply by *gender* of the perpetrator and *type* of intimate relationship. Analyses on the individual level by gender, relationship status, race and other factors are revealing. Social structural and resource factors on the state level related to changing rates also suggest strategies for prevention and intervention.

Risk Factors

Gender Differences

Women are especially at risk of partner homicide. Although men are at higher risk of being killed by an acquaintance or stranger than an intimate, women are more likely to be killed by a current or former spouse or boyfriend than by any other type of assailant (Browne et al., 1999; Greenfield et al., 1998; Langan & Dawson, 1995; Plass & Straus, 1987). Before the mid-1980s, the number of women victims of intimate homicide was not much higher than that of men victims. However, by the 1990s, about three women were killed for every man. Of all partner homicides in recent years, about 70% of the victims are women killed by male partners and 30% are men killed by female partners. The major reason for this increasing gender gap is a substantial decline in the rates of husbands and ex-husbands being killed by wives. A decrease in homicides of wives and ex-wives also has occurred, but the decline is not as dramatic (Browne *et al.*, 1998; Dugan, Nagin, & Rosenfeld, in press; Greenfield *et al.*, 1998). The rate of girlfriends and ex-girlfriends killed by their male partners remained about the same over the past 20 years (Greenfield *et al.*, 1998), although it increased during portions of the time period (Bixenstine, 1996; Browne *et al.*, 1998), with a slight overall increase in the killing of white girlfriends (Greenfield *et al.*, 1998). Browne and Williams (1993) speculate that the increased homicides of unmarried women in the early 1980s may be from the emphasis placed on married women by intervention programs and legal protections. For example, in some states, legal provisions and other services for dating couples lagged behind those for married couples. Alternatively, the informal, ambiguous nature of dating relationships may arouse more fear of abandonment in men, a risk factor described later.

Racial Differences

Black and Native American populations are at particularly high risk for partner homicide, whereas Latino partner homicide rates are below those of black and non-Hispanic whites (for a review see Hampton, Carrillo, & Kim, 1998). Between 1976 and 1997, rates for partner homicides among blacks averaged 5 to 10 times higher than for whites (Greenfield *et al.*, 1998; see also Block & Christakos, 1995; Goetting, 1995; Mercy & Saltzman, 1989; Plass & Straus, 1987). This finding is consistent with high rates of nonfamily homicide (e.g., O'Carroll & Mercy, 1986) and nonlethal family violence among American blacks (Cazenave & Straus, 1979). As in the overall statistics, over the past two decades there has been a steady decrease in partner homicide among blacks, much of it due to a decline in homicides against black partners by black women (Greenfield *et al.*, 1998; Mercy & Saltzman, 1989; Rosenfeld, 1997).

A number of explanations exist for the relatively high rate of lethal and nonlethal family violence by blacks. An earlier theory that blacks constitute a subculture that accepts violence has been largely disproven by studies that include other explanatory variables. As Hampton (1987) pointed out, black homicide rates are much more highly associated with social structural factors—especially poverty and level of employment—than with ethnicity itself. Centerwall (1995) found that the higher rates of black partner homicide in one city disappeared after controlling for household crowding, a proxy for low socioeconomic status (SES). Similar findings exist for nonlethal partner violence, where low income and occupational status explains higher rates for blacks (Cazenave & Straus, 1979). Black women may become scapegoats for the frustration felt by black men in a society that promises opportunities for success but discriminates racially (Harvey, 1986; White, 1985). Ecological models that include the stress of urban living and high-risk environments in addition to poverty also have been proposed (Hampton, 1987). A recent review indicated that social instability and change within a community also are stronger risk markers than poverty (Hampton, Carrillo, & Kim, 1998).

Social response to nonlethal violence may also be a factor. Black women may be reluctant to rely as much on the criminal justice system for protection and are especially vulnerable to violence because of racism and poverty (Harvey, 1986; Hawkins, 1987). Hawkins linked the devaluation of black life in America and the reluctance of a dominant society to aid victims to high mortality rates in the black community. A lack of medical help, for example, can make the difference between serious injury and death.

Prior Assaults

Because Supplementary Homicide Reports do not contain information about the prior interactions of specific couples, no national estimates are available on the number of partner homicides that involve a history of physical assault or threat prior to the lethal incident (Browne, 1997). However, more detailed studies of homicides with smaller samples indicate that a significant proportion of partner homicides by women occur in response to an assault, a history of assault, or threats (e.g., Browne, 1987; Chimbos, 1978; Daly & Wilson, 1988; Daniel & Harris, 1982; Goetting, 1987; Kellerman, Rivara, Rushforth, & Banton, 1993; Rosenfeld, 1997; Totman, 1978; Wilbanks, 1983). In an examination of prosecution cases, women were four times more likely than men to have faced a weapon or been assaulted at or around the time of the murder (Langan & Dawson, 1995). Both clinical and research studies document a history of physical assaults by men who eventually kill their female intimates (e.g., Campbell, 1992; Crawford & Gartner, 1992; Dutton & Kerry, 1996; Wolfgang, 1958). The escalation or a high frequency of violence may be additional risk markers for partner homicide (Browne, 1987; Kellerman et al., 1993; Straus, 1996). Stalking and harassment by men also may be precursors of homicides by men (e.g., Browne, 1986; Meloy, 1998) or by women in response to threatening behaviors by current or former male partners (e.g., Campbell, 1992; Wilson & Daly, 1995).

Motives

Empirical findings strongly suggest a self-defense motive for many women perpetrators of partner homicide. As far back as Wolfgang's (1958) classic study of criminal homicide in Philadelphia, the importance of self-defense in partner homicides by women was noted. In analyzing police and court records, Wolfgang found that at least 60% of husbands killed by their wives had "precipitated" their own deaths; that is, they were the first to use physical force, strike blows, or threaten with a weapon, compared to only 9% of wife victims (Wolfgang, 1958). These figures were based on "provocation recognized by the courts" and do not necessarily reflect the number of wives who had actually experienced physical abuse or threat from their partners.

Studies of abused women who kill indicate that they often feel hopelessly trapped in a desperate situation from which they see no avenue of safe escape (e.g., Browne, 1987; Hamilton & Sutterfield, 1997; Totman, 1978). Compared with other battered women, battered women who kill are more likely to be unemployed (Goetting, 1995; Roberts, 1996), to have less social support (Dutton, Hohnecker, Halle, & Burghardt, 1994), to suffer more frequent assaults and receive more severe injuries (Browne, 1987; Gillespie, 1989), to be raped by their partners (Browne, 1987), to use less violence against their partners (O'Keefe, 1997), to be threatened with death by their partners, and to believe their lives are in danger (Browne, 1987; O'Keefe, 1997). The homicide occurs as part of an attempt to stop their partner from harming them or a child any further, to prevent an attack they believe to be imminent and life-threatening, or during a violent assault (Browne, 1986, 1987; Dugan, Nagin, & Rosenfeld, in press; Grant, 1995; Jurik & Winn, 1990; Maguigan, 1991). In one study of intimate homicide, women reported a much higher level of fear than men who killed women partners (Stout & Brown, 1995). Mann (1992) also found that women often reported a self-defense motive (32% men to 57% women in two cities), but she interpreted these reports as "excuses" by the women (Mann, 1988). However, based on evidence of prior assaults, threats, and physical injuries, judges and juries seem generally to believe that such homicides are in self-defense or that there were strong mitigating circumstances. Women are more likely than men to be screened out of prosecution because of self-defense or, if tried, to have lower conviction rates and shorter prison sentences when convicted (Langan & Dawson, 1995).

In contrast to the predominance of a self-defense motive for women, empirical and clinical studies indicate that men's motives appear to revolve more around jealousy or the imminent or actual termination of a relationship (Barnard, Vera, Vera, & Newman, 1982; Block & Christakos, 1995; Cazenave & Zahn, 1992; Goetting, 1995; Stout, 1993; Wilson et al., 1995). Self-defense is estimated to be 7 to 10 times less frequent for husbands than for wives (Campbell, 1981; Wolfgang, 1958). As illustrated by the opening vignette, there is growing evidence that separation or the threat of separation is a significant precipitant of partner homicides by men (Campbell, 1981; Wilson & Daly, 1993; Wilson, Johnson & Daly, 1995).

Wilson and colleagues contend that this is due to the perception among some men that they are entitled to control the lives of their wives or girlfriends. Indeed, early psychiatric evaluations of men who killed women partners (Barnard et al., 1982) indicated that the precipitating event in male-perpetrated partner homicide was usually some type of perceived rejection on the part of the woman. Separation or threat of separation was especially threatening, being interpreted by the men to represent "intolerable desertion, rejection, and abandonment" (p. 278). In killing their wives, men believed they were responding to an offense against them: the woman leaving. Other studies found both estrangement and jealousy as reasons for the killing of wives (e.g., Campbell, 1981; Crawford & Gartner, 1992; Goetting, 1995). Campbell (1981) placed these men's jealousy within the context of a patriarchal culture. She reviewed studies linking "machismo" culture with greater violence toward women and contended that, "Because women are considered the possession of men in patriarchy, real or imagined sexual infidelity is the gravest threat to male dominance" (p. 78). Estrangement homicides by men were also characterized in one study (Ontario, 1974–94) by offenders who were unemployed (75% vs. 59%), had a criminal record (71% vs. 55%), and used a gun (41% vs. 30%) (Dawson & Gartner, 1998).

Male-perpetrated partner homicides often occur soon after separation. Recent data suggest that about *half* of estrangement homicides occur within 2 months of separation, and almost all occur within a year. For example, Stout (1993) found that over half (60%) of estrangement killings occurred within 1 month; 90% were within 1 year; Wallace (1986) found nearly half (47%) within 2 months and 76% within a year; Wilson and Daly (1993) found half within 2 months and 87% within a year. These studies indicate that the time period immediately following leaving an abusive mate may be an especially dangerous time for a woman. However, homicides by male partners also may occur months or even years after the couple are separated or divorced.

Types of Abusers

Although there are some common patterns, men who perpetrate partner homicides vary on ethnic, socioeconomic, and behavioral dimensions. Even in studies of men who perpetrate nonlethal violence toward women intimates, there are many differences between perpetrators. Some studies of *nonlethal* cases show distinctions among men who batter that seem to relate types of abuse they perpetrate with different types of childhood experiences and with resulting attachment and personality disorders (Holtzworth-Munroe & Stuart, 1994). For example, severe physi-

cal abuse in childhood is empirically linked with antisocial traits, generalized aggression, alcoholism, and severe violence against an intimate
partner in adulthood (Saunders, 1995). However, severe violence by a man
against his partner may not be the best predictor of partner homicide. This
antisocial type may be the most intimidating and controlling, but his "dis-
tancing" attachment style may help him let go of intimate relationships
more easily than other types of personalities. The borderline/dysphoric
type, on the other hand, is an individual who experienced emotional
rejection in childhood and developed an "anxious" attachment style and
the greatest fear of abandonment (see Dutton, 1998). He is more likely to
have a history of suicide attempts and help seeking and, while he may be
quite psychologically abusive, his physical abuse in the relationship often
is not severe (Saunders, 1992). Although much empirical work remains to
be done, it is the borderline/dysphoric batterer who appears most at risk
to kill his partner. Stout's (1993) study of men incarcerated for the murder
of their women partners gave support to this link; men who killed their
partners reported more emotional abuse (witnessing violence, alcoholic
parents) than physical abuse in their childhoods. Humphrey and Palmer
(1982) found more childhood losses among men who killed their partners
than among extrafamilial killers or nonviolent men.

Suicidality

Homicide–suicide occurs in only a small proportion of homicide
cases. Men are more likely to kill themselves following the commission of a
partner homicide than are women (e.g., Block & Christakos, 1995; Cooper
& Eaves, 1996). Homicide–suicide is much more likely in cases of partner
femicide than non-partner femicide (Moracco, Runyan, & Butts, 1998).
When considering only partner homicides by men, homicide–suicides
comprise a substantial minority of cases: 15% in Chicago (Block & Christakos, 1995); 27% in North Carolina (using medical records and law enforcement officer interviews (Morton, Runyan, Moracco, & Butts, 1998);
24% in Canada (Daly & Wilson, 1988); 32% (plus 12% serious suicide
attempt) in British Columbia (Cooper & Eaves, 1996); 19% in Philadelphia
(Wolfgang, 1967); and 26% in one Florida county (Wilbanks, 1983) [ave. =
24%]. As found with other intimate homicides by men, the perpetrator
typically develops suspicions about his partner's infidelity, real or imagined, and the triggering event is often her withdrawal or estrangement
(e.g., Cooper & Eaves, 1996; Danson & Soothill, 1996; Marzuk, Tardiff, &
Hirsch, 1992). Only a small percentage of cases seem to involve "mercy
killings," in which the woman is in declining health and there is little prior
conflict (Morton, Runyan, Moracco, & Butts, 1998). In a detailed analysis of

the impact of loss and jealousy on male-perpetrated partner homicide, Rasche (1988) found that men who killed because their relationship ended were more likely to commit suicide after the homicide, whereas men who killed out of jealousy were more likely only to kill their partners.

Alcohol and Other Drugs

Alcohol and other drugs have long been associated with violent crime, and intimate homicide is no exception. Associations have been found in national FBI data (e.g., Kellerman et al., 1993), city data (e.g., Goetting, 1995), pretrial studies (e.g., Browne, 1987), and surveys of prosecutors' records (e.g., Langan & Dawson, 1995). Here again, there are gender differences. For example, in a survey of prosecutors' records, 66% of husband perpetrators and 37% of wife perpetrators had been using alcohol at the time of the homicide, and 22% of the husband perpetrators— but only 3% of the wife perpetrators—had used illegal drugs (Langan & Dawson, 1995). Similar findings were found in one state's review of medical examiner data and interviews with police investigators (Smith, Moracco, & Butts, 1998).

However, a high correlation with alcohol or other drug use does not mean that substance abuse directly causes lethal aggression (Gondolf, 1995). Although studies of nonlethal partner violence find that men who are violent toward women partners are more likely to abuse alcohol or other drugs than are nonabusive men (Bennett, 1995), alcohol does not seem to have a disinhibitory effect on a physiological level; rather, it may have an association with violence because of other factors such as macho attitudes, constricted information-processing ability, or a socially supported excuse or "time-out" from sanctions. Abusive men with alcohol or drug problems do attack their wives more frequently, are more apt to inflict serious physical injuries on their partners, and are more likely to assault their partners sexually than abusers without a history of substance abuse (e.g., Frieze & Browne, 1989). Thus substance abuse may increase the risk that a seriously injurious or fatal incident will occur.

Firearms

While the majority of those murdered by an intimate are killed by a firearm, the 20-year decline in intimate homicides is paralleled by a decline in such homicides committed with firearms—from 71% in 1976 to 61% in 1996 (Greenfield et al., 1998). Firearm assaults in the family are 12 times more likely to result in death than non-firearm assaults (Saltzman, 1992). Here there are either no gender differences or greater use of firearms by women in the family (e.g., Goetting, 1995; Smith, Moracco, & Butts, 1998). Studies suggest that women may have more need of firearms to defend themselves and equalize the strength differences between themselves and their partners (e.g., Chimbos, 1978). Compared to battered women who do not kill, women who kill intimate partners also had greater access to their partners' guns (Roberts, 1996).

Risks to Others

One cannot assume that only the partner will die in a partner homicide incident. As in LaQuana's murder, family members are sometimes injured or killed as well. Although the rates are low, in about 4% of cases in which men kill their intimate partners, they also kill others (Block & Christakos, 1995; Langan & Dawson, 1995; Wilson, Daly, & Danielle, 1995). In one small sample study of multiple killings by men, 38% of the other victims were children, 35% were people attempting to protect the woman or help her to leave (relatives and friends), and 29% were perceived sexual rivals (Block & Christakos, 1995). Conversely, less than 1% of women who kill partners also kill others as a part of the homicide incident (Block & Christakos, 1995; Langan & Dawson, 1995; Wilson, Daly, & Danielle, 1995).

Because of the differences in motives and behaviors of women and men perpetrators, we will present cases of both female- and male-perpetrated partner homicide.[2] Risk factors for lethal—and severe nonlethal—partner violence will be highlighted and discussed in a following section. Each case illustrates only *some* of the possible risk factors, and the reader is cautioned that there is no single type of partner homicide offender.

Case Description 1: A Man Who Killed His Wife

His friends and relatives described Steve as quiet, gentle, and kind. What mattered most to him were his children, his small business, and his home in the country. He believed that he stood to lose all three of these if his divorce became final. Steve and Sally had been married for 8 years and had two children, ages 6 and 8, at the time of the incident. They had met at a meeting of Amnesty International. Sally was attracted to Steve by his gentleness and good looks. She could not see his insecurities and his tendency to become dependent on and possessive of women. He worked as a nurse for a school department and she was a special education teacher. The early years of their marriage were stressful but exciting for both of them. Having a child right away and paying off school debts was difficult, but they shared many

[2]These two case examples had many facts changed in order to hide the identities of the families.

dreams and worked toward fulfilling them. They built a home in the country and started a business raising goats and selling goat cheese.

The seeds for conflict and for Steve's sense of threat, however, were planted early in the relationship. Sally had more education and made more money than Steve did. Despite his liberal views about new roles for women, the disparity would sometimes aggravate him. He wanted to quit his job to expand their business into a full-time operation. Sally was frightened that their income would be too little and gave him ultimatums about leaving him if he followed through with his plans. He took this as a put-down of his abilities. He also felt she was abandoning him and their dreams.

Another common argument concerned what they each thought was best for the children. The rigidity of Steve's upbringing surfaced at these times. His temper flashed if the children did not eat the "right" food or complete their homework on time. The strictness of his own father could be seen in him. He hated the way his father had treated him; he was frequently made to feel "small" when he did not live up to expectations, and his father had threatened him with a belt. Yet Steve found that he sometimes acted the same way as his father had. Steve's anger doubled whenever he felt that Sally's parents were interfering in their lives, especially with the raising of their children. He never felt accepted by his in-laws because he did not share their religious background.

Occasionally when they argued, Steve would yell at Sally. At first he only raised his voice, but later he would call her names like "stupid" or "bitch" and accuse her of marrying him only for his paycheck or in order to have children. Although Steve's yelling was infrequent, when combined with his much greater size, he intimidated Sally. She became more passive in hopes that his outbursts would stop. Steve learned that a hard stare or storming out of the house was enough for him to get his way. Secretly, Sally began to wonder if she should leave him. She finally developed enough courage to ask for a temporary separation, explaining that it could get their marriage back on track. Steve reacted by begging her not to "throw him out." He held her by the shoulders and shook her. He stopped suddenly and they were both surprised by what he had done. He cried and apologized, saying that he would never touch her again.

A week later, when they were talking alone in the bedroom, Sally again told Steve that she thought it would be best if they separated temporarily. She said that she felt extremely tense near him, that he was sullen all the time, and that he needed help. He again grabbed her by the shoulders and said that he could not leave, his "whole life was here." His fear changed to rage and he began to choke Sally. He pushed her onto the bed shouting, "No! No! No!" The shouting brought the children to the door and he stopped. He left the house quickly and called later to say he was moving out. Sally obtained a restraining order to keep him away. A preliminary divorce hearing established that Steve was allowed to visit the children twice a week.

In his desperation to maintain the relationship, Steve violated the restraining order several times. The judge found him in contempt of court. At the time, however, there were no criminal penalties for such a violation. One time, after dropping the children off, Steve yelled to Sally through the window that he had a gun in the car and would kill her and burn down the house if she did not take him back. On another occasion, Sally let him in the house, thinking that would lower the risk of violence. She told him she was going ahead with the divorce. Steve carried her into the bedroom, slapped her, and raped her. Sally went to the local battered women's shelter with the children and stayed for a week. The police took no action because marital rape was not a criminal offense at the time. They also felt that, by letting Steve into the house, Sally was partly responsible for the violence.

About a month before the divorce, while returning the children, Steve pushed his way into the house, beat Sally up, and attempted to rape her. To her, the sexual violence was his statement that she belonged to him and that she would not get away. She felt totally degraded. Sally went to the police and told them she wanted the violence stopped. But because she said she did not want Steve to go to jail, they took no action. They were also tired of her "complaining"; her fear made her seem abrasive and shrill at times.

As the divorce date approached, Steve's violence escalated. On one occasion, he shoved Sally against a wall so hard that she struck her head. Another time he held her arms so tightly that they were bruised for a week. He called her repeatedly at home and at work, either to plead with her or threaten her. Her attorney and co-workers saw her bruises and difficulty walking due to beatings and rapes. They called the police and prosecutor and asked them to take action but were told there was insufficient evidence for arrest. Sally's spirit collapsed and she told a counselor that she felt resigned to more violence, including her own death. She considered relocating to another state but feared she could not get as good a job there; she also did not want to take the children away from their relatives.

Two days before the divorce, Steve brought the children home from a visit and made a last attempt to reconcile. Sally became frightened that he would become violent again and screamed at him to leave. She went toward the phone. Steve got there first and tore it off the wall. Sally ran into the garage and was headed for the car when Steve caught her. He struck her repeatedly on the head with a board that he picked up from the floor. When he saw she was no longer breathing, he went to the neighbors and told them to call the police because someone had killed his wife.

This case illustrates some of the structural components of relationships in which husbands kill their wives, the psychology of the offender and victim, and the responses of social agencies. These dynamics will be discussed later in the chapter. The next case is an example of a woman who killed her husband. This case illustrates the motive of self-defense, noted previously as a common motive among women who kill their partners.

Case Description 2: A Woman Who Killed Her Husband

Nicole met Gary when she was 27, a few months after an acrimonious divorce from her first husband. She had two small children and was feeling overwhelmed and vulnerable. Gary was warm and charming and quickly became involved with the details of her life. They dated for 6 months before living together, and were married by the time they had known one another a year. Gary had a family by a previous marriage; they resided in another state and Nicole knew very little about them.

The first incidents of physical aggression occurred when Nicole and Gary had been dating 5 months. They were at a party at which another man repeatedly asked Nicole to dance, although she refused each time. Gary drank quite a bit that night. (Nicole discovered later that he also used amphetamines daily.) As they left the party, he turned and hit her in the stomach with his fist, asking if she wouldn't rather leave with her "new friend." He apologized by the time they reached home, and the next day he admitted that he was mainly frightened by how much he had come to care about her and how deeply he wanted her to be his. Gary didn't drink heavily during the rest of their courtship, and there were no further assaults. He was the most affectionate man Nicole had ever known, and his involvement with her and the children seemed an invaluable support.

The next assault occurred about 4 months after their wedding. Nicole had been in a car accident in which she was thrown into the windshield, and she was hospitalized for head and facial injuries. Gary became jealous of the male doctors and angry about the length of her hospital stay. The tension was exacerbated because Nicole did not have adequate health insurance and bills were mounting quickly. After Nicole returned home, Gary was still upset and on edge. This assault was triggered when Nicole had her mother drive her to a doctor's appointment while Gary was at work. Gary returned home early that day and found that Nicole was not at home. When Nicole and her mother returned, he was waiting. He demanded to know where she had been and refused to believe her story of going to the doctor. He ripped the bandages from her forehead and chin and accused her of spending his money on plastic surgery so that she could look beautiful for other men. Gary dragged Nicole into the bathroom and began to hit her repeatedly with the back of his hand. The assault ended when Gary realized that Nicole was bleeding. He became concerned and gentle, washing her injured face with his hands, applying ice, reassuring her that everything would be alright.

Nicole went to her mother's with the children the next day. However, she was unable to come up with enough money for a deposit and first month's rent on an apartment and was frightened about her medical bills. Gary confessed that he had been taking amphetamines and made an appointment at the mental health center for counseling. He told Nicole that his first wife had left him for another man and attributed his irrational fears to his past bad experiences. Nicole and the children returned home, although against Nicole's better judgment. She was withdrawn and depressed for several months, and Gary attributed the next assault to her refusal to "forgive" him and meet his sexual needs.

Arguments in the relationship usually started over the children or over sex. As the marriage went on, Gary assumed a father role with the children, establishing rules and disciplining them harshly for infractions. He over-ruled Nicole on her decisions and accused her of attempting to turn the children against him. Although initially they adored him, the children began to fear Gary, and would jump up on the couch and sit very still when they heard his truck turning into the driveway at night. They called this "being good." When Gary got upset, he became very verbal, escalating from lectures to accusations. Verbal abuse quickly turned into physical violence. Nicole couldn't reason with Gary once an assault began. He would suddenly stop himself, become concerned over Nicole's injuries, and tell her how important she was to him. The next day he would be loving and contrite, and the household would be peaceful for a few weeks until his anger escalated again.

After the first year of marriage, Gary also became sexually abusive. Sexual attacks typically began late at night when Nicole had fallen asleep. These assaults were severe and often involved the use of other violence as well. Nicole nearly always sustained injuries. She began to suffer from sleep disorders and stomach cramps, and eventually developed ulcers. During these assaults, Gary would sometimes verbally fantasize about sex with his ex-wife's daughter. After his death, Nicole found out that charges had been filed against him for sexual molestation and for assault of his first wife but had been dropped when he left the relationship. Gary also had fantasies about killing his first wife. Nicole became increasingly afraid.

As Gary's violence became more severe, Nicole became desperate. She called the police for help if she could reach a phone during an assault. She also left Gary several times. However, her leaving or attempts to gain help only seemed to make things worse. Gary shifted his homicide fantasies about his ex-wife to threats against Nicole. He warned her that he could find her wherever she went, and that he would kill her if she tried to leave him or called the police again. He came after her the few times she left, and her family was so frightened by his behavior that Nicole quit turning to them for help. The police did not arrest Gary when they were called to the house, since he was always gone by the time they arrived, although they did transport her to the hospital several times when she needed treatment. Nicole felt that her love for Gary had ended, and she wanted only to find safety for herself and her children. She talked to the prosecutor about pressing charges or filing for divorce, but gave up when she found that Gary would remain free in the community during the long months it would take for legal action to be completed. His threats were so severe that Nicole was sure she would be killed if she took action.

The most severe assault occurred when Nicole attempted to talk with Gary about separation. Gary became furious and attacked her, beating her over the head with a heavy vase. A neighbor intervened and the police were called. Gary was jailed and Nicole was hospitalized. This time Nicole agreed to file charges, and after she left the hospital, found an apartment for herself and the children. She filed for divorce and obtained a restraining order. However, upon his release from jail, Gary followed the children home from school and quickly learned their location. Several times he intimidated her daughter into letting him into the apartment and then refused to leave when Nicole got home. Nicole attempted to have the restraining order enforced, but the police informed her it was no longer valid because the daughter had allowed him on the premises. Although Gary was not assaultive during this period, Nicole lived in constant fear.

When Gary won weekly visitation rights in the divorce settlement, Nicole took the children and left the state. It took Gary months, but he quit his job and found them. Nicole was ill and had been unable to find steady employment, and the children were falling behind in school. Gary just moved in and Nicole felt she didn't have the strength to fight back. He found work quickly and began to pay the bills, insisting that Nicole stay home and regain her strength. Assaultive incidents were infrequent now. Nicole told herself she'd build her strength up and try again.

Gary lost his job after 3 months, and the only work Nicole could find was on the swing shift. Gary's drinking increased, as did his verbal abuse. Increasingly, much of this was directed toward the children. Nicole was especially worried about her daughter Sarah, who had become withdrawn and silent, rarely leaving her room unless Gary made her come out and join the family. One night Nicole came home at midnight to find her daughter hiding in the garage. Sarah was crying and disheveled and admitted that Gary had been sexually abusing her but had threatened to kill her if she told. It was Friday night. Nicole promised her that they would be gone by Monday, before she had to be alone with Gary again. She and the children spent the weekend making what plans they could with Gary in the house.

Gary always spent Sundays playing pool at a favorite bar. As soon as he left the house Sunday, Nicole called a friend from work to come over and pick up the children. They packed as much as they could while they waited. When the friend arrived, Nicole loaded the children and their belongings in the car, insisting they get to safety immediately. She stayed behind for just a few minutes to pack legal papers and gather some things for herself. Nicole was barely back in the house when she heard Gary's pickup truck pull into the driveway. He slammed on the brakes and ran toward the door, yelling that she had better let him in. He had never come home that early on a Sunday. Nicole realized he must have been watching the house all along; maybe he had overheard their planning.

Nicole fastened the chain lock and ran toward the kitchen to call the police, but Gary was in a rage and was already forcing the door. Gary's .22 was in the hall closet. Nicole dialed 911 and then grabbed the gun and ran back toward the front window. She hoped that if Gary saw her with the gun it would hold him off until help arrived. As the chain lock gave way, Nicole backed up into the dining room, facing Gary but holding the gun toward the floor. She told him that she had called the police and that they would be there any minute, but he still came toward her, raging at her about leaving, grabbing a suitcase that was standing in the living room, and throwing it aside, flushed red in his anger. He kept saying, "You've had it now!"—a phrase Nicole remembered preceding the beating with the vase. Gary picked up a dining room chair, held it over his head and came toward her, and Nicole lifted the gun and fired once. Gary died at 10 o'clock that evening, and Nicole was arrested and charged with his murder.

   This case illustrates some dynamics of homicide in which a woman kills a mate in self-defense on the basis of her assessment of danger from previous assaults and threats against herself or her children and the failure of repeated attempts to attain safety.

Medical Issues

   Among professionals who are in a position to detect and prevent partner homicide, medical practitioners are especially pivotal. As Browne (1992) noted, the medical community—along with the criminal justice system—is the most likely to see women victims and thus constitutes a front line of identification and intervention. Failure to identify and intervene in cases of violence by intimates is costly to society, because assaults between intimates tend to be repeated over time, produce more injuries than assaults by strangers, and lead to both acute and chronic physical and mental health problems in survivors (Browne, 1992). However, medical settings often fail to identify violence by intimate partners as the source of physical injuries or secondary physical problems. Straus (1986) noted that medical settings can become more active in identifying high-risk cases and in promoting public health campaigns to reduce risk factors, and suggested that the public's trust in the medical field makes it well-positioned to be effectively involved. Case identification can occur in all types of medical health settings.

   The surgeon general of the United States began a public health campaign in the 1980s to combat family violence by making public pronouncements and supporting physician training. In 1992, the American Medical Association established that domestic violence is sufficiently prevalent to justify screening all women in medical and mental health settings. The American Medical Association, the American Nurse's Association, the American College of Emergency Physicians, the American College of Obstetricians and Gynecologists, the American Academy of Family Physicians, and other health organizations all have made responding to interpersonal violence a major priority. Screening instruments, curricula, and accreditation guidelines have been developed to improve the delivery of care to victims and sensitize practitioners to the scope and dynamics of violence between intimates (Campbell, 1998; Warshaw, & Ganley, 1995). Public health researchers also have taken the lead in researching possible connections between firearm possession, homicide, and suicide (e.g., Cummings, Koeopsell, Grossman, Savarino, & Thompson, 1997).

Even with these advances, most practitioners infrequently ask about violence unless protocols are in place. When asked about these silences, practitioners describe patients' unwillingness to disclose on this sensitive topic, their own feeling of helplessness about responding to disclosures, and a fear of opening a "Pandora's box" (Sugg & Inui, 1992). However, research indicates that victims are most successfully identified by asking direct and specific questions (Feldhaus, Kozial-McLain, Amsbury, Norton, Lowenstein, & Abbot, 1997) and that these questions can be successfully asked in a variety of medical settings (e.g., Warshaw & Ganley, 1995; Ashur, 1993). Important roles exist for all levels of health-care and mental health–care providers in identifying individuals with past and current family violence histories and in offering appropriate services and referrals to patients and their families. (See Browne, 1992, pp. 3188–3189 for specific AMA guidelines and recommendations.) Special roles for social workers and nurses in medical settings have recently been described (Boes, 1998).

Legal Issues

Legal and Extralegal Alternatives for Abused Spouses

Although women's greatest risk of lethal and nonlethal assault is from their current and former partners, societal protections from partner assaults are still relatively recent. Before the mid-1970s, assaults against wives were considered only misdemeanors in most states, even if the same assault would have been classified as a felony if perpetrated against a stranger or acquaintance. Police were not empowered to arrest on misdemeanor charges, and emergency restraining orders were not available or lacked provisions for enforcement (Browne & Williams, 1989). Only in the late 1970s were legal protections and shelters for battered women and their children established (Schechter, 1982).

By the early 1980s, shelters and legal alternatives were available in most of the 50 states, although such protections still vary widely by jurisdiction in content and implementation. Almost all states now have enhanced provisions for arrest, emergency and long-term restraining orders, crisis lines, and emergency shelters. Interestingly, the decline in partner homicide rates over the past 20 years shows some correlation with the establishment of protections for women faced with violent and assaultive mates. For example, Browne and Williams (1989)—in analyzing national homicide data for the years of 1976–1984—noted over a 25% decline in the rates of women killing male partners over that time period, and found that those states having more domestic violence laws and other resources (e.g., shelters, crisis lines, support groups) for battered women had lower rates of partner homicides by *all* women. The presence of resources for intimate violence was related to the overall sharp decline in partner homicides. Stout (1989) conducted a state-by-state analysis of partner homicides by men for 1980–1982 and found lower rates associated with more shelter services and a greater number of domestic violence statutes (e.g., injunctions, warrantless arrests, domestic violence as separate offense). Stout (1992) also found that the number of women serving in state legislatures was related to lower rates of intimate homicide by male partners. Among state laws related to lower homicide rates by males were fair employment practices, equal pay, equality of public accommodations and housing, and civil injunction relief for victims of abuse (Stout, 1992). Dugan, Nagin, and Rosenfeld (in press) found similar results to these two studies in their analysis of partner homicides from 1976 to 1992 in the 29 largest U.S. cities. Decreased homicides were related to more hotlines and help accessing services, but the relationship with women's economic status was not strong. However, studies have not found a correlation between rates of men killing female intimates and the number of programs for men who batter (Browne & Williams, 1989; Stout, 1989).

The availability and use of personal protection or restraining orders has grown steadily throughout the past 20 years. Most states have criminalized the violation of such orders, and many give police officers the authority to arrest without a warrant given probable cause that a violation has occurred. However, there are doubts about the effectiveness of these orders. For example, although many female stalking victims obtain such orders (28%), the majority of the orders are violated (75%: Harrell, Smith, & Newmark, 1993; 69%: Tjaden & Thoennes, 1998). Sherman (1992) has called the system a "cruel hoax" for promising protection that cannot be delivered. He contends that restraining orders are often weakly enforced. Even when they are enforced, they do not seem to work well in chronic or severe cases (Sherman, 1992; Grau, Fagan, & Wexler, 1984; Harrell & Smith, 1996).

Legal Sanctions as Deterrence

Police training in family crisis intervention that occurred in the early 1970s claimed to reduce the incidence of family homicide (e.g., Bard, 1970). However, further analyses of these studies showed inconclusive results (Elliot, 1989; Liebman & Schwartz, 1973). Deterrence of nonlethal violence through arrest at the misdemeanor level was compared with interventions consisting of police mediation or separation of the couple in a random trial experiment in the early 1980s (Sherman & Berk, 1984). In this study, arrest appeared to be more effective in deterring further nonlethal aggression. Partly as a result of these findings, many police departments adopted pro-arrest or mandatory arrest policies. However, recent attempts to replicate the experiment in five sites indicate that arrest is generally not more effective in reducing recidivism than other police actions (Fagan & Browne, 1994; Garner, Fagan & Maxwell, 1995). Arrest seems to work most effectively as a deterrent with perpetrators who are married and employed (Sherman, 1992).

Most criminal justice strategies—restraining orders, arrest, prosecution, short jail sentences—are based on the assumption that an offender who has physically assaulted or threatened an intimate partner will rationally weigh the costs and benefits of any future assaultive actions. Yet for many men who kill, fear of abandonment or intense feelings of rage and desperation, as described earlier, cloud rationale decision making (Fagan, 1996). Past legal standards in the United States in themselves may have contributed to men feeling justified in taking extreme action toward female partners when the partners are separated from them or appear to be involved intimately with another. Historically, women have been viewed as the property of their husbands and under their husband's control (Schechter, 1982). Traditionally, courts were reluctant to intervene between a man and his wife or to "usurp" a man's authority over members of his household (e.g., Dobash & Dobash, 1979; Weitzman, 1981; Fagan & Browne, 1994). In cases of intimate homicide, there is a long legal and cultural tradition of viewing men's violence as being in "the heat of passion." For example, for many years, men—but not women—were sometimes legally excused for the killing of an unfaithful mate because it was done in the "heat of passion" (Coker, 1992). Today, no American jurisdiction legally allows a husband to strike his wife, and physical attacks and threats by intimate partners are taken much more seriously. However, attitudes from the past may linger about violence as being primarily "out of control" behavior.

Expert Evidence at Trial

It has only been since the late 1970s that the self-defense plea has been applied to cases in which a woman kills an intimate partner in defense of herself or a child. Prior to that, women often pleaded temporary insanity in women-perpetrated partner homicide cases (see Schneider & Jordan, 1978; Sonkin, 1987; Thyfault, 1984; Walker, Thyfault, & Browne, 1982). In general, self-defense is defined as *the justifiable use of a reasonable amount of force against an adversary, when an individual reasonably believes that he or she is in immediate danger of being seriously hurt or killed and that the use of such force is necessary to avoid this harm.* This perception—and the decision on how much force is needed to avert the danger—need only be reasonable, even if it later turns out to be wrong (e.g., LaFave & Scott, 1972). For women faced with violence and threat in their intimate relationships, a successful application of the self-defense plea involves presenting evidence as to the reasonableness of the woman's perception that her partner could and might cause her severe harm, and her belief that she needed to take her defense into her own hands at the time the incident occurred. Having been physically assaulted or threatened by the abuser in the past is not a defense for homicide in itself; such a history is relevant only as it contributes to the woman's belief at the time of the homicide that she is in serious danger.

When women defend themselves against violent partners, the preparation of a comprehensive defense may make the difference between acquittal and long prison terms. Indeed, in the past decade, some governors have granted clemency to incarcerated battered women because they did not have the benefit of expert testimony at their trials (Gagne, 1998). Nicole was charged with first-degree murder in the shooting death of her ex-husband Gary. She went to trial pleading self-defense and used an expert witness to testify to the effects of the violence, threats, and repeated failed attempts to gain safety by fleeing or using legal resources on her perception that she was in immediate lethal danger and had to protect herself. Nicole was acquitted (although such acquittals are still rare), and she and the children returned to her family, although both she and her daughter suffered from severe depression. Guidelines now exist to help attorneys and expert witnesses prepare a case and interview the individuals involved (National Institute of Justice, 1996; Galliano & Nichols, 1988). Expert testimony has typically centered on the concept of a battered woman syndrome or battered spouse syndrome. This testimony describes a constellation of perceptions, responses, and long-term effects of abuse that characterize many women victims of a partner's violence and help place in a larger empirical context the circumstances and facts of a particular case.

Most court rulings now allow testimony on battered woman syndrome but have restricted experts giving opinions about the "ultimate issue" of a woman's state of mind at the time of the killing. Recently, problems with the battered woman syndrome have been pointed out, including its lack of emphasis on the social causes of women's entrapment with violent mates and a lack of scientific consensus on its definition (National Institute of Justice, 1996). However, jurors still appear to need information from an expert witness on several features of self-defense homicide cases, even if they are not subsumed under a "syndrome."

Empirical studies indicate that even contemporary jurors often are ill-informed about key dynamics of violence between men and women partners (Dodge & Greene, 1991). For example, jurors may have difficulty understanding why a battered woman might stay in a relationship that involves severe violence and abuse. Empirical evidence on the dangers of *leaving* a violent and threatening mate, such as that presented in the earlier part of this chapter, and the fact that separation may sharply escalate the danger faced by an abused woman, is helpful in underscoring the reasonableness of a woman's fears of retaliation if she leaves. Problems are most likely to arise if the woman does not fit the stereotype of a "good" victim. In one vignette study, if the woman was portrayed as a "bad" or dysfunctional wife or mother, she had a greater chance of being convicted, even if the levels of assault and threat she faced were held constant (Follingstad, Brondino, & Kleinfelter, 1996).

Social and Family Issues

Many social and family issues associated with partner homicide were present in the two case descriptions. We will highlight a few of those issues here.

Social Issues

Too often, social agencies that could balance the power between the couple consider the violence a "private matter," part of a domestic squabble to which the two partners contribute equally. Fortunately, the community in which the case of Steve and Sally took place has seen some changes in the criminal justice response. The state now has a law that makes marital rape and restraining-order violations criminal offenses. There is a mandatory arrest law for spousal battery, and the local prosecutor does not usually drop complaints at the request of the victim. There is also a special detectives unit trained to deal with sexual and domestic crimes. Although these responses have not been conclusively shown to prevent homicide, there is growing evidence that a coordinated community response—e.g., law enforcement agencies, abuser programs, victim services, and health care—provides the most effective strategy for lowering rates of nonlethal violence (e.g., Murphy, Musser, & Maton, 1998). However, it is not enough for health, mental health, police, and social service providers to be trained to identify and respond to victims of assault; public education is needed to change attitudes about male privilege and appropriate responses (Stark & Flitcraft, 1996).

A potential social response to partner homicide is illustrated by the events following Sally's death. This case was plea-bargained from first- to second-degree murder, and a guilty plea was entered. At Steve's sentencing hearing, a psychiatrist testified that violence was very uncharacteristic of the defendant. However, the psychiatrist used limited and biased accounts of events in the marriage because he relied primarily on Steve's story. He also stated that Steve had been pushed to the "breaking point" by Sally's "taunting." This tendency to blame women victims of crime rather than the perpetrators, especially victims who were intimately involved with their attackers, is still sometimes found in our disciplines of law and mental health.

Steve was sentenced to 10 years in prison but was released after only 3 years. While he was in prison, the children lived with his parents. Upon his release, he was awarded custody of the children. Apparently, the decision makers viewed the murder as caused by Steve's emotional distress and the victim's behavior and did not think that more prison time would act as a specific or general deterrent. They also did not seem to take into account the emotional trauma that Steve caused the children by repeatedly physically abusing and threatening their mother and then killing her. The emotional abuse suffered by children in violent marriages is now well documented (e.g., Edleson, 1999). Unfortunately, however, there is little in the way of research or policy regarding children who survive domestic homicide.

Family Issues

The homicide cases presented also illustrate some of the factors arising from the family of origin and the nuclear family. Gary's early history contained both loss and exposure to severe violence. Gary's mother died when he was only 9 years old; he idealized her and said they had been quite close. His father was extremely strict and abusive. He battered Gary's mother, his stepmother, and Gary. In spite of this, Gary admired his father and emulated him, even in his choice of a profession. Steve's harsh upbringing also was a risk marker of husband-to-wife violence (Hotaling & Sugarman, 1986), especially of severe violence (Saunders, 1995). Sally's greater educational attainment, although not much greater than Steve's, was another risk marker (Hornung, McCullough, & Sugimoto, 1981). Her status was likely to threaten the traditional sex-role beliefs of Steve's upbringing. Their different religious backgrounds were another such indicator (Hotaling & Sugarman, 1986). The case of Steve and Sally also illustrates some of the relationship dynamics of wife abuse, not all of which end in murder. Despite the man's wish for a nonviolent, egalitarian marriage on a cognitive level, the structure and stresses of the marriage brought out this socially reinforced "need" for control. In both of the histories presented, the controlling behavior of the men was a repetition of what they had experienced as children. This behavior further alienated their wives, who eventually sought either temporary or permanent separation when they were not able to negotiate change in the relationship. Over time, the negative spiral accelerated, with the men seeking more control and the women seeking escape from escalating abuse and danger.

Assessing Psychopathology and the Risk of Homicide

A common reaction to descriptions of brutality by men against their female partners is to think of the perpetrator as mentally "deranged." What else would explain such severe violence or a gruesome murder by someone who professed to love the victim? However, measures of psychopathology in themselves are not very good predictors of dangerousness and usually need to be combined with environmental indicators (Monahan, 1996). Large, well-controlled studies of psychopathology with perpetrators of partner homicide have yet to be conducted. A review of prosecutor records showed that 11% of the husbands and 15% of the wives studied were reported to have had a history of mental illness, but details about the type of diagnosis were lacking (Langan & Dawson, 1995). In one small-sample study, the profile of men who killed their wives was very similar to that of men who killed strangers, although the latter group had a greater tendency toward psychopathic traits and impulsivity (Kalichman, 1988). The psychopathic deviate scale was the most elevated in both groups. The majority (69%) of women who killed their partners did not have significant scale elevations. In-depth case studies often report some form of dissociate reaction among perpetrators as well (Berkman, 1980; Blinder, 1984). However, standardized measures are rarely used in these studies.

If men who kill their partners are similar to men who assault without killing, then they are unlikely to suffer from severe mental disorders. In a Minnesota Multiphasic Personality Inventory (MMPI) study of men who assault female intimates, abusive men were characterized as irritable, erratic, and unpredictable. They demonstrated signs of being distrustful of others, were isolated and severely alienated, and had excessive concerns about their own masculinity (Bernard & Bernard, 1984). Studies of nonlethal violence by men indicate that they have a range of personality disorders, but disorders related to severe violence (Saunders, 1995) may not be the same as disorders related to lethal violence.

Predicting Risk for Partner Homicide

In an effort to predict relationships at risk for lethal violence, several lethality checklists have been developed. Some common behavioral and background characteristics have been identified among men who are killed by their female intimates. In a multivariate analysis comparing battered women who killed their partners with those who had not, Browne (1987) found seven variables that distinguished the homicide from the nonhomicide groups: (a) frequency of assault by the man, (b) severity of the woman's injuries, (c) frequency and severity of sexual assault, (d) frequency of the man's intoxication, (e) the man's drug or alcohol use, (f) the man's threats to kill the woman and others, and (g) suicide attempts or threats by the woman. Many of these same factors were found in a study by O'Keefe (1997). By the end of their relationships, women who killed their mates often were experiencing frequent and severe attacks from men who were also sexually assaulting them, drinking heavily and/or abusing other drugs, and threatening to kill them or others. The case of Nicole and Gary illustrates all of these variables to some extent. Crucial factors include the severity of the assaults and threats and the effectiveness of the woman's attempts to gain help or stop the violence. Repeated failed attempts to attain safety produce desperation in a victim and a sense of "being on one's own with the danger" when a life-threatening incident seems imminent.

Because most of the women in the studies believed they were about to be killed, the same risk factors may apply to men who kill women intimates. Campbell (1986; Stuart & Campbell, 1989) relied on this logic when developing the initial version of her danger assessment instrument for use with battered women. It is a 15-item checklist that correlates significantly and moderately with the severity of violence and injuries reported by battered women and distinguishes among different groups of battered women as expected (e.g., emergency room setting versus community; Campbell, 1995). In addition to the factors listed by Browne (1987), Campbell asked women about the presence of guns in the home, whether their partners were violent outside the home, whether the partner controlled all aspects of the woman's life, and whether their income was below the poverty level.

Other risk assessment checklists and instruments are under development. The MOSAIC-20 (de Becker, 1997) emphasizes the role of woman's intuition. A recent study confirms that women's prediction of severe violence was as accurate as a list of factors from Campbell's checklist and other risk factors (Weisz, Tolman, & Saunders, 2000). Hart (1990) provides a list of factors to consider in assessing lethality. In addition to many of the factors found in Campbell's danger assessment instrument, she includes depression in the offender and fantasies of homicide. Straus (1996) developed "criteria for identifying life-threatening risk (LTR) among violent men" from findings of the second National Family Violence Survey. Of the 17 factors associated with the perpetration of severe violence, those most unique to this list include physical abuse of a child, attitudes supporting wife abuse, injuring pets, property destruction, and police involvement. Again, it should be pointed out that "severe violence" and lethality may have a different set of predictors. Bixenstein (1996) relied on several of these sources in constructing a list of 45 risk factors for lethal spouse abuse, which he lists in descending order. His list is unique in two other ways: (1) it includes demographic indicators such as race, age, cohabitation; and (2) it includes 10 variables that can be assessed with standardized measures (e.g., empathic ability, antisocial traits, paranoid ideation).

Even if we know precursors of violence, it remains difficult to predict homicide because it is a rare event.[3] For example, a review of records for spousal homicide in Detroit and Kansas City in the mid-1970s revealed that in nearly every case police had been called to the home at least once in the 2 years before the homicide (Breedlove, Kennish, Sandler, & Sawtell, 1976). However, one needs to consider the large number of police calls that do *not* result in homicide. Sherman (1992) reports one analysis showing that the risk of homicide is less than 1 in 1,000 at homes with prior police calls, and increases only to 3 in 1,000 with nine or more calls. The early studies of police calls also are limited because they refer to calls to "residences" and do not analyze gender differences. Building accurate prediction models is difficult even among severe cases of partner violence, because even severe assaults rarely end in death. About 108,000 men and an equal number of women had a gun or knife used against them by an intimate partner in 1985 (based on a sample of predominantly nonpoor respondents), yet partner homicides represented less than 2% of this figure (Straus & Gelles, 1990). Sherman and his associates found that none of the 110 Milwaukee cases involving guns and threats of death by intimates ended in homicide over a 22-month period (Sherman, Schmidt, Rogan, & DeRiso, 1991). *Post hoc* analyses of cases in which a partner homicide has occurred, although helpful in identifying general risk factors, still do not account for why only a few cases of those with similar risk factors result in lethal violence.

[3]Rosen (1954) first pointed out the problem of predicting rare events. A highly accurate prediction formula may identify most of the "true positives" but may not be useful because of the exceedingly high rate of "false positives" it also selects. Thus, the science of predicting the most dangerous forms of behavior is still rudimentary and may never be very good (Monahan, 1996).

Treatment Options

Therapists from a variety of disciplines seem unprepared to assess dangerousness in violent families. For example, most therapists did not suggest appropriate interventions in response to a written case description with many signs of danger (Harway & Hansen, 1993). Even when told that the case had a lethal outcome, only a small percentage focused on the problems of the perpetrator; many focused primarily on the underlying dynamics of the couples.

Once a practitioner is able to detect some of the risk factors for lethality, there may be a legal or ethical obligation to warn or protect potential victims. Most state laws mandate practitioners to warn or protect victims if lethal violence is believed to be imminent. The landmark court decision establishing the duty to warn potential victims involved a woman who was killed by her boyfriend (*Tarasoff v. Regents of U. of Calif.*, 1997). The court found that the boyfriend's therapists had failed to warn his victim after they had determined that he posed serious danger as a result of his psychological condition. The court stated that therapists are expected to: "(1) exercise a reasonable degree of skill, knowledge, and care ordinarily possessed and exercised by members of their profession; (2) having exercised such a reasonable degree of skill, therapists who find that a patient poses a serious danger of violence to others bear a duty to exercise reasonable care to protect the foreseeable victim of such danger" (pp. 438–439). Many court cases subsequent to Tarasoff also involved women in danger from intimate male partners. However, detection skills, lethality assessment, and possible protective action apply also to battered women who appear homicidal.

Sonkin and Ellison (1986) reviewed duty to warn court cases as they evolved and noted that courts gradually broadened the scope of practitioners' duty. Some recent rulings take the definition of potential victim beyond an identifiable victim and include the potential for physical and mental harm to family members and the general public (Koocher, 1988). These court actions have been curtailed, however, by laws in over 10 states (American Psychological Association, 1988). For example, a California law granted therapists immunity from lawsuit unless "the patient has communicated a serious threat of violence against a reasonably identifiable victim" (Sonkin & Ellison, 1986, p. 206).

In many states, therapists must try to inform the victim and the police of a serious threat. Clinicians were at first concerned that the rulings would create a reluctance to treat dangerous patients and that patients, upon hearing of the duty to warn, would drop out of treatment. Apparently, such consequences have not occurred (McNeill, 1987). McNeill points out some of the benefits of the ruling that clinicians often overlook. For example, when the principle case (*Tarasoff v. Regents of the U. of Calif.*, 1974) went before the court for a rehearing, the court broadened the options for psychotherapists. The duty to warn was broadened to the duty to protect, which means that detaining a client for observation becomes an option. McNeill encourages therapists to inquire about clients' violent propensities and any history of violence as an indicator of future violence. She suggests that the following indicators be considered:

- The extent to which the client appears to have a plan as distinguished from a fantasy.
- The specificity with which the client describes the plan.
- Whether the client has targeted a victim or a victim is reasonably foreseeable with knowledge in the therapist's possession.
- Whether triggering events are attached to the plan that will cause the client to activate it upon the occurrence of some conditions.
- Whether a dramatic or sudden change in the client's circumstance has occurred, such as divorce, loss of job, infidelity of spouse, romantic rejection, failure in an educational setting, humiliation caused by a known person, or death of a loved one.
- Whether any steps have been taken to execute the plan, such as purchasing a weapon or other dangerous material, buying an airplane ticket to visit the intended victim, saving money toward the objective, sending threats to the victim directly or through third parties, or performing minor acts as a prelude to an intended "grand finale."

Typically, treatment does not follow perpetrators into a prison setting once an intimate homicide has occurred. Men who abuse their partners and are incarcerated for homicide or attempted homicide are usually not ordered by courts to receive treatment for their violence. Even if they are, few states have prison-based programs (Center for Effective Public Policy, 1997). As in the case of Steve, the homicide is seen as an isolated "act of passion" that will never occur again. These men often make model prisoners; treatment referrals are more likely to be made for individuals who are aggressive while incarcerated. Some perpetrators also refuse treatment because they fear that any information they reveal will be used against them in an appeals process and will lengthen their time in prison.

Women incarcerated for killing their partners also have critical needs for intervention and support. Many suffer from posttraumatic stress disorder, panic disorder, and depression as a result of the violence they have experienced as well as the aftermath of the lethal incident. Many also lose custody of and even contact with their children as a result of the incident and their incarceration. A number of communities have established advocacy programs for these women (e.g., Bauschard, 1986). Support groups in prisons can be sponsored by corrections counselors, community shelters, mental health centers, or other entities. A major need of these women is to have their emotional, physical, and sexual abuse experiences validated (Grant, 1995) and to deal with the multiple losses involved in the homicide incident and its consequences. Even though their abuser is dead, women survivors may continue to fear him and to evidence posttraumatic stress disorder and other acute and chronic emotional and physical conditions. For women whose relationships with an abusive partner involved extreme levels of control, isolation, and invasions of privacy, the realities of prison life—including pat and body-cavity searches, middle-of-the-night bed checks, the potential for sexual assault, the necessity to follow all orders immediately, and the complete loss of privacy and freedom—may parallel aspects of earlier traumas.

Finally, more attention needs to be directed toward helping the children who survive these tragedies. Little is known about the suffering they endure. If studies of nonlethal violence are a guide, then there is reason for grave concern about the potential for boys in these families to become violent later in life. Two potent risk factors (as in Gary's case) are combined: being exposed to violence in childhood (Hotaling & Sugarman, 1986) and the sudden, traumatic loss of a parent (Humphrey & Palmer, 1982). The immediate and long-term emotional turmoil child survivors of parental homicide experience is likely to be great. In addition to the effects of the sudden traumatic loss of a parent and the effects of physical or sexual abuse they themselves may have suffered from the abuser, they may experience guilt that they did not somehow prevent the killing and may have split loyalties between their parents or surviving relatives if they hear differing accounts of who was to "blame."

Summary

In this chapter, we described the extent and trends of homicide between intimate partners, synthesized available empirical evidence on motives and risk factors, and presented two cases that illustrate some common dynamics involved when a spouse or lover takes the life of his or her partner. We stressed the differing rates, background characteristics, and motives of women and men perpetrators of partner homicide and discussed some legal, social, and treatment issues. Empirical studies across localities and types of populations indicate that there are clear differences between the motives of men and women, with women more likely to commit partner homicide in response to violence and threat by male intimates and men more likely to perpetrate homicide in response to jealousy or separation. Although the decrease in intimate homicide over the past quarter-century is promising and is related to legal and social resources for nonlethal aggression, this decrease has been much greater for the killing of male than of female intimates.

The ability to prevent any particular person from committing homicide may remain a difficult task, because homicide is a relatively rare event. Although clinicians are obligated to warn and protect potential victims in some circumstances, the science of risk prediction is in its infancy. The discovery of risk markers, however, can lead to prevention programs on a social and family level that will decrease all forms of partner violence, including its most extreme form, intimate homicide. Finally, it will be through the lessons taught to the children in our present generation, through example and words, that the most effective prevention will take place.

References

American Psychological Association. (1988, June). New laws limiting duty to protect (John Bales) (p. 18). *APA Monitor*. Arlington, VA: Author.

Ashur, M. L. (1993). Asking about domestic violence: Safe questions. *Journal of the American Medical Association, 269*, 2367.

Bard, M. (1970). *Training police as specialists in family crisis intervention*. Washington, DC: U.S. Government Printing Office.

Barnard, G. W., Vera, H., Vera, M. I., & Newman, G. (1982). Til death do us part: A study of spouse murder. *Bulletin of the American Academy of Psychiatry and the Law, 10*, 271–280.

Bauschard, L. (1986). *Voices set free. Battered women speak from prison*. St. Louis, MO: Women's Self-Help Center.

Bennett, L. W. (1995). Substance abuse and the domestic assault of women. *Social Work, 40*, 760–771.

Berkman, A. S. (1980). The state of Michigan versus a battered wife. *Bulletin of the Menninger Clinic, 44*, 603–616.

Bernard, J. L., & Bernard, M. L. (1984). The abusive male seeking treatment: Jekyll and Hyde. *Family Relations, 33*, 543–547.

Bixenstine, V. E. (1996). Spousal homicide. In H. V. Hall (Ed.), *Lethal violence 2000*. Kamuela, HI: Pacific Institute for the Study of Conflict and Aggression.

Blinder, M. (1984). The domestic homicide. *Family Therapy, 11*, 185–198.

Block, C. R., & Christakos, A. (1995). Intimate partner homicide in Chicago over 29 years. *Crime and Delinquency, 41*, 496.

Boes, M. E. (1998). Battered women in the emergency room: Emerging roles for the ER social worker and clinical nurse specialist. In A. R. Roberts (Ed.), *Battered women and their families: Intervention strategies and treatment programs* (2nd ed., pp. 205–229). New York: Springer.

Breedlove, R. K., Kennish, J. W., Sandler, D. M., & Sawtell, R. K. (1976). Domestic violence and the police: Kansas City. In Police Foundation (Ed.), *Domestic violence and the police* (pp. 23–33). Washington, DC: Police Foundation.

Browne, A. (1986). Assault and homicide at home: When battered women kill. In M. J. Saks & L. Saxe (Eds.), *Advances in applied social psychology* (pp. 57–79). Hillsdale, NJ: Erlbaum.

Browne, A. (1987). *When battered women kill.* New York: Free Press.

Browne, A. (1992) Violence against women: Relevance for medical practitioners. *Journal of the American Medical Association, 267,* 3184–3189.

Browne, A. (1997). Violence in marriage: Until death do us part? In A. P. Cardarelli (Ed.), *Violence between intimate partners: Patterns, causes, and effects* (pp. 48–69). Needham Heights, MA: Allyn & Bacon.

Browne, A., & Williams, K. R. (1989). Exploring the effect of resource availability and the likelihood of female-perpetrated homicides. *Law and Society Review, 23,* 75–94.

Browne, A., & Williams, K. R. (1993). Gender, intimacy, and lethal violence: Trends from 1976 through 1987. *Gender and Society, 7,* 78–98.

Browne, A., Williams, K. R. & Dutton, D. G. (1999). Homicide between intimate artners: A 20-year review. In M. D. Smith & M. A. Zahn (Eds.), Homicide: A sourcebook of social research. Thousand Oaks, CA: Sage.

Campbell, J. C. (1981). Misogyny and homicide of women. *Advances in Nursing Science/Women's Health, 3,* 67–85.

Campbell, J. C. (1986). Nursing assessment for risk of homicide with battered women. *Advances in Nursing Science, 8,* 36–51.

Campbell, J. C. (1992). If I can't have you, no one can: Power and control in homicide of female partners. In J. Radford & D. E. H. Russell (Eds.), *Femicide: The politics of woman killing* (pp. 99–113). Boston: Twayne Publishers.

Campbell, J. C. (1995). Prediction of homicide of and by battered women. In J.C. Campbell (Ed.), *Assessing dangerousness: Violence by sexual offenders, batterers, and child abusers* (pp. 96–113). Thousand Oaks, CA: Sage.

Campbell, J. C. (1998). *Empowering survivors of abuse.* Thousand Oaks, CA: Sage.

Cazenave, N., & Straus, M. A. (1979). Race, class, network embeddedness and family violence. *Journal of Comparative Family Studies, 10,* 281–300.

Cazenave, N. A., & Zahn, M. A. (1992). Women, murder, and male domination: Police reports of domestic homicide in Chicago and Philadelphia. In E. C. Viano (Ed.), *Intimate violence: Interdisciplinary perspectives* (pp. 83–96). Washington, DC: Hemisphere Publishing.

Center for Effective Public Policy. (1997, October). Findings from the batterers' intervention focus group: Recommendations to the Violence Against Women Grants Office Corrections Program Office. Silver Springs, MD: National Institute of Corrections.

Centerwall, B. S. (1995, June). Race, socioeconomic status, and domestic homicide. *Journal of the American Medical Association, 273,* 1755–1758.

Chimbos, P. D. (1978). *Marital violence: A study of interspousal homicide.* San Francisco: R & E Associates.

Coker, D. K. (1992). Heat of passion and wife killing: Men who batter/men who kill. *Review of Law and Women's Studies, 2,* 71–130.

Cooper, M., & Eaves, D. (1996). Suicide following homicide in the family. *Violence and Victims, 2,* 99–112.

Crawford, M., & Gartner, R. (1992). *Woman killing: Intimate femicide in Ontario 1974–1990.* Toronto: Woman's Directorate, Ministry of Social Services, Government of Ontario.

Cummings, P., Koeopsell, T. D., Grossman, D. C., Savarino, J., & Thompson, R. S. (1997). Association between the purchase of a handgun and homicide or suicide. *American Journal of Public Health, 87,* 974–978.

Daly, M., & Wilson, M. (1988). *Homicide.* New York: Aldine de Gruyter.

Daniel, A. E., & Harris, P. W. (1982). Female homicide offenders referred for pretrial psychiatric examination: A descriptive study. *Bulletin of the Academy of Psychiatry and Law, 10*, 261–269.

Danson, L., & Soothill, K. (1996). Murder followed by suicide: A study of the reporting of murder followed by suicide in *the Times*, 1887–1990. *Journal of Forensic Psychiatry, 7*, 310–322.

Dawson, J. M., & Langan, P. A. (1994). *Murder in families*. Washington, DC: U.S. Department of Justice, Office of Justice Programs.

Dawson, M., & Gartner, R. (1998). Differences in the characteristics of intimate femicides. *Homicide Studies, 2*, 378–399.

de Becker, G. (1997). *The gift of fear: Survival signals that protect us from violence*. Toronto: Little Brown.

Dobash, R. E., & Dobash, E. (1979). *Violence against wives*. New York: Free Press.

Dodge, M., & Greene, E. (1991, Winter). Juror and expert conceptions of battered women. *Violence and Victims, 6*, 271–282.

Dugan, L., Nagin, D., & Rosenfeld, R. (in press). Explaining the decline in intimate partner homicide: The effects of changing domesticity, women's status, and domestic violence resources. *Homicide Studies*.

Dutton, M. A., Hohnecker, L. C., Halle, P. M., Burghardt, K. J. (1994, October). Traumatic responses among battered women who kill. *Journal of Traumatic Stress, 7*, 549–564.

Dutton, D. G., & Kerry, G. (1996). *Modus operandi and psychological profiles of uxoricidal males*. Unpublished study, Department of Psychology, University of British Columbia.

Dutton, D. G.. (1998). *The abusive personality: Violence and control in intimate relationships*. New York, NY: The Guilford Press.

Edleson, J. L. (1999). Children's witnessing of adult domestic violence. *Journal of Interpersonal Violence, 14*, 839–870.

Elliot, D. S. (1989). Criminal justice procedures in family violence crimes. In L. Ohlin & M. Tonry (Eds.), *Family violence: Crime and justice, a review of research* (Vol. 11, pp. 427–480). Chicago: University of Chicago Press.

Fagan, J. (1996). *The criminalization of domestic violence: Promises and limits*. Washington, DC: National Institute of Justice, Office of Justice Programs, U.S. Department of Justice.

Fagan, J., & Browne, A. (1994). Violence between spouses and intimates: Physical aggression between women and men in intimate relationships. In A. Reiss & J. A. Roth (Eds.), *Understanding and preventing violence. Vol. 3: Social Influences* (pp. 115–292). Washington, DC: National Academy Press.

Feldhaus, K., Koziol-McLain, J., Amsbury, H., Norton, I., Lowenstein, S., & Abbott, J. (1997). Accuracy of three brief screening questions for detecting partner violence in the emergency department. *Journal of the American Medical Association, 277*, 1357–1361.

Follingstad, D. R., Brondino, M. J., & Kleinfelter, K. J. (1996, September). Reputation and behavior of battered women who kill their partners: Do these variables negate self-defense? *Journal of Family Violence, 11*, 251–267.

Frieze, I. H., & Browne, A. (1989). Violence in marriage. In L. Ohlin & M. Tonry (Eds.), *Family violence* (pp. 163–218). Chicago: University of Chicago Press.

Gagne, P. (1998). *Battered women's justice: The movement for clemency and the politics of self-defense*. New York: Twayne.

Galliano, B., & Nichols, M. (1988). Mental health professional as expert witness: Psychosocial evaluation of battered women accused of homicide or assault. *Journal of Interpersonal Violence, 3*, 29–41.

Garner, J., Fagan, J., & Maxwell, C. D. (1995). Published findings from the NIJ spouse assault replication program: A critical review. *Journal of Quantitative Criminology, 8*, 1–29.

Gartner, R. (1990). The victims of homicide: A temporal and cross-national comparison. *American Sociological Review, 55,* 92–106.

Gillespie, C. K. (1989). *Justifiable homicide: Battered women, self-defense, and the law.* Columbus: Ohio State University.

Goetting, A. (1987). Homicidal wives. *Journal of Family Issues, 8,* 332–341.

Goetting, A. (1995). *Homicide in families and other special populations.* New York, NY: Springer Publishing.

Gondolf, E. W. (1995). Alcohol abuse, wife assault, and power needs. *Social ervice Review, 69,* 274–284.

Grant, C. A. (1995). Women who kill: The impact of abuse. *Issues in Mental Health Nursing, 16,* 315–326.

Grau, J., Fagan, J., & Wexler, S. (1984). Restraining orders for battered women: Issues of access and efficacy. *Women and Politics, 4,* 13–28.

Greenfeld, L. A., Rand, M. R., Craven, D., Klaus, P. A., Perkins, C. A., Ringel, C., Warchol, G., Maston, C., & Fox, J. A. (1998, March). *Violence by intimates: Analysis of data on crimes by current or former spouses, boyfriends, and girlfriends.* Washington, DC: U.S. Department of Justice, Bureau of Justice Statistics.

Hamilton, G., & Sutterfield, T. (1997). Comparative study of women who have and have not murdered their abusive partners. *Women and Therapy, 20,* 45–55.

Hampton, R. L. (1987). Family violence and homicide in the black community: Are they linked? In R. L. Hampton (Ed.), *Violence in the black family* (pp. 135–156). Lexington, MA: Lexington Books.

Hampton, R. L., Carrillo, R. & Kim, J. (1998). Violence in communities of color. In R. Carrillo & J. Tello (Eds.), *Family violence and men of color* (pp. 1–30). New York: Springer.

Harrell, A. V., & Smith, B. E. (1996). Effects of restraining orders on domestic violence victims. In E. S. Buzawa & C. G. Buzawa (Eds.), *Do arrests and restraining orders work?* (pp. 214–242). Thousand Oaks, CA: Sage.

Harrell, A. V., Smith, B. E., & Newmark, L. (1993). *Court processing and the effects of restraining orders for domestic violence victims* [Final report to the State Justice Institute]. Washington, DC: The Urban Institute.

Hart, B. (1990). Assessing whether batterers will kill. Pennsylvania Coalition Against Domestic Violence. http://www.mincava.umn.edu/hart/lethali.htm.

Harvey, (1986). Homicide among young black adults: Life in the subculture of exasperation. In D. F. Hawkins (Ed.), *Homicide among black Americans* (pp. 153–157). Lanham, MD: University Press of America.

Harway, M., & Hansen, M. (Eds.). (1993). Therapist perceptions of family violence. *Battering and family therapy: A feminist perspective* (pp. 42–53). Thousand Oaks, CA: Sage.

Hawkins, D. F. (1987). Devalued lives and racial stereotypes: Ideological barriers to the prevention of family violence among blacks. In R. L. Hampton (Ed.), *Violence in the black family* (pp. 189–206). Lexington, MA: Lexington Books.

Holtzworth-Munroe, A., & Stuart, G. L. (1994). Typologies of male batterers: Three subtypes and the differences among them. *Psychological Bulletin, 116,* 476–497.

Hornung, C. A., McCullough, B. C., & Sugimoto, T. (1981). Status relationships in marriage: Risk factors in spouse abuse. *Journal of Marriage and the Family, 43,* 675–692.

Hotaling, G. T., & Sugarman, D. B. (1986). An analysis of risk markers in husband to wife violence: The current state of knowledge. *Violence and Victims, 1,* 101–124.

Humphrey, J. A., & Palmer, S. (1986). Stressful life events and criminal homicide. *Omega: Journal of Death and Dying, 17,* 299–308.

Jurik, N., & Winn, R. (1990). Gender and homicide: A comparison of men and women who kill. *Violence and Victims, 5,* 227–242.

Kalichman, S. C. (1988). MMPI profiles of women and men convicted of domestic homicide. *Journal of Clinical Psychology, 4,* 847–853.

Kellermann, A. L., & Mercy, J. A. (1992). Men, women, and murder: Gender-specific differences in rates of fatal violence and victimization. *Journal of Trauma, 33,* 1–5.

Kellermann, A. L., Rivara, F. P., Rushforth, N. B., & Banton, J. G. (1993). Gun ownership as a risk factor for homicide in the home. *New England Journal of Medicine, 329,* 1084–1091.

Koocher, G. P. (1988). A thumbnail guide to "duty to warn" cases. *Clinical Psychologist, 41,* 22–25.

LaFave, W. R., & Scott, A. W., Jr. (1972). *Handbook of criminal law.* St. Paul, MN: West Publishing.

Langan, P. A., & Dawson, J. M. (1995). *Spouse murder defendants in large urban counties.* Washington, DC: U.S. Department of Justice, Bureau of Justice Statistics.

Liebman, D., & Schwartz, J. (1973). Police progress in domestic crisis intervention: A review. In J. Snibbe & H. Snibbe (Eds.), *The urban policeman in transition* (pp. 421–472). Springfield, IL: Charles C. Thomas.

Maguigan, H. (1991). Battered women and self-defense: Myths and misconceptions in current reform proposals. *University of Pennsylvania Law Review, 140,* 379–486.

Mann, C. R. (1988). Getting even? Women who kill in domestic encounters. In S. L. Johann & F. Osanka (Eds), *Representing ... battered women who kill* (pp. xxi., 393, 8–26). Springfield, IL: Charles C. Thomas.

Mann, C. R. (1992). Female murderers and their motives: A tale of two cities. In E. Viano (Ed.) *Intimate violence: Interdisciplinary perspectives* (pp. 73–81). New York: Hemisphere.

Marzuk, P. M., Tardiff, K., & Hirsch, C. S. (1992). The epidemiology of murder–suicide. *Journal of the American Medical Association, 267,* 3179–3183.

McNeill, M. (1987). Domestic violence: The skeleton in Tarasoff's closet. In D. J. Sonkin (Ed.), *Domestic violence on trial: Psychological and legal dimensions of family violence* (pp. 197–217). New York: Springer.

Meloy, R. (1998). *The psychology of stalking: Clinical and forensic perspectives.* San Diego, CA: Academic Press.

Mercy, J. A., & Saltzman, L. E. (1989). Fatal violence among spouses in the United States, 1976–1985. *American Journal of Public Health, 79,* 595–599.

Michigan Domestic Homicides, October 1995–September 1996 [http://comnet.org/dvp/victims.html].

Monahan, J. (1996). Violence prediction: The past twenty and the next twenty years. *Criminal Justice and Behavior, 23,* 107–119.

Moracco, K. E., Runyan, C. W., Butts, J. D. (1998). Femicide in North Carolina, 1991–1993. *Homicide Studies, 2,* 422–446.

Morton, E., Runyan, C., Moracco, K. E., & Butts, J. D. (1998). Partner homicide–suicide involving female homicide victims. A population based study in North Carolina, 1988–1992. *Violence and Victims, 13,* 91–106.

Murphy, C. M., Musser, P. H., & Maton, K. I. (1998). Coordinated community intervention for domestic abusers: Intervention system involvement and criminal recidivism. *Journal of Family Violence, 13,* 263–284.

National Institute of Justice. (1996). *The validity and use of evidence concerning battering and its effects in criminal trials: Report responding to Section 40507 of the Violence Against Women Act.* Washington, DC: U.S. Department of Justice Office of Justice Programs.

O'Carroll, P. W., & Mercy, J. A. (1986). Patterns and recent trends in black homicide. In D. F. Hawkins (Ed.), *Homicide among black Americans* (pp. 29–42). Lanham, MD: University Press of America.

O'Keefe, M. (1997). Incarcerated battered women: A comparison of battered women who killed their abusers and those incarcerated for other offenses. *Journal of Family Violence, 12,* 1–19.

Plass, P. S., & Straus, M. A. (1987, June). *Intra-family homicide in the United States: Incidence, trends, and differences by region, race and gender.* Paper presented at the Third National Family Violence Conference, University of New Hampshire, Durham.

Rasche, C. (1988, November). *Domestic murder–suicide: Characteristics and comparisons to non-suicidal mate killing.* Paper presented at the 40th annual meeting of the American Society of Criminology, Chicago.

Roberts, A. R. (1996, September). Battered women who kill: A comparative study of incarcerated participants with a community sample of battered women. *Journal of Family Violence, 11,* 291–304.

Rosen, A. (1954). Detection of suicidal patients. *Journal of Consulting Psychology, 18,* 397–403.

Rosenfeld, R. (1997). Changing relationships between men and women: A note on the decline in intimate partner homicide. *Homicide Studies, 1,* 72–83.

Saltzman, L. (1992). Weapon involvement and injury outcomes in family and intimate assaults. *Journal of the American Medical Association, 267,* 3042.

Saltzman, L., Mercy, J. A., Rosenberg, M. L., Elsea, W. R., Napper, G., Sikes, R. K., & Waxweiler, R. J. (1990). Magnitude and patterns of family and intimate assault in Atlanta, Georgia, 1984. *Violence and Victims, 5,* 3–18.

Saunders, D. G. (1992). A typology of men who batter: Three types derived from cluster analysis. *American Journal of Orthopsychiatry, 62,* 264–275.

Saunders, D. G. (1995). Prediction of wife assault. In J. C. Campbell (Ed.), *Assessing dangerousness: Violence by sexual offenders, batterers, and child abusers* (pp. 68–95). Newbury Park, CA: Sage.

Schecter, S. (1982). *Women and male violence.* Boston: South End Press.

Schneider, E. M., & Jordan, S. B. (1978). Representation of women who defend themselves in response to physical or sexual assault. *Family Law Review, 1,* 118–132.

Schuller, R. A., & Hastings, P. A. (1996). Trials of battered women who kill: The impact of alternative forms of expert witness. *Law and Human Behavior, 20,* 167–187.

Scott, P. D. (1974). Battered wives. *British Journal of Psychiatry, 125,* 433–441.

Sherman, L. W., & Berk, R. A. (1984). The specific deterrent effect of arrest for domestic assault. *American Sociological Review, 49,* 261–272.

Sherman, L. W. (1992). *Policing domestic violence: Experiments and dilemmas.* New York: Maxwell Macmillan International.

Sherman, L. W., Schmidt, J. D., Rogan, D. P., & DeRiso, C. (1991). Predicting domestic homicide: Prior police contact and gun threats. In M. Steinman (Ed.), *Woman battering: Policy responses* (pp. 73–93). Cincinnati, OH: Anderson Publishing.

Smith, P. H., Moracco, K., & Butts, J. D. (1998). Partner homicide in context: A population-based perspective. *Homicide Studies, 2,* 400–421.

Sonkin, D. J. (1987). The assessment of court-mandated male batterers. In D. J. Sonkin (Ed.), *Domestic violence on trial* (pp. 174–196). New York: Springer.

Sonkin, D. J., & Ellison, J. (1986). The therapist's duty to protect victims of domestic violence: Where have we been and where are we going. *Violence and Victims, 1,* 205–214.

Stark, E., & Flitcraft, A. (1996). *Women at risk: Domestic violence and women's health.* Thousand Oaks, CA: Sage.

Stawar, T. L. (1996). Suicidal and homicidal risk for respondents, petitioners, and family members in an injunction program for domestic violence. *Psychological Reports, 79,* 553–554.

Stout, K. D. (1989, Summer). Intimate femicide: Effects of legislation and social services. *Affilia, 4,* 21–27.

Stout, K. D. (1992). "Intimate femicide?" An ecological analysis. *Journal of Sociology and Social Welfare, 19,* 29–50.

Stout, K. D. (1993). Intimate femicide: A study of men who have killed their mates. *Journal of Offender Rehabilitation, 19,* 81–94.

Stout, K. D., & Brown, P. (1995, Summer). Legal and social differences between men and women who kill intimate partners. *Affilia, 10,* 194–205.

Straus, M. A. (1986, June). Domestic violence and homicide antecedents. *Bulletin of the New York Academy of Medicine, 62,* 446–465.

Straus, M. A. (1996). Identifying offenders in criminal justice research on domestic assault. In E. Buzawa (Ed.), *Do arrests and restraining orders work* (pp. 14–29). Thousand Oaks, CA: Sage.

Straus, M. A., & Gelles, R. (1990). *Physical violence in American families: Risk factors adaptations to violence in 8,145 families.* New Brunswick, NJ: Transaction Publishers.

Stuart, E. P., & Campbell, J. C. (1989). Assessment of patterns of dangerousness with battered women. *Issues in Mental Health Nursing, 10,* 245–253.

Sugg, N. K., & Inui, T. (1992). Primary care physicians' response to domestic violence: Opening the Pandora's box. *Journal of American Medical Association, 267,* 3157–3160.

Tarasoff v. Regents of the University of California. (1974). 118 Cal. Rptr. 129, 529 P 2d 553.

Thyfault, R. K. (1984). Self-defense: Battered women syndrome on trial. *California Western Law Review, 20,* 485–510.

Tjaden, P., & Thoennes, N. (1998, April). *Stalking in America: Findings from the national violence against women survey.* Washington, DC: U.S. Department of Justice, National Institute of Justice Centers for Disease Control and Prevention.

Totman, J. (1978). *The murderess: A psychological analysis of violent behavior.* San Francisco: R & E Research Associates.

Walker, L. E., Thyfault, R. K., & Browne, A. (1982). Beyond the juror's ken: Battered women. *Vermont Law Review, 7,* 1–14.

Wallace, A. (1986). *Homicide: The social reality.* Sydney: New Wales Bureau of Crime and Statistics.

Warshaw, c. & Ganley, A (1995). *Improving the health care response to domestic violence: A resource manual for health care providers.* San Francisco: Family Violence Prevention Fund.

Weisz, A. N., Tolman, R. M., & Saunders, D. G. (2000). Assessing the risk of severe domestic violence: The importance of survivors' predictions. *Journal of Interpersonal Violence, 15,* 75–90.

Weitzman, L. (1981). *The marriage contract: Spouses, lovers and the law.* New York: Free Press.

White, E. C. (1985). *Chain chain change: For black women dealing with physical and emotional abuse.* Seattle, WA: Seal Press.

Wilbanks, W. (1983). The female homicide offender in Dade County, Florida. *Criminal Justice Review, 8,* 9–14.

Wilson, M., & Daly, M. (1993). Spousal homicide risk and estrangement. *Violence and Victims, 8,* 3–17.

Wilson, M., Daly, M., & Daniele, A. (1995). Familicide: The killing of spouse and children. *Aggressive Behavior, 21,* 275–291.

Wilson, M., Johnson, H., Daly, M. (1995) Lethal and nonlethal violence against wives. *Canadian Journal of Criminology: Special Issues: Focus on the Violence Against Women Survey, 37*(3), 331–361.

Wolfgang, M. E. (1958). *Patterns in criminal homicide.* New York: Wiley.

Wolfgang, M. E. (1967). A sociological analysis of criminal homicide. In M. E. Wolfgang (Ed.), *Studies in homicide.* New York: Harper & Row.

Index